CLINICAL EFFICACY OF POSITRON EMISSION TOMOGRAPHY

DEVELOPMENTS IN NUCLEAR MEDICINE
Series editor Peter H. Cox

Cox, P.H. (ed.): Cholescintigraphy. 1981. ISBN 90-247-2524-0

Cox, P.H. (ed.): Progress in radiopharmacology 3. Selected Topics. 1982. ISBN 90-247-2768-5

Jonckheer, M.H. and Deconinck, F. (eds.): X-ray fluorescent scanning of the thyroid. 1983. ISBN 0-89838-561-X

Kristensen, K. and Nørbygaard, E. (eds.): Safety and efficacy of radiopharmaceuticals. 1984. ISBN 0-89838-609-8

Bossuyt, A. and Deconinck, F.: Amplitude/phase patterns in dynamic scintigraphic imaging. 1984. ISBN 0-89838-641-1

Hardeman, M.R. and Najean, Y. (eds.): Blood cells in nuclear medicine I. Cell kinetics and bio-distribution. 1984. ISBN 0-89838-653-5

Fueger, G.F. (ed.): Blood cells in nuclear medicine II. Migratory blood cells. 1984. ISBN 0-89838-654-3

Biersack, H.J. and Cox, P.H. (eds.): Radioisotope studies in cardiology. 1985. ISBN 0-89838-733-7

Cox, P.H., Limouris, G. and Woldring, M.G. (eds.): Progress in radiopharmacology 1985. 1985. ISBN 0-89838-745-0

Cox, P.H., Mather, S.J., Sampson, C.B. and Lazarus, C.R. (eds.): Progress in radiopharmacy. 1986. ISBN 0-89838-823-6

Heiss, W.-D., Pawlik, G., Herholz, K. and Wienhard, K. (eds.): Clinical efficacy of positron emission tomography. 1987. ISBN 0-89838-898-8

Clinical efficacy of positron emission tomography

Proceedings of a workshop held in Cologne, FRG, sponsored by the Commission of the European Communities as advised by the Committee on Medical and Public Health Research

edited by

W.-D. HEISS, G. PAWLIK, K. HERHOLZ and **K. WIENHARD**

Max-Planck-Institute for Neurological Research, Cologne, F.R.G.

1987 SPRINGER-SCIENCE+BUSINESS MEDIA, B.V.

Distributors

for the United States and Canada: Kluwer Academic Publishers, P.O. Box 358, Accord Station, Hingham, MA 02018-0358, USA
for the UK and Ireland: Kluwer Academic Publishers, MTP Press Limited, Falcon House, Queen Square, Lancaster LA1 1RN, UK
for all other countries: Kluwer Academic Publishers Group, Distribution Center, P.O. Box 322, 3300 AH Dordrecht, The Netherlands

Library of Congress Cataloging in Publication Data

```
Clinical efficacy of positron emission tomography.

  (Developments in nuclear medicine)
  Workshop held Oct. 23-25, 1986.
  Includes bibliographies.
  1. Tomography, Emission--Evaluation--Congresses.
I. Heiss, W.-D. (Wolf-Dieter)  II. Commission of the
European Communities.  III. Series.  [DNLM: 1. Brain--
radionuclide--congresses.  2. Heart--radionuclide--
congresses.  3. Lung--radionuclide--congresses.  4. Soft
Tissue Neoplasms--radionuclide--congresses.  5. Tomography,
Emission Computed--congresses.  W1 DE998KF /
WL 141 C6408 1986]
RC78.7.T62C55  1987      616.07'572         87-13984
```

ISBN 978-94-010-8002-6   ISBN 978-94-009-3345-3 (eBook)
DOI 10.1007/978-94-009-3345-3
EUR 10972 EP

Book information

Publication arranged by: Commission of the European Communities, Directorate-General Information Market and Innovation, Luxembourg

Copyright/legal notice

Neither the Commission of the European Communities nor any person acting on behalf of the Commission is responsible for the use which might be made of the following information.

BIOMEDICAL ENGINEERING IN THE EUROPEAN COMMUNITY
MEDICAL RESEARCH PROGRAMME OF THE EEC

The European Community involvement in the field of Medical Research started in 1978 with the first Medical Research Programme containing 3 concerted action projects. Since then, it extended to about 34 projects presently and about 72 projects proposed within the 4th Medical Research Programme due to start in 1987.

Community objectives have concentrated on the prevention of illness and disability, the early detection of disease and rehabilitation.

The criteria applied for the selection of projects are:
- the topic should be of importance to Community as a whole;
- the topic should have practical importance, in particular from a social and economic point of view;
- on scientific grounds: either the project should need to be implemented jointly or at least could be carried out much more effectively on a Community basis than separately in each Member State.

The Medical Research Programme is executed in form of "concerted actions", which means that the Commission of the European Communities provides funds for the co-ordination of research. The research itself is funded entirely from national sources.

Within the framework of selected projects, the Commission of the European Communities facilitates collaboration in the following way:
1) By awarding a contract to a project leader, who is responsible for co-ordination and contact between participating centers;
2) By providing funds for the exchange of scientific personnel and materials and for scientific meetings;
3) By funding centralized facilities, such as computing and statistical services, and publications which arise from concerted actions.

The management of this programme is undertaken by a General Concerted Action Committee (GCAC) and by Concerted Action Committees (COMACs).

The present study was conducted under the auspices of COMAC-BME, which is responsible for the co-ordination of research in biomedical engineering. Details of the activity of COMAC-BME have been described by Beneken et al., Journal of Medical Engineering & Technology, Vol. 9, No 2, March-April 1985, pages 61-65.

More detailed information can be obtained from:

Commission of the European Communities
Directorate-General XII/F/3
Rue de la Loi, 200
B - 1049 Brussels, Belgium

Brussels, 6 October 1986

TABLE OF CONTENTS

Brain Tumors

FOREWORD

The series of workshops sponsored by the European Communities started with "Methodology of PET" at Hammersmith Hospital, London, in March 1984. This was followed by "Radiochemistry, Methodology and Standardization in PET" at the Service Hospitalier Frédéric Joliot in Orsay, France, in March 1985. Both these meetings were, in the opinion of all participants, great successes, and it was agreed that such work-shops should continue and be organized on the same basis. After these two workshops on the fundamentals of PET, time now is ripe to evaluate the clinical efficacy of PET investigations, and to discuss to what extend the information provided by this high technology and theoretical area has contributed to the understanding of disease mechanisms, leading to immediate clinical applications.

As pointed out in the previous meetings, PET using short-lived radioisotopes produced in an on-line cyclotron is restricted to a few centers. Therefore, the topics studied so far were mainly of scientific interest and clinical problems were dealt with only marginally. Before this costly technique can be spread and new information made accessible to a broader clinical clientele, its clinical value must be demonstrat-ed.

So far, in the majority of studies, the central nervous system was the primary target organ, and PET has contributed a great deal to our understanding of brain physiology and pathology. Also on the heart, a substantial number of studies have been performed in various centers, but the application of PET to this organ is still somewhat limited. Studies of other organs, e.g., the lungs, and of special topics, e.g., cancer, are scarce, and it is still controversial if PET has a special place in the diagnosis or detection of pathophysiologic mechanisms in these organs and diseases.

In the United States, great efforts are being made to broaden clinical applications of PET. These have been supported by high-rank politicians as well as by wide publicity in the media culminating in a special meeting, held under the auspices of the President of the United States (see Issue of J. Nucl. Med. of December 1985).

At present, there are approximately 10 PET centers within the EEC with another 2 groups in Sweden and one developing in Finland. Ten more

PET centers are being planned for the next 2 to 3 years in member countries of the European Communities. Among the existing groups, several are in close contact with clinical facilities or are directly located in a clinical department or a hospital. Therefore, the work done in most of the centers is focussing on clinical problems. Indeed, some of the results have already had clinical impact changing our understanding of disease and patient care.

In order to further develop these clinical applications, more exchange of experience and coordination of research topics is necessary between the EEC groups. One goal is to condense what has been achieved to date and to have this assessed by Senior Clinical Experts who are not directly involved in PET studies. It is with these aims in mind that a proposal was made for the European Communities to sponsor a workshop on "Clinical Efficacy of PET".

The objective of this third workshop was to answer the following:

1. What new information on human disease and its treatment has been provided or is emerging through PET studies ?
2. Are the clinical research questions being addressed truly relevant?
3. Are there other clinical research problems that should be tackled?
4. What is the role of PET as a clinical diagnostic tool?
5. What is the role of PET in proving and quantifying the efficacy of therapy?

To deal with these topics, representatives of the PET centers as well as clinicians primarily not involved in PET studies were invited to participate on a workshop held in Cologne on October 23-25, 1986.

W.-D. Heiss
G. Pawlik
K. Herholz
K. Wienhard

INTRODUCTION

DEMANDS ON POSITRON EMISSION TOMOGRAPHY FOR EXAMPLE IN CLINICAL NEUROLOGY

W.-D. Heiss

Max-Planck-Institut für neurologische Forschung, Cologne, FRG

The diagnosis of neurological disease has been revolutionized by the advance of threedimensional imaging techniques, especially X-ray computed tomography (CT). With this technique it became possible for the first time to visualize the location and size of a lesion in the brain and to discriminate among various types of brain damage, e.g., tumor, infarction or hemorrhage. In many instances, however, CT as a modality to image morphology does not contribute to the understanding of pathophysiologic mechanisms and cannot be applied for the assessment of therapeutic effects on altered physiologic parameters. For that purpose nuclear medicine techniques can be used which are able to estimate various physiologic variables regionally in the brain. As a disadvantage of these modalities imaging function rather than morphology of brain tissue the coarse spatial resolution inherent to all isotope techniques when compared to CT and magnetic resonance imaging (MRI) of protons must be accepted. The main demand on nuclear medicine techniques must therefore be the quantitation of physiologic and pathologic processes which are necessary for the understanding of pathophysiology of lesions visualized by modalities imaging morphology.

Imaging of Morphology

Imaging of morphology is the domain of CT and MRT of protons. With regard to the spatial resolution all nuclear medicine techniques are inferior to those methods. Additionally, the type of a lesion usually cannot be recognized by nuclear medicine techniques which unspecifically show the focal damage. This is especially true for the clinically important diagnosis of intracranial hemorrhage which in all stages is still detected best by CT because the magnetic resonance signal of blood is changing in the course after the hemorrhage (Gomori et al., 1985).

Early infarcts and small ischemic lesions, however, can be detected by MRT when CT still shows normal structures. When disturbances of blood supply do not lead to morphological damage but to functional disturbance

MRT and CT cannot detect a lesion. This focal functional disturbance can be demonstrated by nuclear medicine imaging techniques for flow (e.g., single photon emission tomography - SPECT - of ^{133}Xe, ^{123}J IMP or ^{99m}Tc HM-PAO) or for various metabolic substrates (positron emission tomography - PET - of ^{15}O$_2$ and ^{18}F-deoxyglucose). In these instances isotope techniques demonstrate the correlate of focal neurologic symptoms, but they additionally show the effect of a focal lesion on the function of the whole brain: as described repeatedly (Baron et al., 1981a; Kuhl et al., 1980; Heiss et al., 1983; Pawlik et al., 1985) a focal lesion in the brain leads to functional deactivation in remote morphologically intact structures which are connected to the area of the primary lesion by projection fiber tracts. This effect was most prominent in the cerebellum contralateral to a hemispheric lesion. The extent of this remote functional deactivation is important for non-localized symptoms, e.g., the psycho-organic syndrome or impairment of consciousness and may affect the capability for rehabilitation in patients with acute localized brain lesions.

The multiple ischemic lesions in multi-infarct dementia can best be visualized by MRT, while CT often does not show all the small ischemic infarcts, especially if they are localized in the subcortical white matter. Nuclear medicine techniques show the region of impaired flow and of impaired metabolism, but in subcortical lesions very often not the lesion proper, but cortical regions inactivated by deafferentation have impaired flow or metabolism (Heiss et al., 1986). It might be a question to these techniques if the impairment of mental functions is related to changes in these functional parameters. Multiple lesions with prolonged T_2 in MRT are unspecific and might be due to multiple sclerosis. The differentiation can only be achieved by additional investigations as immunoglobin concentration or oligoclonal antibodies in the spinal fluid (Bewermeyer et al., 1986). I doubt that nuclear medicine techniques could help in this difficult and clinically important differential diagnosis. In degenerative dementia impaired mentation is present long before morphologic changes in CT or MRT are visible. For the diagnosis of early cases of degenerative dementia of the Alzheimer type methods must be applied which show disturbed function before morphology is altered. This may be achieved quantitatively by PET of ^{18}fluorodeoxy-glucose where changes in metabolic rate are typically found in the parietal and parieto-temporal cortex long before atrophy of the cortex is obvious in CT (Chase et al., 1984). This typical distribution of impaired function can also be seen in SPECT but the changes can not be quantified with this technique (Podreka et al., 1986). For the early diagnosis of degenerative dementia and for the differentiation to MID or to depressive syndromes in the aged the functional imaging modalities - SPECT and PET - are better suited than CT and MRT. In contrast to the pattern observed in Alzheimer cases metabolic rate is markedly decreased in the frontal and temporal lobe in Pick's disease.

Verification of suspected Huntington's chorea is also feasible with functional imaging: As shown originally by Kuhl et al. (1982) metabolism in the striate is impaired long before the atrophy of the caudate nucleus can be seen on CT images. Again, this diagnosis which is of utmost importance for the patient and his family can be made early only in PET or SPECT.

The detection of space occupying lesions in the head, especially of intracranial tumors, is the domain of the morphological imaging modalities as CT and MRT, and the value of these techniques for clinical neurology cannot be reached by any other technique. In these instances isotope techniques show unspecifically a lesion and its effect on whole brain function. However, the type and grade of a cerebral neoplasm very often remains obscure. Here again is a clinical demand for accurate diagnosis which could be fulfilled by studies of flow or metabolism: DiChiro et al. (1983) have shown that malignant gliomas have a very high metabolic rate for glucose, while low grade astrocytomas have metabolic rates similar to the white matter. A further differentiation of these results may help to assess the malignancy of an intracranial tumor: This would give an accurate diagnosis without biopsy which often does not reach all parts of a growth with different tissue compartments. This knowledge would help in the planning of appropriate treatment.

Physiology and Pathophysiology

While imaging of morphology is the domain of CT and MRT, imaging of function of brain tissue in the form of various physiologic parameters can only be achieved today by nuclear medicine techniques with sufficient spatial resolution. Distribution of flow and unilateral local changes can be estimated by SPECT of ^{131}J IMP and ^{133}Xe HM-PAO but quantification which is necessary for inter- and intraindividual comparison is still limited with this method. Flow and metabolism can be

quantified regionally by PET under various physiologic conditions
(Phelps et al., 1982). Specific patterns of metabolic activation were
described for the different sensoric modalities and appropriate
metabolic changes were also observed during various tasks, as motoric
movements or automated speech. These studies can be used as a tool for
functional neuroanatomy indicating all the structures involved in simple
or complex tasks. Such studies are not feasible with the morphological
imaging techniques.

   Autoradiography in animal experiments and its clinical correlate
PET have helped our understanding of the pathophysiology of ischemic
brain damage, the final stage of which can only be visualized by CT and
MRT. The cause is always a transient or permanent disturbance of the
tissue supply and only this important step can be demonstrated by flow
estimation with SPECT. PET with the application of several tracers
permits the description of various mechanisms compensating for impaired
blood circulation and of the stages when the metabolic demand of the
tissue cannot be fulfilled leading to irreversible tissue damage: In
cases with decreased circulation due to arterial stenosis the oxygen
extraction fraction and the rate for metabolic substrates is kept to a
normal level by increased blood volume (Gibbs et al., 1984). If blood
supply is critically diminished the extraction fraction is increased and
thereby the metabolic supply of the tissue is guaranteed (Powers et al.,
1984). Both, these instances are fully reversible and permanent deficits
or morphologic lesions do not develop if they are corrected. Only if the
metabolic rate of oxygen (or glucose) drops below a critical level the
structural integrity of the tissue is endangered and permanent lesions
develop. Very often cerebral blood flow is increased above the normal
value at stages after an ischemic attack when the tissue is already
irreversibly damaged. This phemomenon with flow increases above the
metabolic demand was observed long before the PET era and termed luxury
perfusion syndrome (Lassen 1966). In these instances further improvement
of blood flow as induced by pharmaceutical or surgical measures cannot
improve the clinical condition of a patient but such strategies would be
helpful in those cases early after the attack when metabolic demand of
still viable tissue is high and flow is low (misery perfusion syndrome,
BARON et al., 1981b). The uncoupling of the physiologic variables can
also occur for glucose uptake with respect to flow and oxygen
consumption: In conditions with impaired blood flow and decreased oxygen

supply glucose can be accumulated in the tissue (Wise et al., 1983). As a consequence anaerobic glycolysis causes high tissue lactacidosis which additionally aggravates ischemic cell damage. Regions with high uptake of glucose shortly after an attack therefore are principially not protected but may as well be infarcted in later investigations. However, in some instances these hypermetabolic areas if they are in a region of hyperperfusion may survive as viable tissue bridges in necrotic areas. All these pathophysiologic mechanisms which are extremely important for the development of a rational therapy of stroke can only be observed by multiple tracer studies with PET: flow, oxygen consumption, glucose metabolism, and blood volume should be investigated to achieve all the information in a single case necessary for the understanding of the individual pathophysiology, and additional information can be obtained by studying regional intracellular pH with ^{11}C DMO: While in most infarcts pH is low due to lactacidosis in cases with hyperperfusion pH may be shifted to the alkaline range (Yamamoto et al., 1985). It must be shown in larger series if this phenomenon has an effect on prognosis.

Partial epileptic seizures are another condition in which the function of brain tissue is changed locally. Very often underlying morphologic lesions are so small that they cannot be resolved by CT or MRT. While these structures have high metabolism during the functional activation of seizure activity they usually are hypometabolic foci in the interictal periods. These hypometabolic foci can be found in PET glucose studies and are sometimes also visible with SPECT. As shown by Engel et al. (1983) PET is a valuable tool in the selection of cases with partial epilepsies for surgery. With a certain number of cases with partial epilepsy who are not responding satisfactory to drug treatment there is a clinical need for atraumatic diagnostic procedures for the detection and localization of such epileptic foci which may be accessible for surgical treatment.

Etiology

A prerequisite of efficient therapy of a disease is the knowledge of its etiology. In many diseases of the central nervous system etiology is obscure. However, there are some examples that nuclear medicine techniques could help to understand the development of pathologic changes.

The cause of the clinical syndrome of Parkinson's disease can be demonstrated in the decreased concentration of dopaminergic fibers in the striate. These fibers accumulate ^{18}F-dopamin after the injection of ^{18}F-DOPA (Garnett et al., 1983). In Parkinson's disease accentuated on one side the decreased concentration of ^{18}F-dopamin in the putamen is obvious while the caudate still has a high activity of the tracer. The distribution of transmitters or of receptors is altered in a number of diseases, perhaps also in psychiatric disorders, and the description of such changes may help in the exploration of the disorders.

Changes in flow, oxygen consumption, and glucose metabolism are epiphenomena of degenerative diseases whose primary pathogenetic damage is unknown. The changes of metabolism observed in Alzheimer cases may be secondary to impaired function and are in no connection to the primary lesion. Besides changes of transmitter activity - e.g., the cholinergic system originating from the nucleus basalis Meynert - alterations of the cellular protein synthesis could be important for the progressive neuronal damage. Bustany et al. (1983) observed decreases in the incorporation rate of ^{11}C-methionine in the association cortex where the first metabolic and morphologic changes develop.

The altered incorporation rate of amino acids could also help to detect brain tumors or their recurrencies. If the various imaging techniques are compared in malignant tumors (Bergström et al., 1983) the accurate size of a malignant growth is only demonstrated in the PET images obtained after injection of ^{11}C-methionine, while CT and Ga-PET show only the area with destroyed blood-brain barrier and glucose PET indicates the core of the tumor with raised glucose uptake due to anaerobic glycolysis. It was shown by Bustany et al. (1983) that malignant gliomas have an exorbitantly increased incorporation rate for ^{11}C-methionine compared to the moderate increases in low grade astrocytoma. This new field in the early diagnosis of tumors and the assessment of their biologic activity as well as the use of amino acid tracers in the long-term management of tumor patients will be dealt with in several papers. One has to stress that the development in tumor research must also consider the application of labeled nucleotides as already used in animal experiments, e.g., ^{18}F-fluoro-uridine (Crawford et al., 1982) - and of labeled monoclonal antibodies.

Estimation of Prognosis

An estimation of prognosis is important for the planning of the further life of a patient and for the family. The descriptive information of an image alone contains certainly prognostic information in space occupying lesions, as tumors, if the type and grade of the neoplasm can be identified. However, in graded pathologic changes as ischemic stroke a quantifyable parameter may add prognostic information to the description of location and extension of the lesion. With two-dimensional flow studies using ^{133}Xe and the scintillation camera we have demonstrated (Heiss et al., 1977) that there is a significant relationship between flow in the acute stage after ischemic stroke and long-term prognosis. These studies need large numbers of patients - in our study more than 400 stroke patients were entered into the study and 180 could be evaluated - which have not been available with PET investigations. With PET being more and more used in clinical routine the numbers necessary for statistical evaluation will soon be collected, and then more studies can b- performed on changes of various parameters in the course after an ischemic or hemorrhagic stroke and their influence on long-term prognosis. Such studies also form a basis for the follow-up under various therapeutic strategies.

Another example where nuclear medicine techniques are demanded is the distinction of carriers of the disease in Huntington families. In clinical Huntington chorea the decrease of CMRGl in the caudate is obvious. In the family members at risk two groups can be distinguished: those with normal and those with decreased glucose metabolism in the basal ganglia. It is justified to assume that those persons with decreased metabolism in the caudate are the carriers of the disease and will be clinically ill in the later course of their life. This assumption is justified by the observation of the occurrence of clinical symptoms in several of those cases (Kuhl et al., 1982). The carriers are well advised not to have children, while the other members with normal caudate metabolism may lead a normal life without restrictions.

Control of Therapy

The control of treatment, the objective assessment of the efficacy of a therapy, must be based on the definition of a therapeutic goal. The best therapeutic goal is the clinical effect but its verification is extremely time consuming and expensive because it must rely on large numbers of patients from controlled clinical trials often under double blind conditions. If a physiologic variable can be defined which is directly related to the pathogenesis, to the course or to the clinical symptoms of a disease, changes of this variable may be used as therapeutic indicators. Since physiologic variables as flow, glucose metabolism, and oxygen consumption can be quantified by PET this method may have an important role in the control of the efficacy of treatment. However, due to the limited availability of PET for clinical purposes such studies are still scarce and criteria are still not well defined. As examples for this application I would like to report preliminary results of glucose measurements before and after drug application: The first example concerns cases with ischemic infarction in which the acute application of piracetam (12 g as infusion) improved CMRGl in the infarcted and the inactivated brain regions (Heiss et al., 1983). The second example is the effect of long-term treatment in dementia: in cases of MID metabolic rate as well as performance in psychologic tests and daily life activities improved with the treatment, while in Alzheimer cases only vigilance and metabolism in the basal ganglia increased. In many instances however effects of drugs might only be visible when the results of multitracer techniques are compared and many regions are investigated: We have found, for instance, that improvement of performance in Alzheimer cases during treatment with a muscarinergic cholinagonist is not concomitant with a diffuse increase in metabolic rate, but an equalization of the heterogeneity of the regional metabolic rates (Szelies et al., 1986).

Pharmacokinetics

A further field of application of nuclear medicine techniques is the follow-up of the fate and distribution of pharmaceutical agents in individual cases. This approach is helpful in the definition of the place of action of a drug and in the detection of drug-refractory cases. With ^{11}C-diphenylhydantoin it could be shown (Baron et al., 1983) that its distribution in the brain is essential for its effectiveness while impaired resorption of the drug does not lead to sufficient brain tissue concentrations.

When antineoplastic agents used for chemotherapy of brain tumors are labeled (e.g., ^{11}C-BCNU) their selective accumulation in the tumor can be used for imaging the tumor and for the demonstration of their specific penetration into the target tissue which is much higher after intracarotid application (Diksic et al., 1984). A completely new field will be opening up in clinical pharmacology when these PET or SPECT techniques have been introduced into broader clinical application. Additional information on the fate of a drug in the body can be obtained by comparing its accumulation and distribution without and with specific premedication: It is well established that a by-product of the synthesis of meperidine namely MPTP (methyl-phenyl-tetra-hydropyridine) destroys dopaminergic neurons in the central nervous system and thereby causes Parkinson's syndrome. As demonstrated in baboons (Moerlein et al., 1986) ^{11}C labeled MPTP accumulates in dopaminergic fibers and the basal ganglia are imaged as regions of high activity. When the oxydation of MPTP to MPP* is blocked by a monoamino oxydase-inhibitor, however, this accumulation in the basal ganglia does not occur. This result demonstrates directly that the active compound is MPP* which is able to penetrate the blood-brain barrier and then destroys selectively the dopaminergic neurons. Also from this type of studies new fields of application of nuclear medicine techniques can be expected.

REFERENCES
Baron, J.C., Bousser, M.G., Comar, D. et al. 1981a. "Crossed cerebellar diaschisis" in human supratentorial brain infarction. Trans. Am. Neurol. Ass., 105, 549-461.
Baron, J.C., Bousser, M.G., Rey, A. et al. 1981b. Reversal of focal "misery-perfusion syndrome" by extra-intracranial arterial bypass in hemodynamic cerebral ischemia. A case study with 15-0 positron emission tomography. Stroke, 12, 454-459.
Baron, J.C., Rougemont, D., Lebrun-Grandié, P. et al. 1983. Local cerebral blood flow and oxygen consumption in evolving irreversible ischemic infarction. In "Positron Emission Tomography of the Brain" (Eds. W.-D. Heiss, M.E. Phelps). (Springer, Berlin, Heidelberg, New York). pp. 120-125.
Bergström, M., Collins, V.P., Ehrin, E. et al. 1983. Discrepancies in brain tumor extent as shown by computed tomography and positron emission tomography using (68-Ga)EDTA, (11-C)glucose, and (11-C)methionine. J. Comput. Assist. Tomogr., 7, 1062-1066.
Bewermeyer, H., Bamborschke, S., Assheuer, J. et al. 1986. Wertigkeit von Zusatzuntersuchungen zur Sicherung der Diagnose bei multipler Sklerose. Dtsch. Med. Wschr., 111, 1398-1405.
Bustany, P., Henry, J.F., Sargent, T. et al. 1983. Local brain protein metabolism in dementia and schizophrenia: in vivo studies with 11-C-L-methionine and positron emission tomography. In "Positron Emission Tomography of the Brain" (Eds. W.-D. Heiss, M.E. Phelps). (Springer, Berlin, Heidelberg, New York). pp. 208-211.
Chase, T.N., Foster, N.L., Fedio, P. et al. 1984. Regional cortical

dysfunction in Alzheimer's disease as determined by positron emission tomography. Ann. Neurol., 15, S170-S174.

Crawford, E.J., Friedkin, M., Wolf, A.P. et al. 1982. 18-F-5-fluorouridine, a new probe for measuring the proliferation of tissue in vivo. Adv. Enzyme, 20, 3-22.

DiChiro, G., Brooks, R.A., Sokoloff, L. et al. 1983. Glycolytic rate and histologic grade of human cerebral gliomas: A study with (18-F)fluorodeoxyglucose and positron emission tomography. In "Positron Emission Tomography of the Brain" (Eds. W.-D. Heiss, M.E. Phelps). (Springer, Berlin, Heidelberg, New York). pp. 181-191.

Diksic, M., Sako, K., Feindel, W. et al. 1984. Pharmacokinetics of positron-labeled 1,3-Bis(2-chloroethyl) nitrosourea in human brain tumors using positron emission tomography. Cancer Res., 44, 3120-3124.

Engel, J., Kuhl, D.E., Phelps, M.E. et al. 1983. Local cerebral metabolism during partial seizures. Neurology, 33, 400-413.

Garnett, E.S., Firnau, G., Nahmias, C. 1983. Dopamine visualized in the basal ganglia of living man. Nature, 305, 137-138.

Gibbs, J.M., Wise, R.J.S., Leenders, K.L. et al. 1984. Evaluation of cerebral perfusion reserve in patients with carotid-artery occlusion. Lancet, I, 310-314.

Gomori, J.M., Grossman, R.I., Goldberg, H.I. et al. 1985. Intracranial hematomas: Imaging by high-field MR. Radiology, 157, 87-93.

Heiss, W.-D., Herholz, K., Böcher-Schwarz, H.G. et al. 1986. PET, CT, and MR imaging in cerebrovascular disease. J. Comput. Assist. Tomogr., 10, 903-911.

Heiss, W.-D., Ilsen, H.W., Wagner, R. et al. 1983. Remote functional depression of glucose metabolism in stroke and its alteration by activating drugs. In "Positron Emission Tomography of the Brain". (Eds. W.-D. Heiss, M.E. Phelps). (Springer, Berlin, Heidelberg, New York). pp. 162-168.

Heiss, W.-D., Zeiler, K., Havelec, L. et al. 1977. Longterm prognosis in stroke related to cerebral blood flow. Arch. Neurol. (Chic.), 34, 671-676.

Kuhl, D.E., Phelps, M.E., Kowell, A.P. et al. 1980. Effects of stroke on local cerebral metabolism and perfusion: Mapping by emission computed tomography of 18-FDG and 13-NH-3. Ann. Neurol., 8, 47-60.

Kuhl, D.E., Phelps, M.E., Markham, C.H. et al. 1982. Cerebral metabolism and atrophy in Huntington's disease determined by 18-FDG and computed tomographic scan. Ann. Neurol., 12, 425-434.

Lassen, N.A. 1966. The luxury-perfusion syndrome and its possible relation to acute metabolic acidosis localized within the brain. Lancet, II, 1113-1115.

Moerlein, S.M., Stöcklin, G., Pawlik, G. et al. 1986. Regional cerebral pharamcokinetics of the dopaminergic neurotoxin 1-methyl-4-phenyl-1,2,3,6-tetrahydropyridine as examined by positron emission tomography in a baboon is altered by tranylcypromine. Neurosci. Letters, 66, 205-209.

Pawlik, G., Herholz, K., Beil, C. et al. 1985. Remote effects of focal lesions on cerebral flow and metabolism. In "Functional Mapping of the Brain in Vascular Disorders" (Ed. W.-D. Heiss). (Springer, Berlin, Heidelberg, New York, Tokyo). pp. 59-83.

Phelps, M.E., Mazziotta, J., Huang, S.C. 1982. Study of cerebral function with positron computed tomography. J. Cereb. Blood Flow Metabol., 2, 113-162.

Podreka, I., Suess, E., Goldenberg, G. et al. 1986. Initial experience with Tc-99m-hexamethylpropyleneamine oxime (Tc-99m-HMPAO) brain SPECT. J. Nucl. Med., 27, 887-888.

Powers, W.J., Grubb, R.L. Jr., Raichle, M.E. 1984. Physiological responses to focal cerebral ischemia in humans. Ann. Neurol., 16, 546-552.

Szelies, B., Herholz, K., Pawlik, G. et al. 1986. Zerebraler Glukosestoffwechsel bei präseniler Demenz vom Alzheimer-Typ - Verlaufskontrolle unter Therapie mit muscarinergem Cholinagonisten -. Fortschr. Neurol. Psychiat., 54, 356-363, 1986.

Wise, R.J.S., Rhodes, C.G., Gibbs, J.M. et al. 1983. Disturbance of oxidative metabolism of glucose in recent human cerebral infarcts. Ann. Neurol., 14, 627-637.

Yamamoto, Y.L., Hakim, A.M., Diksic, M. et al. 1985. Focal flow disturbances in acute strokes: Effects on regional metabolism and tissue pH. In "Functional Mapping of the Brain in Vascular Disorders" (Ed. W.-D. Heiss). (Springer, Berlin, Heidelberg, New York, Tokyo). pp. 85-105.

B R A I N

Cerebral Vascular Disease

ISCHEMIC STROKE STUDIED BY ^{15}O-LABELED COMPOUNDS: MISERY PERFUSION AND LUXURY PERFUSION

J.C. Baron

Service Hospitalier Frédéric Joliot
CEA, Département de Biologie
Hopital d'Orsay
Orsay, France

The concomittant study of local cerebral blood flow (CBF) and oxygen consumption ($CMRO_2$) by PET and oxygen-15 labeled compounds has led to an improved understanding of the pathophysiological mechanisms of tissue damage and dysfunction in acute stroke patients (Ackerman et al., 1981; Baron, 1985; Frackowiak, 1985; Phelps et al., 1982; Powers and Raichle, 1985).

In this respect, these studies have demonstrated that a diminished perfusion may either represent a state of primary hemodynamic failure, be secondary to depressed oxygen metabolism, or even be in excess of the oxygen demand. Obviously, distinguishing among these 3 situations should be of paramount importance when designing therapeutic attempts at improving outcome.

DEFINITIONS

Primary metabolic depression has been defined as a matched decrease in CBF and $CMRO_2$, in which the normal coupling between perfusion and metabolism is intact. The extent of metabolic depression in areas of gray matter distant from an actual infarct can be considerable. It represents a sign of disconnection that can affect the overlying cortex in cases with lesions of deep gray nuclei and, vice-versa, the deafferented-deefferented cortex with white matter lesions, and the contralateral cortex and cerebellum with supratentorial infarcts (Feeney and Baron, 1986). These effects may underlie some of the clinical expressions of stroke (diaschisis) and may be involved in the long-term recovery process; they may also turn out to be important targets for enhancers of synaptic and metabolic activity.

Primary hemodynamic failure, when sufficiently severe to override autoregulation, manifests itself as a decrease in CBF with a fully or

disproportionately preserved $CMRO_2$. This situation of impaired coupling, which is characterized by a decreased oxygen tissue tension and an
increased oxygen arterio-venous difference and extraction fraction
(OEF), has been termed "misery perfusion". Its presence indicates that
oxygen supply is inadequate relative to oxygen demand, a precarious
state that encompasses both oligemia (mild hypoperfusion with fully
maintained $CMRO_2$) and true ischemia (moderate to severe hypoperfusion
with depressed $CMRO_2$).

The inverse situation, that of oxygen supply in excess of demand,
was recognized by Lassen (1966) long before the advent of PET, as the
cause of the "red veins syndrome", and it was named "luxury perfusion".
It is characterized by an increased oxygen tissue tension and a decreased OEF, and indicates restoration of perfusion in a previously
ischemic tissue. The CBF can be increased, normal, or decreased, but is
consistently in excess of $CMRO_2$, which itself can be normal or depressed, depending on the damage that incurred during previous ischemia.
Luxury perfusion per se may be harmful to the tissue (Siesjö, 1978) and,
hence, may require specific therapy. Anti-ischemic treatment obviously
is of no avail in situations of luxury perfusion.

PET RESULTS AND DISCUSSION
Previous studies

PET studies of acute stroke patients have demonstrated complex
interleaving of these three basic patterns, which is observed not only
in the ultimately damaged area (as defined by late CT scans), but also
in large surrounding zones of brain tissue as well as distant from that
area. Furthermore, rapidly changing patterns have been encountered in
patients studied serially within the first two weeks after their
stroke.

The normal flow-metabolism couple is impaired in over 90% of the
cases studied within the first month of stroke. Areas of misery perfusion are seen in 45 - 57% of the cases studied within 4 days, and only
exceptionally beyond the 12th post-stroke day. During the first 4 days,
areas of luxury perfusion are found in about 40% of cases, while luxury
perfusion within the ultimately necrotic area is the rule between 10 and
40 days after a stroke (Ackerman et al., 1981; Baron, 1985; Lenzi et
al., 1982; Wise et al., 1983). Two studies have demonstrated the transition within a few days from massive misery perfusion, which is a neces-

sary but usually quite transient state in the ischemic process, to luxury perfusion - a process always associated with tissue necrosis (Baron et al., 1983c; Wise et al., 1983).

Early luxury perfusion with hyperemia presumably reflects post-ischemic reactive hyperemia, as it sometimes occurs in ultimately intact brain tissue surrounding the final infarct (Baron et al., 1983b); it is, however, more frequently seen within the core of infarction (Ackerman et al., 1981; Baron, 1985; Baron et al., 1983c; Lenzi et al., 1982). Despite the fact that the $CMRO_2$ values measured with the $^{15}O_2$ continuous-inhalation technique are overestimated in luxury perfusion, if no correction is made for blood pool (Lammertsma et al., 1983; Pantano et al., 1985), it was shown that the former areas have a better preserved $CMRO_2$ than the latter (Baron et al., 1983b). More detailed studies using this improved methodology can now be performed.

On the other hand, instances of early relative luxury perfusion characterized by a low CBF in excess of a profound by depressed $CMRO_2$ presumably reflect the precipitous fall in energy metabolism that occurs within areas irreversibly damaged by ischemia (Wise et al., 1983).

Quite differently, the late phase of luxury perfusion is observed exclusively within necrotic areas showing contrast enhancement on CT (Baron et al., 1983a). It has been suggested to reflect the stage of re-vascularization that characterizes ongoing brain necrosis (Ackerman et al., 1981).

When misery perfusion is observed in acute stroke and the affected tissue ultimately becomes necrotic, local $CMRO_2$ has been generally found dramatically reduced (Baron et al., 1983b, 1983c; Wise et al., 1983). However, it is important to note that large areas of misery per-fusion affecting ultimately viable tissue frequently surround the final infarct. Thus, a state of oligemia-ischemia threatening the involved tissue with irreversible damage, can be seen in humans during the first 4 days of stroke (Ackerman et al., 1981; Baron et al., 1983b). As these facts are reminiscent of "ischemic penumbra", a concept derived from experiments in the subhuman primate (Astrup, 1982), a detailed study of the CBF and $CMRO_2$ values found in these misery perfusion areas was performed (Baron et al., 1983b). "Viable areas" turned out to have bet-ter preserved CBF and $CMRO_2$ than ultimately necrotic areas, with well-delineated threshold values of 11 ml/100g/min and 1.5 ml/100g/min, re-spectively. The latter figure was largely confirmed in PET studies using a different $^{15}O_2$ method, and in patients belonging to other categories of stroke (Powers et al., 1984, 1985a, 1985b).

As viewed by PET, ischemic "penumbra" should conceptually feature depressed $CMRO_2$ (as a corollary of reduced neuronal synaptic activity) and maximally increased OEF (severe misery perfusion), and the involved tissue should demonstrate viability in some instances and ultimate necrosis in others, in accordance with the dynamics of penumbra.

The previous studies either showed well-defined thresholds (Baron et al., 1983b) or did not provide an estimate of final tissue outcome (Wise et al., 1983), leaving unanswered the issue of whether penumbra - and its potential therapeutic correlates - could be actually demonstrated in humans.

In addition, Wise et al. (1983) reported on a patient with massive misery perfusion, in whom the arterial blood pressure was pharmacologically increased: although this increased CBF by a factor of two, it also reduced OEF in the same proportion without altering $CMRO_2$ (Wise et al., 1983). This study has been taken as evidence against the role of reperfusion in acute stroke, but it was performed several days after stroke, and the prevailing $CMRO_2$ and CBF in the core of ischemia were both well below the above mentioned thresholds. (In the surrounding temporal cortex, which also exhibited massive misery perfusion but with only mildly lowered $CMRO_2$, the metabolic rates seemed to increase with induced hypertension).

Present study

We have expanded our initial study (Baron et al., 1983b) and looked at the significance of focal misery perfusion in acute stroke patients (Baron et al., 1986).

From our data bank, we retrospectively selected 24 studies performed in 17 patients between 30 hours and 12 days after onset of completed supratentorial ischemic stroke. They were selected on the grounds of an individually statistically significant ($p<0.05$) focal misery perfusion (Baron et al., 1983b). Quantitative $^{15}O_2$ steady-state studies were carried out using the ECAT II PET camera, with measured attenuation co-efficients (Lebrun-Grandie et al., 1983). The areas showing significant misery perfusion were selected, and were then classified according to spontaneous outcome (using late CT scans at corresponding head levels) as either "necrotic", "viable" (morphologically intact), or "partly necrotic" (both decreased and normal tissue density).

There were 131 regions of interest showing misery perfusion, comprising 101, 10, and 21 regions in the "viable", "partly necrotic", and "necrotic" subgroups, respectively.

The previously described thresholds (Baron et al., 1983b) were recovered, separating "viable" from "necrotic" areas at the CBF and $CMRO_2$ dividing lines of about 11 ml/100g/min and 1.6 ml/100g/min, respectively; the "partly necrotic" areas were randomly distributed on both sides of these lines. There was, however, some overlap of "viable" and "necrotic" areas about these threshold lines.

When expressed as percentage of contralateral homologous areas, the thresholds were $\sim 45\%$ and $\sim 65\%$ for CBF and $CMRO_2$, respectively, with $CMRO_2$ being maintained at close to 100% down to CBF levels of $\sim 55\%$, below this level, there was a linear fall in $CMRO_2$ (Fig. 1).

In addition to these ROIs with normal $CMRO_2$, a large number of ROIs displayed lowered $CMRO_2$, with only mild increases in OEF, testifying to a combination of metabolic depression with superimposed mild oligemia. The OEF vs. CBF plot demonstrated that OEF progressively increased with decreasing CBF, to reach near maximum values (>0.80) at CBF levels of $\sim 8 - 12$ ml/100g/min; with lower CBF values, OEF began to fall, indicating precipitous metabolic failure within ultimately necrotic areas. Ultimately "viable" areas with preserved $CMRO_2$ (>85%) and maximal OEF, indicating a precarious but still fully "compensated" situation, were observed in 5 patients studied between day 2 and day 4 after stroke onset. Only in one patient studied on day 2, $CMRO_2$ was depressed ($\sim 75\%$) at a CBF reduction of approx. 50% and despite maximum OEF (~ 0.85), suggesting impaired neuronal function as a result of inadequate oxygen supply. Since clinical recovery in this patient was excellent, and late CT scans showed no morphological damage in this area, the description would meet the working criteria for ischemic penumbra.

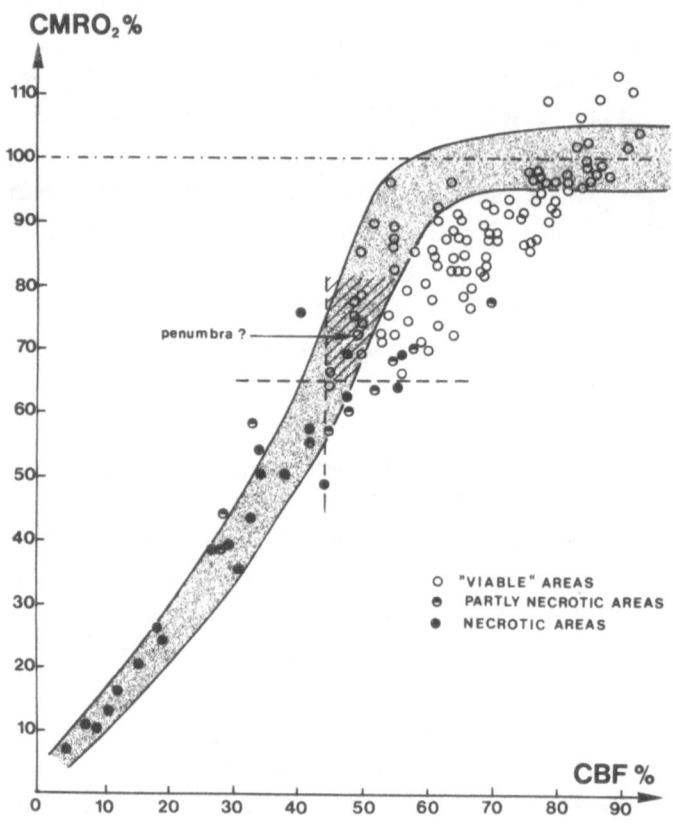

Fig. 1 Plot of local CBF versus local CMRO2, both expressed as
percentages relative to contralateral (healthy) hemisphere, in 131
regions of interest with significant (p<0.05) misery perfusion.
The broken lines represent apparent thresholds separating "viable"
from ultimately necrotic areas. The shaded area represents the
zones of maximally preserved CMRO2, i.e., those areas where the
oxygen extraction fraction is close to 100%; it shows the relationships between CMRO2 and CBF that first allow full preservation of
CMRO2 (oligemia down to a CBF of approx. 55%), followed by a decrease in CMRO2 due to ischemia (55%>CBF>45%) and infarction (CBF<
45%). The hatched zone indicates, where "penumbra" associated with
ultimately viable tissue should presumably be located.

COMMENTS

As discussed earlier (Baron et al., 1983b, 1986), the CBF threshold found is consistent with the infarction threshold reported in unanesthetized monkeys with permanent MCA occlusion (Jones et al., 1981), taking into account the inevitable mixture of gray and white matter in our regional sampling method. The $CMRO_2$ threshold is in agreement with theoretical estimates (Astrup, 1982) but has not been measured in animals.

The decrease in OEF that occurs below the CBF threshold presumably reflects a precipitous decline in energy metabolism heralding irreversible damage, and it is consistent with previous data (Wise et al., 1983).

Above the threshold, the vast majority of areas affected by misery perfusion showed only a mild decrease in CBF and moderately increased OEF. Tissue viability, which was the rule for this pattern of changes, was associated either with preserved $CMRO_2$ (a state of uncomplicated oligemia) or, more unexpectedly, with mildly depressed $CMRO_2$. As this metabolic depression was obviously not the immediate result of inadequate oxygen supply, it may reflect either a superimposed disconnection effect (see above), a selective loss of neurons in a previously "penumbral" area, or a self-protective reaction to ischemia (Astrup, 1982; Mies et al., 1983; Strong et al., 1983).

Ultimately "viable" areas with maximally increased OEF, a situation observed only within 4 days of stroke onset, were detected in 6 patients. In 5, the $CMRO_2$ was fully preserved, indicating that any further drop in CBF would have resulted in a fall in metabolism, and, if too profound and long lasting, in irreversible damage. Only in one patient, a situation of possible penumbra was actually detected. In this patient, the vast majority of the involved areas ultimately escaped frank infarction; a similar case, occurring in the context of vasospasm after subarachnoid hemorrhage, has been reported by Powers et al. (1985). Wise et al. (1983) described another patient with similar PET findings, but in this case, most of the affected tissue progressed to infarction at follow-up. This variable outcome is consistent with the consept of ischemic penumbra, and may be reflected in the overlap of "viable" and "necrotic" areas about the threshold lines (Fig.1) These considerations should stimulate further large-scale PET studies of very early stroke patients, because the definitive demonstration of penumbra in humans may radically alter the prevailing pessimistic view of stroke therapy.

The actual course with time of acute misery perfusion as related to final tissue outcome, to long-standing misery perfusion (Baron et al., 1981; Samson et al., 1985), and to metabolic depression states, also remains to be elucidated.

REFERENCES

Ackerman, R.H., Correia, J.A., Alpert, N.M., et al. 1981. Positron imaging in ischemic stroke disease using compounds labeled with oxygen-15. Arch. Neurol., 38, 537-543.

Astrup, J. 1982. Energy-requiring cell functions in the ischemic brain. J. Neurosurg., 56, 482-497.

Baron, J.C., Bousser, M.G., Rey, A., et al. 1981. Reversal of focal "misery-perfusion syndrome" by extra-intracranial arterial bypass in hemodynamic cerebral ischemia. Stroke, 12, 454-459.

Baron, J.C., Delattre, J.Y., Bories, J., et al., 1983a. Comparison study of CT and positron emission tomography in recent cerebral infarction. AJNR, 4, 536-540.

Baron, J.C., Rougemont, D., Bousser, M.G., et al. 1983b. Local CBF, oxygen extraction fraction (OEF) and CMRO2: prognostic value in recent supratentorial infarction in humans. J. Cereb. Blood Flow Metab., 3, (Supp. 1), 1-12.

Baron, J.C., Rougemont, D., Lebrun-Grandie, P., et al. 1983c. Measurement of local blood flow and oxygen consumption in evolving irreversible cerebral infarction: an in vivo study in man. In "Cerebral Vascular Disease 4" (Eds. J.S. Meyer, H. Lechner, M. Reivich and E.O. Ott). (Excerpta Medica, Amsterdam-Oxford-Princeton). pp. 205-212.

Baron, J.C. 1985. Positron tomography ischemia: a review. Neuroradiol., 27, 509-516.

Baron, J.C., Samson, Y., Bousser, M.G., et al. 1986. Measurements of rCBF and rCMRO2 in acute stroke with PET. In "Acute Brain Ischemia" (Eds. N. Battistini et al.). (Raven Press, New York). pp. 81-87.

Feeney, D.M. and Baron, J.C. 1986. Diaschisis: Progress review. Stroke, 17, 817-827.

Frackowiak, R.S.J. 1985. Pathophysiology of human cerebral ischemia: studies with positron tomography and oxygen 15. In "Brain Imaging and Brain Function" (Ed. L. Sokoloff). (Raven Press, New York). pp. 139-161.

Jones, T.H., Morawetz, R.B., Crowell, R.M., et al. 1981. Thresholds of focal cerebral ischemia in awake monkeys. J. Neurosurg., 54, 773-782.

Lammertsma, A.A., Wise, R.J.S., Heather, J.D., et al. 1983. Correction for the presence of intravascular oxygen 15 in the steady state technique for measuring regional oxygen extraction ratio in the brain. J. Cereb. Blood Flow Metab., 3, 425-431.

Lassen, N.A. 1966. The luxury perfusion syndrome and its possible relation to acute metabolic acidosis localized within the brain. Lancet, 2, 1113-1115.

Lebrun-Grandie, P., Baron, J.C., Soussaline, F., et al. 1983. Coupling between regional blood flow and oxygen utilization in the normal brain; a study with positron tomography and oxygen-15. Arch. Neurol., 40, 230-236.

Lenzi, G.L., Frackowiak, R.S.J. and Jones, T. 1982. Cerebral oxygen metabolism and blood flow in human cerebral ischemic infarction. J. Cereb. Blood Flow Metab., 2, 321-335.

Mies, G., Auer, C.M., Ebhardt, G., et al. 1983. Flow and neuronal density in tissue surrounding ischemic infarction. Stroke, 14, 22-28.

Pantano, P., Baron, J.C., Crouzel, C., et al. 1985. The 15-0 continuous inhalation technique: correction for intravascular signal using C-15-0. Eur. J. Nucl. Med., 10, 387-391.

Phelps, M.E., Mazziotta, J.C. and Huang, S.C. 1982. Study of cerebral function with positron computed tomography. J. Cereb. Blood Flow Metab., 2, 113-162.

Powers, W.J., Grubb, R.L. and Raichle, M.E. 1984. Physiological response to focal cerebral ischemia in humans. Ann. Neurol., 16, 546-557.

Powers, W.J., Grubb, R.L., Baker, R.P., et al. 1985a. Regional cerebral blood flow and metabolism in reversible ischemia due to vasospasm. J. Neurosurg., 62, 539-546.

Powers, W.J., Grubb, R.L., Darriet, D., et al. 1985b. Cerebral blood flow and cerebral metabolic rate of oxygen requirements for cerebral function and viability in humans. J. Cereb. Blood Flow Metab., 5, 600-608.

Powers, W.J. and Raichle, M.E. 1985. Positron emission tomography and its application to the study of cerebrovascular disease in man. Stroke, 16, 361-376.

Samson, Y., Baron, J.C., Bousser, M.G. et al. 1985. Effects of extra-intracranial arterial bypass on cerebral blood flow and oxygen metabolism in humans. Stroke, 16, 609-616.

Siesjö, B.K. 1978. Brain Energy Metabolism. John Wiley, Chichester.

Strong, A.T., Tomlinson, B.E. Verrables, G.S., et al. 1983. The cortical ischaemic penumbra associated with occlusion of the middle cerebral artery in the cat. J. Cereb. Blood Flow Metab., 3, 97-108.

Wise, R.J.S., Bernardi, S., Frackowiak, R.S.J., et al. 1983. Serial observations on the pathophysiology of acute stroke: the transition from ischaemia to infarction as reflected in regional oxygen extraction. Brain, 106, 197-222.

ISCHEMIC DISEASE STUDIED WITH ^{15}O LABELLED COMPOUNDS: METABOLIC AND HEMODYNAMIC DISPARITIES

R.S.J. Frackowiak
MRC Cyclotron Unit, Hammersmith Hospital and
National Hospital for Nervous Diseases, Queen Square
London, U.K.

This article attempts to evaluate how PET may affect the care of patients with ischemic cerebrovascular disease. PET scanning studies of patients with cerebral ischemic disease have been reported in the open literature from 1978 (Baron et al., 1978). Quantitative PET techniques have been described since 1979 for measuring cerebral blood volume (CBV) and cerebral metabolic rate of glucose (CMRGlu) (Phelps et al., 1979; Reivich et al., 1979), and 1980 for cerebral blood flow (CBF) and cerebral metabolic rate of oxygen (CMRO$_2$) (Frackowiak et al., 1980). Since then PET scanning has advanced technically and new methods for measuring a variety of physiological variables have been described or refined (Phelps et al., 1986). The work to date has been confined to relatively few centres around the world and has therefore been oriented very largely in the direction of research rather than routine diagnostic use. A considerable amount of new insight has been obtained over the last 7 years which makes it now possible to classify patients with cerebrovascular disease in physiological as well as clinical terms. These advances with those in anatomical and structural diagnosis made by CT and NMR scanning and digital subtraction angiography now provide the practicing clinician with a very considerable armamentarium for analysing the precise problems of the individual patient, and planning the most appropriate management.

It has been clear for many years that clinical classifications alone are poor in differentiating the diverse pathologies that underlie the common ischemic syndromes. The PET studies to be described in this chapter show that there is also a wide variety of pathophysiological states underlying similar clinical presentations. The knowledge of these patterns and their reliable detection should have a profound influence on choices of medical and/or surgical therapy of patients with ischemic syndromes.

ACUTE ISCHAEMIA AND CEREBRAL INFARCTION

What has been elucidated in human cerebral ischemic pathophysiology
with PET so far? The study of energy metabolism in acute ischaemia has
been fruitfully pursued by a number of PET groups (Frackowiak, 1985a).
There have not been many studies in terms of numbers of patients, but
most agree on the substance of the observations if not always their
interpretation. This section will summarise the main findings to date.

Perfusion

An important aspect of the study of ischaemia is an appreciation of
the relationship between the supply of the essential energy substrates,
glucose and oxygen and demand for them by the cerebral tissues (Jones et
al., 1985; Kuhl et al., 1980). This can be done regionally with PET by
reference to the fractional arterio-venous extraction of the substrate
into the tissue from the perfusing blood. The extraction of glucose is
normally about 10% and that of oxygen 40%. There is therefore a greater
reserve of glucose than oxygen in the blood stream, hence oxygen becomes
the first limiting substrate when perfusion fails. PET can be used to
clearly image ischaemia and to measure its depth and extent. Ischaemia
occurs when the supply of energy substrates becomes limiting to metabolism. Patients with recent ischemic strokes have been studied and invariably, if studied early enough after the ictus, show a focally raised
region of fractional oxygen extraction (OER) (Wise et al., 1983). The
OER is highest the earlier the study is performed and values approaching
100% extraction have been recorded. In the regions of brain exhibiting
focally increased levels of oxygen extraction, CBF is very low and invariably below 15 ml/100ml/min. Oxygen metabolism though also focally
depressed is relatively preserved. In other words the uncoupling of CBF
and $CMRO_2$ expressed by the rise in OER to maximal levels is primarily
due to a profound drop in perfusion. The regional changes of perfusion
invariably occupy recognisable territories of cerebral arteries.

Metabolism

The changes in $CMRO_2$ are more heterogeneous in the very earliest
phases. Cerebral cortex has relative preservation of $CMRO_2$ and hence
higher OER values than basal nuclei and deep white matter. This appears
to be a time dependent process. In patients studied sequentially, the
regions of high oxygen extraction show progessive decline in the value

of the OER, most commonly to frankly subnormal levels, sometimes as low
as 5 - 10%. Patients studied more than 3 days after their stroke almost
invariably show a focally depressed OER in the diseased cerebral region
affected by ischaemia. A low OER is a second and specific form of flow-
metabolism uncoupling. It explicitly implies that the low OER region
requires proportic tely less oxygen than normal brain, despite considerably impaired perfusion (CBF) which might, viewed alone, lead to
the erroneous conclusion that the hypoperfused region was still
ischemic. In fact the brain, previously subjected to an acute episode of
ischaemia, is now relatively overperfused in relation to its residual
metabolic requirements. The area of low CBF has the pathophysiological
characteristics of an infarct. Any region of brain which has depressed
metabolic activity and yet does not use all the oxygen available to it
can no longer be considered capable of normal metabolic activity. The
likeliest cause for this is cell death, i.e. infarction (Frackowiak and
Wise, 1983).

Thresholds

The metabolic and perfusion thresholds for infarction in terms of
depth and duration of ischaemia remain imprecisely known though some
preliminary, largely extrapolated data are available in the literature
(Lenzi et al., 1982; Powers et al., 1985). The period of supranormal
oxygen extraction may last hours, a considerable proportion of this at
submaximal levels so that the actual ischemic episode may be very short.
The time course of maximal oxygen extraction is still imprecisely understood, acute sequential studies in patients with very early ischaemia are
now needed, with clear documentation of subsequent functional outcome.
Such studies may have a considerable impact on defining early prognostic
features of ischemic disease.

Infarction

The progression from a state of ischaemia (i.e. high OER and relatively greater depression of CBF than $CMRO_2$), to one of infarction
with low OER and $CMRO_2$, has also been studied. This is a remarkably
quick process, which as alluded to above, may evolve with a different
time course in different tissues. It has been observed that the OER of
subcortical tissues tends to be lower than that of cortex even in the
earliest stages of the ischemic stroke. One explanation is that the

degree of ischaemia resulting from a drop in perfusion pressure in a major cerebral or cranial artery is not the same in the deep tissues, where superficial and deep perforating arterial territories meet, as in the cortex. This is not substantiated by the PET data which show that the level of perfusion is the same in the two territories even when very early measurements are made (the earliest a patient has been studied after a stroke is 90 min). Another explanation is that certain neuronal populations are more susceptible to ischemic cell death than others. There is some evidence in the experimental literature that this may be so.

The fall in OER which is almost invariably seen in stroke patients may be due to two causes. The CBF may rise in a region of infarction, perhaps as a result of disobliteration of an artery so that perfusion is re-established through a dysautoregulated region of brain. The increase in flow through a region incapable of any increase in metabolic activity because of established cell death will show a fall in the fractional extraction of oxygen, because this represents the relationship between the two variables. On the other hand, in some instances, the fall in OER has been shown to be due to a further fall in metabolic activity of the region without much apparent change in perfusion. This further fall in $CMRO_2$ may be due to delayed cell death, or alternatively a further episode of ischaemia occurring in the same territory in between the two measurements. Again there are precedents in the experimental literature for the occurrence of delayed cell death in, for example, specific neuronal populations in the hippocampus.

Chronic, submaximal OER elevation

With time, as the infarction matures, the OER tends to revert to normal. In certain instances, particularly when the infarct has been large, a chronically depressed OER is observed. Such regions invariably have very low residual metabolic activity. Very rarely the progression to a state of low OER in the very early stages of the stroke does not occur. In these patients an elevation of OER, which is considerably less than maximal and usually of the order 55 - 70% is seen as long as four days after the onset of symptoms. One would expect on physiological grounds that these patients have a special risk of further ischemic events. Attempts at altering perfusion pressure in the phase of submaximally elevated oxygen extraction are limited. A patient with TIAs with persistently, though submaximally raised oxygen extraction which normalised on extracranial-intracranial arterial bypass surgery has been described (Baron et al., 1981a). A few cases of reversion of elevated oxygen extraction to normal in patients with ischemic episodes and extensive extracranial occlusive disease have also been reported following endarterectomy or extra-intracranial bypass surgery (Gibbs et al., 1985). We have also had the opportunity of studying such a patient suffering from a profound right hemiplegia and aphasia which came on three days before her first PET examination. She was found to have an area of low $CMRO_2$ throughout the territory of the middle cerebral artery, but uncharacteristically the OER was still elevated at 60% or so. We attempted to raise perfusion by medical means and did so quite successfully, but no change in $CMRO_2$ occurred and therefore a fall in OER was produced. In an attempt to see whether a delayed improvement might occur, perfusion was medically maintained for over 24 hours. Again no change in $CMRO_2$ or function was noted and OER remained low. When the CBF was allowed to fall back to natural levels, unsustained by medication, the OER rose back to the previously elevated, though submaximal levels and again no change in $CMRO_2$ was noted. These passive changes of perfusion through a dysautoregulated, pressure dependant vascular bed had no effect on the underlying level of metabolism, which was detemined by the population of neurones surviving the initial ischemic event. Perfusion was just sufficient to maintain this level of metabolism but with little reserve, and presumably any further fall in perfusion pressure would have caused a further ischemic event. These rare cases of impaired perfusion reserve are more common in patients presenting with transient ischemic events or minor strokes from major cervical artery occlusions as will be described below. There have been no reported studies in patients with evolving infarction and the earliest stages of evolving stroke, secondary to acute carotid occlusion have not been studied. Treatment of patients with drugs designed to suppress metabolism lend themselves to study as does objective monitoring of the primary aim of therapy and the metabolic result. The question of metabolic activity as a prognostic factor and its accuracy in indicating cell death, as well as the correlation of degrees of disability with residual metabolic levels and patterns of disturbance remain to be investigated (Sokoloff, 1981).

Reversible metabolic deficits

The sequence of events in transient ischemic attacks is largely un-explored. It is not clear whether patients with TIA have a completely reversible metabolic deficit, or whether the changes are so restricted in space or degree that no clinical deficit is clinically obvious, but limited neuronal death occurs. This latter scenario would have major im-plications on the therapeutic attitude to patients with TIA, and on the understanding of intellectual decline known to be associated with cere-bral ischemic disease. There is also the question of cerebral functional recovery. Acute observations with sequential follow-up to assess if fo-cally depressed metabolism is ever reversible are urgently required. Samson and his colleagues have recently suggested that revascularisation surgery in the context of a normal OER and hence absence of ischemia may in certain circumstances lead to an augmentation of metabolic activity in the reperfused territory. The reasons for this are not at all clear and are explained with difficulty in the context of the pathogenic mechanisms described above (Samson et al., 1985).

Diaschisis

Various other phenomena have been described in patients after acute cerebral infarction whose clinical significance is not always clear. The most dramatic and frequently observed phenomenon is that termed "crossed cerebellar diaschisis". This appears to be a transneural effect with de-pression of contralateral cerebellar metabolism in patients with cere-bral infarcts. The depression is not on a vascular, ischemic basis be-cause the relationship between CBF and $CMRO_2$ remains quite normal. The depression may come on in the earliest days after the stroke, or some days later. The phenomenon may be reversible and may have an association with the size and/or position of the supratentorial infarction. This phenomenon was first recognised by Baron and his colleagues at Orsay (Baron et al., 1981b). They feel that it represents a functional de-activation of the crossed cerebellar hemisphere as a result of inter-ruption of cortico-ponto-cerebellar connections by the infarction. The phenomenon has now also been described in other supratentorial patho-logies. The status of other forms of diaschisis is less certain. Claims that the contralateral cerebral hemisphere also undergoes some functional deactivation are on less certain ground. Our own data, recently re-evaluated, show that when patients with strokes are compared to normal subjects, the contralateral cerebral hemisphere shows a 15% lower metabolism. However, if the comparison is made with subjects who are arteriopaths who have a similar profile of stroke risk-factors as the patients, but who have never suffered a clinical episode of cerebral ischemia, then no difference can be demonstrated. This suggests that neuronal loss due to subclinical ischemic events can occur and may confuse the interpretation of distant metabolic effects seen in patients with acute cerebral infarction (Wise et al., 1986).

The study of the natural history of ischemic stroke suggests a very pessimistic outlook therapeutically, both in terms of tissue rescue and salvage. The time course of true cerebral ischemia is very short and for any therapy to be effective it must be applied at a time of maximal pathophysiological disturbance which is also the time at which revascularisation therapy carries greatest risk. Our attention will therefore now shift to studies of at-risk states for stroke and the assessment of patients in whom prophylactic treatment designed to prevent further episodes of ischaemia is being considered.

PREVENTION OF ISCHEMIA

The pathophysiology of cervical occlusive disease has been studied in a number of laboratories and permitted the description of the normal homeostatic mechanisms which help to prevent ischaemia when perfusion pressure falls. These studies have centred on haemodynamic mechanisms as well as energy metabolism. The cerebral circulation normally exhibits autoregulation, which means that CBF is independent of blood pressure over a wide range. The maintenance of blood flow at these constant levels, dictated by metabolic requirements rather than moment to moment fluctuations of systemic pressure, is accomplished by alteration of the calibre of the cerebral resistance vessels. Reciprocal vasodilatation in the face of hypotension results in an appropriate fall in peripheral resistance which counteracts the fall in cerebral perfusion pressure, hence flow is maintained constant. Conversely, a rise in blood pressure is counterbalanced by vasoconstriction and an augmentation of peripheral resistance. Studies in patients with cervical occlusive disease have demonstrated pathophysiological patterns which indicate the breakdown or exhaustion of these normal homeostatic haemodynamic mechanisms (Gibbs et al., 1984).

Perfusion reserve

The first pattern is of vasodilatation manifesting as a focal increase of CBV in the territory of the occluded artery. Examination of
patients with occluded cervical arteries has shown that CBV asymmetries
are always such that the higher CBV is on the side of the occlusion.
Group analysis has failed however to find a critical CBV which dis-
criminates occluded from patent arterial territories. The reason for
this is that CBF and CBV are inter-related variables. Normally there is
a reasonably linear relationship between the two. Thus occlusions which
cause little change in perfusion pressure because of excellent collaterals will show no change in flow and litte change in CBV. If the
perfusion pressure falls more markedly, vasodilatation will be pronouncend but flow may remain normal. The fall in perfusion pressure may
be so marked that maximal vasodilatation and the consequent fall in
peripheral resistance will be insufficient to maintain CBF (Frackowiak,
1985). From the above, it is apparent that the ratio of CBF to CBV should
vary as a function of local perfusion pressure. When perfusion pressure
falls, the ratio CBF/CBV should fall, even outside the limits of autoregulation. Our studies with patients have demonstrated focal changes
of CBF/CBV as predicted. The ratio has high discriminant value between
territories of patent carotids, those which are occluded in isolation,
those which are occluded with contralateral stenoses and those with
bilateral occlusions (Lenzi et al., 1982). Patients with symptoms
suggestive of a haemodynamic component to their ischemia, e.g. posturally
related amaurosis contralateral to limb symptoms, or watershed territory
infarcts on CT, show the severest decreases in the CBF/CBV ratio. In fact
this ratio represents the reciprocal of the cerebral vascular transit
time, that is the mean flow velocity of blood in the regional cerebral
circulation. The lower the ratio, the slower the flow velocity and the
longer the residence time, which is what one would predict in a
circulation which is maximally vasodilated and where the perfusion
pressure is low.

Oxygen carriage reserve

The correlation of this index of the haemodynamic status of the circulation with the OER has shown a striking relationship. The progressive
fall in CBF/CBV accompanying increasing severity of cervical occlusive
disease is associated with no change in OER until a threshold value is

reached when further haemodynamic compromise is accompanied by an increase in oxygen extraction. This threshold represents the point of
maximal vasodilatation and the exhaustion of the perfusion reserve which
is the first line of defence against energy failure when vascular
occlusion occurs. It is at this stage that CBF begins to fall. Many
patients, particular those with previous symptomatic strokes or TIA have
lower than normal baseline flow. However this is matched to the residual
metabolic function and the OER is normal. In the case of haemodynamic
decompensation CBF begins to fall and the brain now has only the oxygen
reserve preventing energy failure and loss of function. Patients with
low CBF/ CBV and submaximal elevations of OER represent 10 - 15% of the
patients with cervical occlusive disease studied by Gibbs. These
patients were also those with the most advanced disease anatomically and
who on careful questioning exhibited clinical features suggestive of
haemodynamic ischaemia. Haemodynamic failure was extremely uncommon in
patients with unilateral carotid occlusion, some occlusive component in
at least one of the other three arteries was found in all those showing
focal increases in OER. It is therefore possible to distinguish patients
who only have impaired haemodynamics and to quantify its severity with
the CBF/CBV ratio. Secondly, patients can also be identified who are in
more precarious physiological state because their haemodynamic reserve
is exhausted and they also show an increase in focal OER. These patients
have local, pressure passive circulations and are calling on their
oxygen reserve as the last defence against onset of ischemia. The two
homeostatic mechanisms seem to act in series preventing any fall in
$CMRO_2$ and hence disturbance of function.

Revascularisation

Patients studied before and two or more months after revascularisation therapy by EC-IC bypass surgery have demonstrated an invariable rise
in the CBF/CBV ratio if the anastomosis is patent. The OER falls if it
is raised pre-operatively, though per-operative infarction has occurred
in a few such patients. This is not altogether surprising given that
these patients are in the most precarious physiological state, which
highlights once more the paradox that those most likely to benefit from
prophylactic revascularisation are also those most likely to suffer
peri-operative strokes. A final consistent observation, based on comparatively few studies, is that the operation of endarterectomy appears

more successful hemodynamically than EC-IC bypass. Patients subjected to endarterectomy showed a significant postoperative increase in CBF as well as an increase in the CBF/CBV ratio. In all these studies except one, there was no change in $CMRO_2$ post-operatively, as would be expected from the submaximal OER.

CONCLUSION

PET is a method of great versatility. It is based on the use of tracers and is a technique capable of making non-invasive regional measurements of tracer concentrations (Phelps et al. 1986). The range of physiological, biochemical and pharmacological variables available for study is at the moment small, though each year sees the reporting of new PET based methods with both new and old tracers. The field of energy metabolism and haemodynamics is now amenable to extensive exploration with well validated methods for measuring the essential variables of CBF, CBV, $CMRO_2$, CMRGlu, OER, GER, the CBF/CBV and the metabolic ratio.

Advances in PET camera design are making the precision of the measurements finer. Spatial definition and localisation are becoming much better defined with multislice, high resolution tomographs. The procedure remain laborious and expensive and consequently it is important that some of the insights resulting from PET studies should be translated into clinical practice through the use of more ubiquitous and readily available techniques. Attempts at developing stress tests of the cerebral circulation by noting the response of CBF or CBV to inhaled CO_2 or a vasodilator have been tried with some success in an attempt to assess the haemodynamic status of patients who might be candidates on pathophysiological as opposed to purely clinical grounds for revascularisation therapy.

REFERENCES

Baron, J.C., Comar, D., Bousser, M.G., et al. 1978. Etude tomographique, chez l'homme du debit sanguin et de la consommation d'oxygen du cerveau par inhalation continue d'oxygen-15. Rev. Neurol., 134, 545-556.
Baron, J.C., Bousser, M.G., Rey, A., et al. 1981a. Reversal of focal "misery-perfusion syndrome" by extra-intracranial arterial bypass in haemodynamic cerebral ischaemia. Stroke, 12, 454-459.

Baron, J.C., Bousser, M.G., Comar, D., et al. 1981b. Crossed cerebellar diaschisis in human supratentorial brain infarction. Trans. Amer. Neurol. Assoc., 105, 459-461.

Frackowiak, R.S.J. 1985a. Pathophysiology of human cerebral ischaemia: studies with positron tomography and oxygen-15. In "Brain Imaging and Brain Function" (Ed. L. Sokoloff). (Raven Press, New York).

Frackowiak, R.S.J. 1985b. The pathophysiology of human cerebral ischaemia: a new perspective obtained with positron tomography. Quat. J. Med., 57, 713-727.

Frackowiak, R.S.J., Lenzi, G.L., Jones, T., et al. 1980. Quantitative measurement of regional cerebral blood flow and oxygen metabolism in man during 15-O and positron emission tomography: Theory, procedure and normal values. J. Comput. Assist. Tomogr., 4, 727-736.

Frackowiak, R.S.J. and Wise, R.J.S. 1983. Positron tomography in ischaemic cerebrovascular disease. Neurol. Clinics, 1, 183-201.

Gibbs, J.M., Wise, R.J.S., Mansfield, A.O., et al. 1985. Cerebral circulatory reserve before and after surgery for occlusive carotid disease. J. Cereb. Blood Flow Metab., 5, (Suppl. 1), S19-S20.

Gibbs, J.M., Wise, R.J.S., Leenders, K.L., et al. 1984. Evaluation of cerebral perfusion reserve in patients with carotid artery occlusion. Lancet, 1, 310-314.

Gibbs, J.M., Wise, R.J.S. and Legg, N.J. 1983. Progress in emission tomographic studies in acute stroke and in patients with carotid occlusion: pathophysiology of cerebral ischaemia and diminished perfusion reserve. In " Progress in Stroke Research II". (Eds. R.M. Greenhalgh and R.F. Clifford). (F. Pitman Publication, London). pp. 214-226.

Jones, T., Wise, R.J.S., Frackowiak, R.S.J., et al. 1985. Uncoupling of flow and metabolism in infarcted tissue. In "Functional Mapping of the Brain in Vascular Disorders" (Ed. W.-D. Heiss). (Springer-Verlag, Berlin). pp. 43-58.

Kuhl, D.E., Phelps, M.E., Kowell, A.P., et al. 1980. Effects of stroke on local cerebral metabolism and perfusion: Mapping by emission computed tomography of 18-FDG and 13-NH-3. Ann. Neurol., 8, 47-60.

Lenzi, G.L., Frackowiak, R.S.J. and Jones, T. 1982. Cerebral oxygen metabolism and blood flow in human cerebral ischemic infarction. J. Cereb. Blood Flow Metab., 2, 321-335.

Phelps, M.E., Huang, S.C., Hoffman, E.J., et al. 1979. Tomographic measurement of cerebral blood volume with 11-C labelled carboxy-haemoglobin. J. Nucl. Med., 20, 328-334.

Phelps, M.E., Mazziotta, J.C., and Schelbert, H. (Eds.) 1986. Positron emission tomography and autoradiography: Principles and applications for the brain and heart. (Raven Press, New York).

Powers, W.J., Grubb, R.L., Darriet, D., et al. 1985. Cerebral blood flow and cerebral metabolic rate of oxygen requirements for cerebral function and viability in humans. J. Cereb. Blood Flow Metab., 5, 600-608.

Reivich, M., Kuhl, D., Wolf, A., et al. 1979. The 18-F-fluorodeoxy-glucose method for the measurement of local cerebral glucose utilisation in man. Circ. Res., 44, 127-137.

Samson, Y., Baron, J.C. Bousser, M.G., et al. 1985. Effects of extra-
    intracranial arterial bypass on cerebral blood flow and oxygen
    metabolism in humans. Stroke, 16, 609-614.
Sokoloff, L. 1981. Localisation of functional activity in the central
    nervous system by measurement of glucose utilisation with radio-
    active deoxyglucose. J. Cereb. Blood Flow Metab., 1, 7-36.
Wise, R.J.S., Bernardi, S., Frackowiak, R.S.J, et al. 1983. Serial
    observations on the pathophysiology of acute stroke: The transi-
    tion from ischaemia to infarction as reflected in the regional
    oxygen extraction. Brain, 106, 197-222.
Wise, R.J.S., Gibbs, J.M., Frackowiak, R.S.J., et al. 1986. No evi-
    dence for transhemispheric diaschisis after human cerebral in-
    farction. Stroke, in press.

BRAIN GLUCOSE METABOLISM AND BLOOD FLOW
IN ISCHEMIC STROKE

G. Pawlik, W.-D. Heiss, K. Wienhard, I.R. Hebold, P. Ziffling,
W. Staffen, K. Herholz, R. Wagner
Max-Planck-Institut für neurologische Forschung
and
Universitäts-Nervenklinik - Division of Neurology
Cologne, FRG

The etiology of brain infarction is clearly multifactorial, and it is generally accepted that numerous interacting mechanisms determine the ultimate fate of brain tissue subjected to critical focal ischemia - whether it turns into frank necrosis, remains morphologically intact but functionless, or resumes normal physiologic activities after a while. Moreover, there is little doubt that the clinical signs and symptoms of ischemic stroke cannot be related to the ischemic focus alone. Much of the resulting deficit, e.g., the often severely disabling "organic brain syndrome", must be attributed rather to secondary deactivation of structurally unaltered tissue suddenly deprived of its established neuronal input.

To date, animal experiments have provided a wealth of detailed knowlegde about various aspects of brain ischemia, but despite great efforts, they did not furnish a unifying stroke model. Therefore, aside from clinical purposes of routine diagnosis, basic stroke research in humans continues to be both a necessity and a challenge, and positron emission tomography (PET), owing to its capability of quantitative physiological imaging in three dimensions, would appear to be just the right tool. Using ^{15}O-labeled tracers, numerous PET studies have attempted to elucidate the complex relationships between the hemodynamics and oxygen metabolism in ischemic stroke; significant observations were reviewed by Baron (1987) and Frackowiak (1987). However, corresponding data on brain blood flow and glucose metabolism are scarce, and previous comparative studies comprised small, heterogeneous series of patients (Kuhl et al., 1980; Baron et al., 1982, 1985; Wise et al., 1983; Celesia et al., 1984). Considering the close relationships between neuronal function, local glucose utilization and blood flow established in normal conditions, their changes in ischemic stroke deserve better characterization. Therefore, it is the purpose of this contribution to summarize our major findings obtained with PET and ^{18}F-labeled tracers of brain glucose metabolism and blood flow in a larger group of selected stroke patients representing the full spectrum of disease stages, infarct locations and sizes.

PATIENTS AND METHODS

Forty patients (25 men, 15 women) aged 55.9 ± 13.68 years (mean $\pm$ SD), with an ischemic stroke verified by the clinical course as well as by magnetic resonance imaging (MRI) and/or X-ray computed tomography (CT) performed at about the same time as PET, were studied in a resting condition between a few hours and three years (median interval 3 weeks) after acute onset of symptoms. Approximately two hours apart, they underwent paired PET measurements, first of brain blood flow on 7 trans-axial slices, then of brain glucose utilization on 14 transaxial slices, using a four-ring positron camera (Scanditronix PC 384) with a spatial resolution of 7.8 mm in the scanning plane and 11 mm in the axial direction. The applied tracer methods, (^{18}F)-methyl fluoride (MF) for blood flow, 2 (^{18}F)-fluorodeoxyglucose (FDG) for glucose metab-olism, scanning procedures and image processing are elsewhere described in detail (Heiss et al., 1984, Pawlik et al. 1987). Local blood flow rates were estimated from concurrently computed clearance rate constant and lambda maps (Koeppe et al., 1985), glucose utilization rates were calculated with rate constants adjusted for the measured tissue activi-ties according to the $k_{1,3}$-optimization procedure (Wienhard et al., 1985), both methods requiring less stringent assumptions about the tracer behavior in abnormal tissue. Standardized regional quantitation was achieved using an interactive mapping program (Herholz et al., 1985); a categorical region matching and block shifting procedure (Pawlik et al., 1986) provided optimum comparability both among subjects and between the hemodynamic and metabolic data of the same patient. Statisti-cal inferences were based on exact nonparametric testing or on univariate analysis of variance with degrees of freedom adjusted according to Huynh and Feldt (1976).

RESULTS AND DISCUSSION
Sensitivity

It is well-known that, in ischemic stroke, the differential sensitivity of the various modern tomographic imaging techniques depends on the time since ictus. While PET, MRI, and CT have comparably high true-positive rates at the chronic disease stage, their respective yields differ the most at early times after onset (Heiss et al., 1986): PET usually becomes positive as soon as clinical symptoms develop; T_2-weighted MR images may show an ischemic lesion approximately four hours after onset of symptoms; only rarely becomes CT positive within less than 12 hours, but it has its merits particularly for the early distinction between ischemic and hemorrhagic stroke. At later stages, MRI of proton density generally provides the best anatomical definition of the ultimate infarct. Among the available PET methods, metabolic imaging seems to be suited best for the early detection of ischemic lesions, i.e., at a time when regional blood flow behaves somewhat unpredictably (see below); in chronic infarction, blood flow and metabolic images mostly yield similar results.

Our experience with more than 300 FDG-PET studies in ischemic stroke does not support the notion derived from a small series of comparative FDG and ^{15}O measurements (Wise et al., 1983) of a clearly inferior sensitivity of the FDG method in early cerebral infarcts because in situations where oxygen consumption and extraction were low, glucose metabolism was normal or only mildly impaired. When using late CT or MRI to define the area of infarction, on early PET scans we always found significantly decreased or increased glucose utilization rates in that region, at times occurring in clusters side by side. Therefore, the sensitivity of FDG-PET is close to 100% - at least for lesions involving gray matter ischemic lesions confined to white matter may sometimes not be detected by PET because of poor image contrast. Occasionally, we observed rather unexpected failures of MRI as demonstrated in Fig. 1.

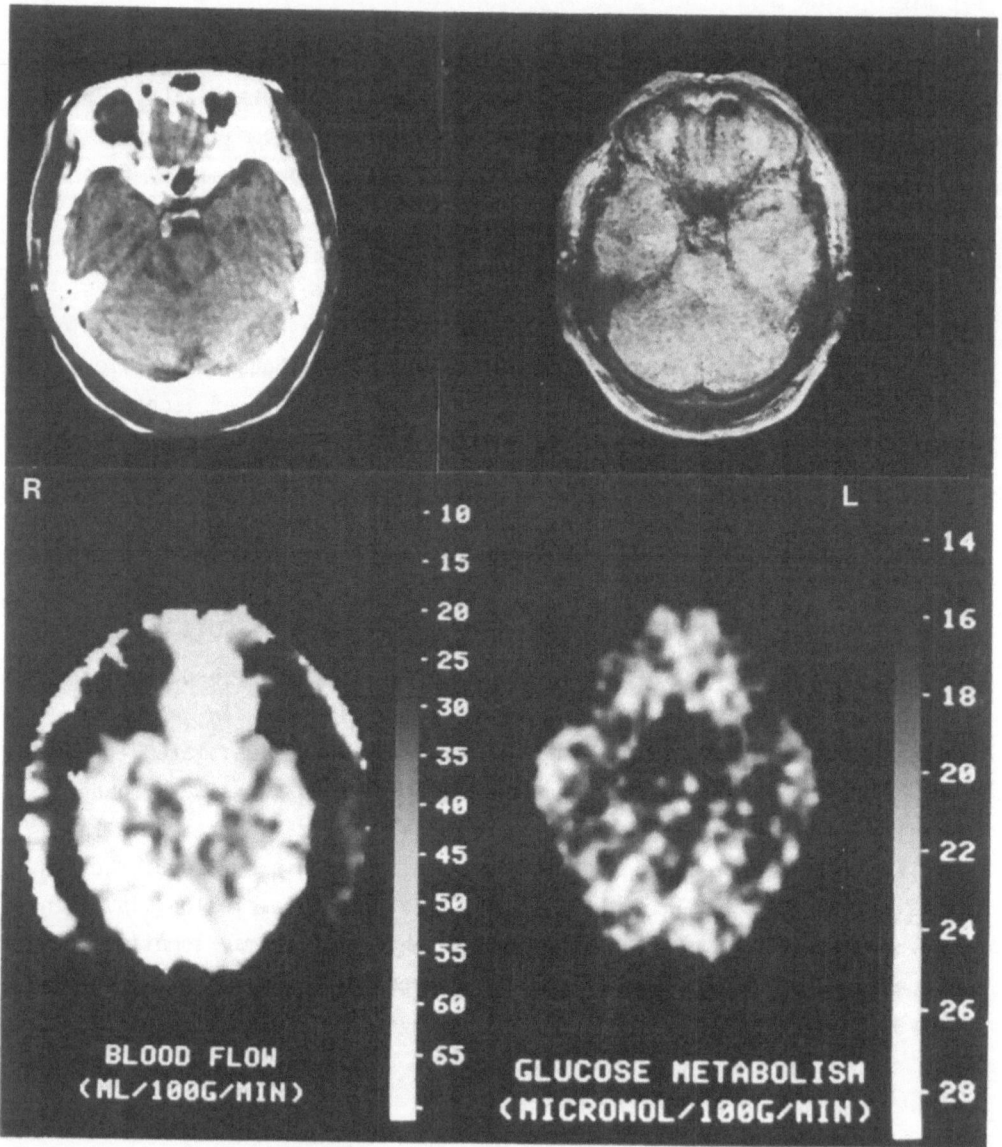

Fig. 1   X-ray CT (upper left), spin echo magnetic resonance
(upper right), and PET (lower row) images showing the upper pons
of a 65-year-old patient, 11 days after right pontine infarction.
While CT (low-density area), local blood flow (hyperperfusion)
and glucose consumption (hypometabolism) are clearly abnormal,
MRI is rather inconspicuous. (Proton density images did not
reveal any abnormality either.)

Functional deactivation and reserve

Long before the introduction of PET, it has been well recognized that a focal brain lesion commonly causes transneural depression of function in more or less distant brain regions normally receiving significant input from or via the injured area. This phenomenon, called "diaschisis" by v. Monakow (1911), was recently reviewed in the light of modern PET findings (Pawlik et al., 1985b; Feeney and Baron, 1986), which therefore are summarized here only in brief.

Apparently, almost any ischemic stroke, depending on the location, size, and completeness of infarction, causes functional deactivation of morphologically unaltered brain tissue according to a chracteristic pattern. These remote effects can be separated into a direct (or asymmetric) and an indirect (or global) component. Direct effects are the predominant feature of supratentorial infarcts involving gray matter. As illustrated in Fig. 2, there usually is some distinct metabolic depression of ipsilateral cerebral cortex, subcortical white matter, basal ganglia, thalamus, upper brainstem, and of contralateral lower brainstem and cerebellum.
Indirect deactivation, by contrast, is charactistic of infratentorial infarcts (Fig. 3).

While a marked organic brain syndrome or a decreased level of consciousness are hardly ever missing in stroke patients with significant global deactivation, even severe direct effects are often masked by the overlying gross neurologic deficit related to the infarct region. However, it is this functional deactivation that one can hope to reverse by treatment with activating drugs (Heiss et al., 1983), specific training, and other rehabilitation measures. Unfortunately, the natural history of diaschisis, its determinants and potential modifiers, are still insufficiently understood because of the small number of stroke victims repeatedly studied by PET at longer intervals (Beil et al., 1985). Some of our cases demonstrate that remarkable functional recovery is indeed possible - even when the infarct is large (Fig. 4).

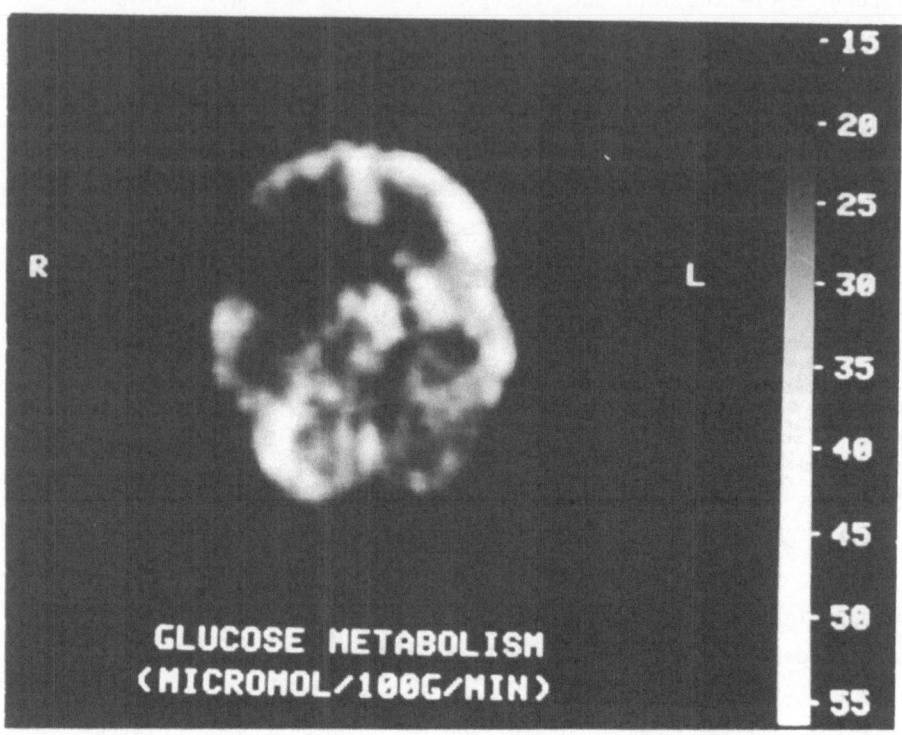

GLUCOSE METABOLISM
(MICROMOL/100G/MIN)

Fig. 2   Oblique PET slice across frontal lobes, basal ganglia, thalami, brainstem, and cerebellum (25° section no.11 according to Matsui and Hirano, 1978) of a 44-year-old patient, 22 days after typical right MCA infarction (size 43 cm³ as estimated from CT) involving frontal and temporal cortex and underlying white matter. Note the path of asymmetrical deactivation down to the left cerebellar hemisphere, and the comparatively minor decrease in global glucose consumption.

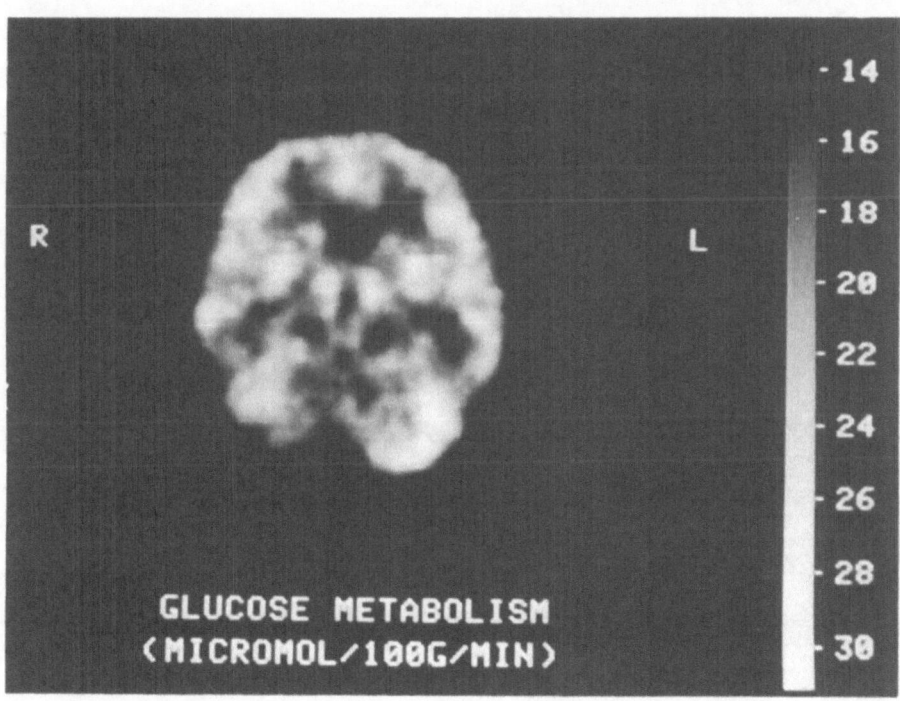

Fig. 3   Oblique PET slice (section similar to Fig. 2) of a 57-year-old patient, 24 days after right inferior cerebellar infarction, showing little asymmetrical deactivation of morphologically intact structures, but severe global metabolic depression.

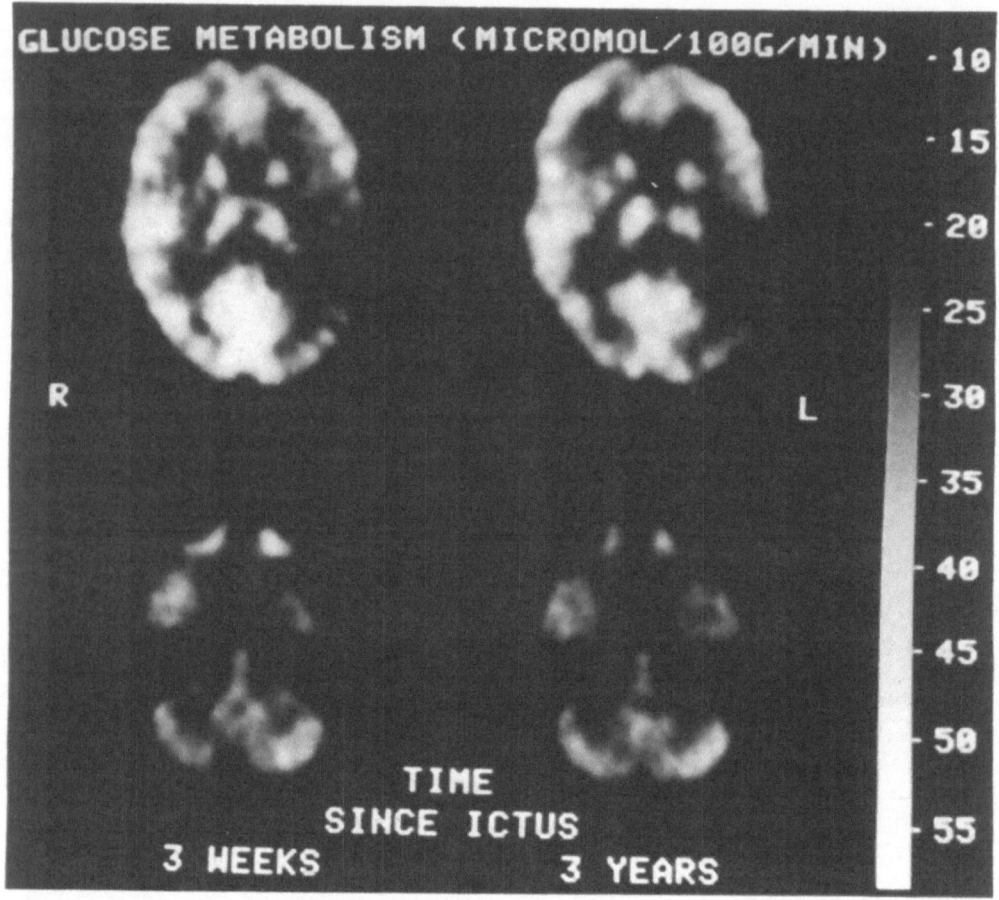

Fig. 4   Characteristic transaxial PET slices across the cerebellum and cerebrum, respectively, of a 49-year-old patient with left temporoparietal infarction (size 39 cm³ as estimated from CT), three weeks and three years after acute onset of stroke symptoms. At the time of the first PET study, when direct and indirect deactivation was marked, there were severe neuropsychological and mild sensori-motor symptoms. Three years later, functional deactivation was mini-mal, and the patient had made an almost full clinical recovery, the residual deficit consisting only of a mild lack of initiative.

An interesting alternative to PET measurements at long post-stroke intervals may be paired PET studies of the functional reserve capacity in the postacute phase, with one PET session in a normal resting state and the other in a condition of physiologic activation. Fig. 5 illustrates the usefulness of this approach in an exemplary case from our series of stimulation studies in aphasics (Pawlik et al., 1985, 1987a). It is conceivable that the results of truly functional studies like these, which are possible only with PET, may have a direct bearing on the routing of therapy.

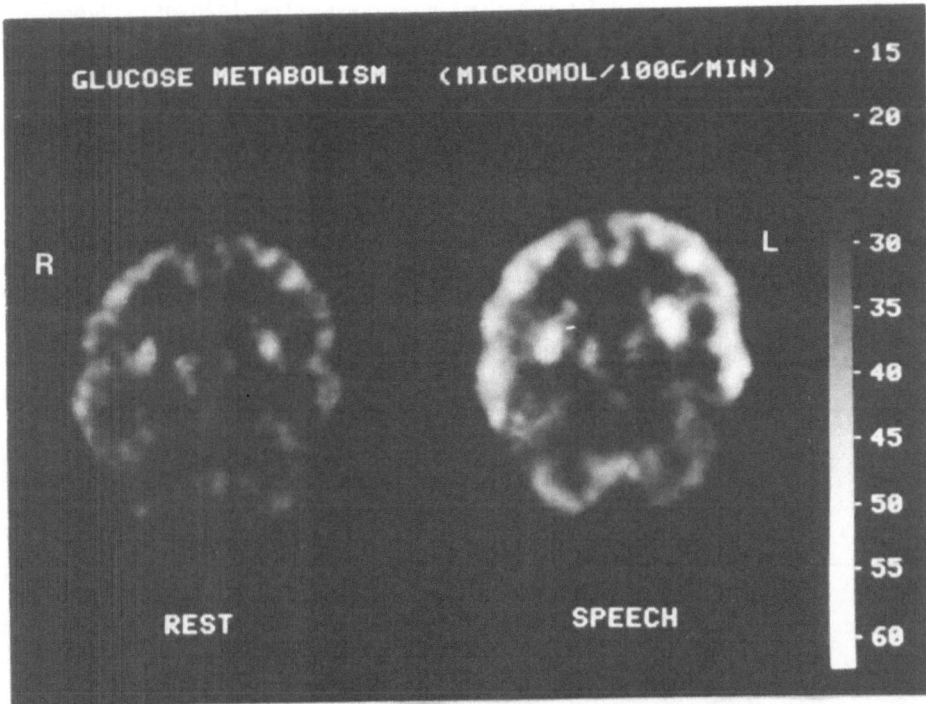

Fig. 5   Corresponding oblique PET slices (30° section no. 13 according to Matsui and Hirano, 1978) of a 50-year-old patient with mixed aphasia due to left insular infarction, studied both at rest 13 days after onset of stroke symptoms and, two days later, during spontaneous speech. Note the remarkable global increase with minor compensation of direct deactivation - except in the cerebellum, where asymmetries are inverted according to the pattern characteristic of the chosen paradigm.

Glucose metabolism/blood flow relationships

The hemodynamic and metabolic averages, as well as the arterio-
venous difference for glucose and the glucose extraction fraction (GEF)
measured in the infarcted region, the cerebrum and cerebellum, respectively, are summarized in Table 1. Both blood flow and glucose consumption rates differed significantly ($P<0.0001$) among the smaller, morphologically intact brain regions, but they were rather similar in the
whole cerebral and cerebellar hemispheres. In the cerebrum, functional
depression was proportionate for blood flow and glucose utilization,
while in the cerebellum contralateral to the infarct, the flow reduction
was slightly more pronouncend than the hypometabolism ($P<0.05$). Even
when considering only the contralateral cerebral and ipsilateral cerebellar hemispheres, there was a significant ($P<0.0001$) difference in
regional GEF, with the lowest value in thalamus ($14.8 \pm 6.47\%$), followed by cerebellum ($15.1 \pm 5.18\%$), striatum ($16.2 \pm 6.30\%$), cerebral
cortex ($17.4 \pm 6.63\%$) and white matter ($18.7 \pm 6.15\%$). Baron et al.
(1985) also found a higher GEF in white matter as compared with gray
matter.

TABLE 1   Regional blood flow & glucose metabolism in 40 patients with
ischemic stroke, 3 weeks (median) after onset of symptoms (mean $\pm$ SD)

Region	rCMRglc (μmol/100g/min)	rCBF (ml/100g/min)	glucose A-V difference (μmol/ml)	glucose extraction fraction (%)
Ischemic lesion	17.2 ± 4.76	23.3 ± 11.06	0.88 ± 0.438	16.1 ± 7.97
Ipsilateral cerebrum	30.1 ± 6.97	34.2 ± 9.54	0.93 ± 0.290	17.2 ± 6.18
contralateral	32.6 ± 6.48	37.2 ± 9.42	0.93 ± 0.280	17.1 ± 6.20
Ipsilateral cerebellum	32.3 ± 6.86	41.2 ± 10.22	0.82 ± 0.238	15.1 ± 5.18
contralateral	28.9 ± 6.33	35.8 ± 9.72	0.86 ± 0.259	15.7 ± 5.42

When PET studies were grouped by the time interval since onset of
stroke symptoms, significant differences among regions emerged (P<0.05)
with respect to their disease stage-dependent pattern of GEF (Fig. 6).
In the infarct area, GEF was highest within three days of the ictus,
while in all other regions; it was lowest at that stage; up to two
weeks, GEF was highest in the contralateral cerebral hemisphere and
lowest in the ischemic lesion. Subsequent changes of GEF were remarkable
only in the infarct, where again an increase was noted that may be
related to the glycolytic activity of white cells, which by that time
usually have infiltrated the necrotic tissue in significant numbers.

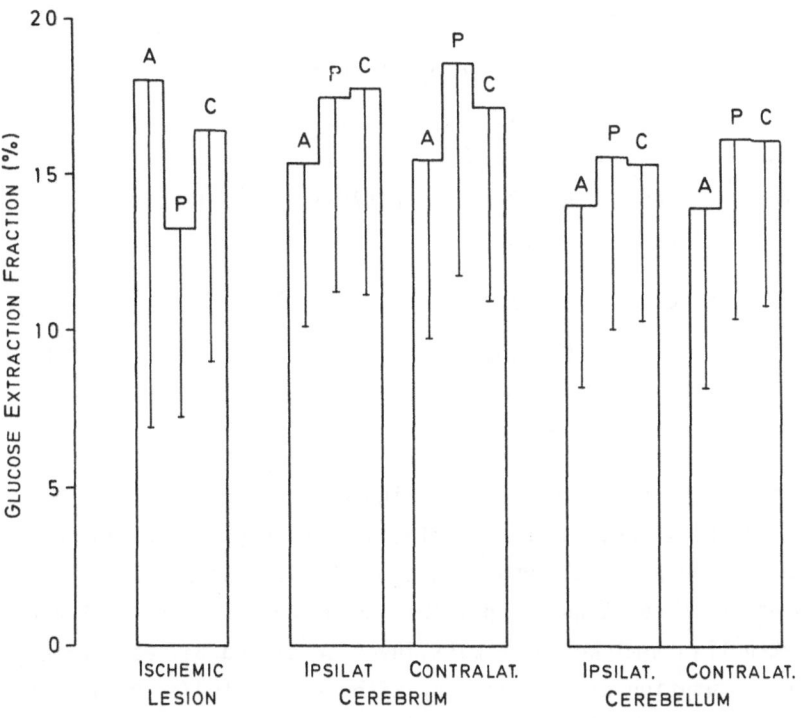

Fig. 6   Regional glucose extraction fraction at the acute (A,
first three days, n = 8), postacute (P, day 4 - 14, n = 8), and
chronic (C, more than two weeks, n = 24) stage of ischemic stroke.
Columns indicate mean values, the error bars one standard
deviation.

The above data are regional averages only and, therefore, do not fully represent the observed metabolic-hemodynamic relations - particularly in the injured region. In order to overcome this problem of data reduction, FDG- and MF-PET images were compared by visual inspection with respect to any obvious uncoupling of blood flow and glucose consumption anywhere in the infarcted area, regardless of the individual absolute level. The results of this very sensitive procedure are given in Table 2, demonstrating significant (P<0.05) pattern changes with time.

TABLE 2   Relationship between local glucose consumption rates (1CMRGlc) and local blood flow (1CBF) in ischemic brain lesions.

	Days after onset of symptoms			
	1 - 3	4 - 14	>14	all
1CMRglc < 1CBF	4 (50%)	6 (75%)	5 (20.8%)	15 (37.5%)
1CMRglc ≈ 1CBF	1 (12.5%)	2 (25%)	13 (54.2%)	16 (40%)
1CMRglc > 1CBF	3 (37.5%)	0 (0%)	6 (25%)	9 (22.5%)
Σ	8 (100%)	8 (100%)	24 (100%)	40 (100%)

P < 0.05 by Freeman-Halton Test

At the acute stage, normal coupling was the exception; at the chronic stage, it was the rule. Relative hyperglycolysis was not observed in the postacute phase, where relative luxury perfusion was prominent, thus refuting the possibility of an early cerebral pseudo-hypermetabolism mimicked by a mass invasion of phagocytes with high glucose consumption as suggested by Wise et al. (1983). Remarkably, in all the three cases with glucose utilization in excess of blood flow during the acute phase of infarction, local metabolic rates were raised significantly above normal values, and all ended up with large defects as illustrated in Fig. 7.

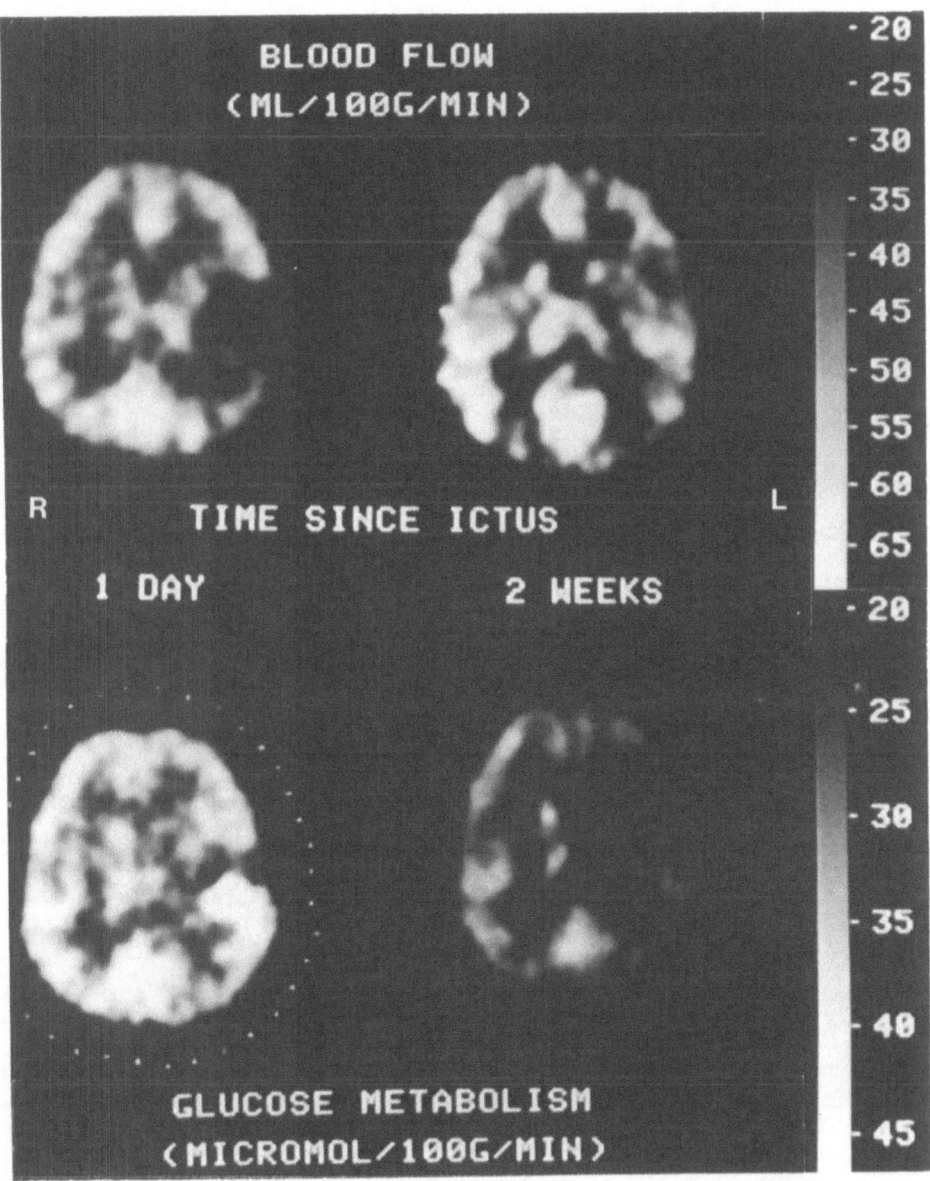

Fig. 7   Blood flow and glucose metabolic maps of a 41-year-old
patient with large left MCA infarction and poor prognosis, one
day and two weeks, respectively, after acute onset of stroke symptoms. Note the inverse temporal behavior of the two physiological
variables.

Patients with early relative hyperperfusion, however, mostly had a
more favorable clinical outcome as exemplified by Fig. 8.

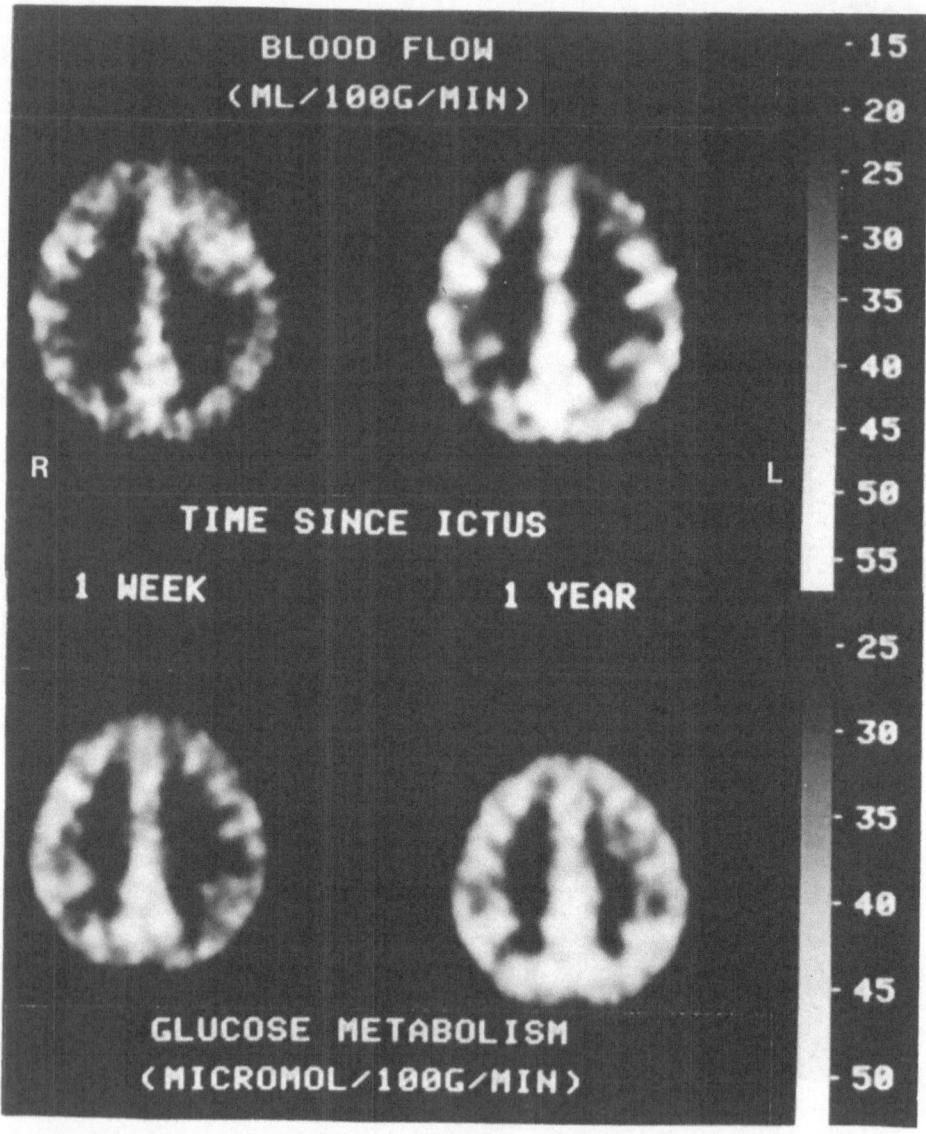

Fig. 8   Blood flow and glucose metabolic maps of a 50-year-old
patient with left frontal infarction and eventually good functional
recovery, one week after acute onset of symptoms and a year later.
Note the initial functional deactivation concurrent with focal
luxury perfusion, and the subsequent normalization of glucose metabolism and blood flow - except for a small frontal focus of residual
ischemia.

CONCLUSIONS

The described findings support the view that basic clinical research commonly has both prospective and immediate effects. On the one side, by advancing the understanding of more general disease mechanisms, it can provide the rationale of prognosis and of future therapies, on the other, there often is an immediate, if inconspicuous influence on the actual clinical management of a patient under study.

In neurology, maybe more than in other medical specialities, efficacious therapeutic action and prognosis require comprehensive knowledge of complex individual functional relationships. This is just the kind of information PET makes available, and therefore this technology derives its clinical efficacy at least as much from the indiviudal results of continuous systematic research activities, as from clear-cut solutions to specific diagnostic problems. Among the modern imaging techniques, PET undoubtedly has its place, and it is not least in ischemic stroke that PET features specific advantages, e.g., repeatable, quantitative multivariate studies of distinct pathophysiologic processes. In this respect, the various established PET tracer methods yield somewhat complementary information, with measurements of glucose metabolism and blood flow certainly covering major aspects.

REFERENCES

Baron, J.C. 1987. Ischemic stroke studied by 15-0-labeled compounds: Misery and luxury perfusion. In "Clinical Efficacy of PET" (Eds. W.-D. Heiss, G. Pawlik, K. Herholz, K. Wienhard). (Martinus Nijhoff Publ., Dordrecht). in press.

Baron, J.C., Lebrun-Grandie, P. Collard, P., et al. 1982. Noninvasive measurement of blood flow, oxygen consumption and glucose utilization in the same brain locus in man by positron emission tomography. J. Nucl. Med., 23, 391-399.

Baron, J.C., Rougemont, D., Samson, Y., et al. 1985. The local interrelationships of cerebral oxygen consumption and glucose utilization in normals and in ischemic stroke patients. In " The Metabolism of the Human Brain Studied with Positron Emission Tomography" (Eds. T. Greitz, D.H. Ingvar, L. Widen). (Raven Press, New York). pp. 377-385.

Beil, C., Rackl, A., Pawlik, G., et al. 1985. Correlative clinico-metabolic follow-up study of cerebral deactivation in ischemic stroke. J. Neurol., 232, (Suppl. 1), 57.

Celesia, G.G., Polcyn, R.E., Holden, J.E., et al. 1984. Determination of regional cerebral blood flow in patients with cerebral infarction. Use of fluoromethane labeled with fluorine-18 and positron emission tomography. Arch. Neurol., 41, 262-267.

Feeney, D.M. and Baron, J.C. 1986. Diaschisis. Stroke, 17, 817-830.

Frackowiak, R.S.J. 1987. Ischemic disease studied with 15-O labelled compounds: Metabolic and haemodynamic disparities. In "Clinical Efficacy of PET" (Eds. W.-D. Heiss, G. Pawlik, K. Herholz, K. Wienhard). (Martinus Nijhoff Publ., Dordrecht). in press.

Heiss, W.-D., Herholz, K., Böcher-Schwarz, H.G., et al. 1986. PET, CT, and MR imaging in cerebrovascular disease. J. Comput. Assist. Tomogr., 10, 903-911.

Heiss, W.-D., Ilsen, H.W., Wagner, R., et al. 1983. Remote functional depression of glucose metabolism in stroke and its alteration by activating drugs. In "Positron Emission Tomography of the Brain" (Eds. W.-D. Heiss and M.E. Phelps). (Springer-Verlag, Berlin-Heidelberg-New York). pp. 162-168.

Heiss, W.-D., Pawlik, G., Herholz, K., et al. 1984. Regional kinetic constants and cerebral metabolic rate for glucose in normal human volunteers detemined by dynamic positron emission tomography of (18-F)-2-fluoro-2-deoxy-D-glucose. J. Cereb. Blood Flow Metab., 4, 212-223.

Herholz, K., Pawlik, G., Wienhard, K., et al. 1985. Computer assisted mapping in quantitative analysis of cerebral positron emission tomograms. J. Comput. Assist. Tomogr., 9, 154-161.

Huynh, H. and Feldt, L.S. 1976. Estimation of the Box correction for degrees of freedom from sample data in randomized block and split-plot designs. J. Ed. Stat., 1, 69-82.

Koeppe, R.A., Holden, J.E., Ip, W.R. 1985. Performance comparison of parameter estimation techniques for the quantitation of local cerebral blood flow by dynamic positron computed tomography. J. Cereb. Blood Flow Metab., 5, 224-234.

Kuhl, D.E., Phelps, M.E., Kowell, A.P., et al. 1980. Mapping local metabolism and perfusion in normal and ischemic brain by emission computed tomography of 18-FDG and 13-NH3. Ann. Neurol., 8, 47-60.

Matsui, T. and Hirano, A. 1978. An Atlas of the Human Brain for Computerized Tomography. (Fischer, Stuttgart).

Pawlik, G., Heiss, W.-D., Beil, C., et al. 1987a. Three-dimensional patterns of speech-induced cerebral and cerebellar activation in healthy volunteers and in aphasic stroke patients studied by positron emission tomography of 2(18F)-fluorodeoxyglucose. In "Cerebral Vascular Disease 6" (Eds. J.S. Meyer, H. Lechner, M. Reivich, E.O. Ott). (Excerpta Medica, Amsterdam-New York-Oxford). in press.

Pawlik, G., Wienhard, K., Beil, C., et al. 1987b. Noninvasive quantitative mapping of brain blood flow in ischemic stroke by dynamic positron emission tomography of (18F)-methyl fluoride. Stroke, in press.

Pawlik, G., Heiss, W.-D., Herholz, K., et al. 1985a. Positron emission tomographic study of variations in brain glucose metabolism related to spontaneous speech. J. Neurol., 232, (Suppl. 1), 227.

Pawlik, G., Herholz, K., Beil, C., et al. 1985b. Remote effects of focal lesions on cerebral flow and metabolism. In "Functional Mapping of the Brain in Vascular Disorders" (Ed. W.-D. Heiss). (Springer-Verlag, Berlin-Heidelberg-New York). pp. 59-83.

Pawlik, G., Herholz, K., Wienhard, K., et al. 1986. Some maximum
    likelihood methods useful for the regional analysis of dynamic
    PET data on brain glucose metabolism. In "Information Processing
    in Medical Imaging" (Ed. S.L. Bacharach). (Martinus Nijhoff Publ.,
    Dordrecht). pp. 298-309.
von Monakow, C. 1911. Lokalisation der Hirnfunktionen. J. Psychol.
    Neurol., 17, 185-200.
Wienhard, K., Pawlik, G., Herholz, K., et al. 1985. Estimation of local
    cerebral glucose utilization by positron emission tomography of
    (18F)2-fluoro-2-deoxy-D-glucose: A critical appraisal of optimi-
    zation procedures. J. Cereb. Blood Flow Metab., 5, 115-125.
Wise, R., Rhodes, C., Gibbs, J., et al. 1983. The relationship between
    oxygen metabolism and glucose utilization in early cerebral
    infarcts. J. Cereb. Blood Flow Metab., 3, (Suppl. 1), S580-S581.

PET STUDIES IN INTERNAL CAROTID OCCLUSION PATIENTS: BASE-LINE HEMODYNAMIC AND METABOLIC ALTERATIONS; EFFECTS OF SURGICAL REVASCULARIZATION AND INDUCED ARTERIAL HYPERTENSION

Y. Samson[1,2], J.C. Baron[1,2]

[1]Service Hospitalier Frédéric Joliot, Dept. de Biologie,
Commissariat à l'Energie Atomique, Orsay, France
[2]Clinique des Maladies du Système Nerveux
Service du Pr. Laplane, Hopital La Salpêtrière, Paris, France

Alterations of the regional cerebral blood flow (CBF), oxygen extraction (OEF) and oxygen utilization ($CMRO_2$) have been reported in several positron tomographic studies of patients with internal carotid artery (ICA) occlusion (Baron et al., 1981; Gibbs et al., 1984, 1985; Samson et al., 1985a,b; Powers et al., 1984a, 1984b). This paper summarizes our findings in such patients. For practical purposes, focal and bilateral (diffuse) functional abnormalities will be discussed separately, although they may be superimposed in individual patients.

I. Focal alterations
Misery-perfusion

Baron et al. (1981) reported the case of a patient with a left ICA occlusion and related hemodynamic TIAs. At the ^{15}O PET study, a regional decrease of CBF with an increase of OEF was found in the left posterior watershed area. Clinical symptoms were alleviated by a successful extra-intracranial arterial (EC-IC) bypass. The post-operative PET study was normal. This pattern of functional abnormality (CBF decrease and simultaneous OEF increase) was termed misery-perfusion (MP). It was considered as a reversible hemodynamic alteration due to a decrease of the cerebral perfusion pressure (CPP) below the lower threshold of the CBF autoregulation. This interpretation has since received confirmation in PET studies from different centers (Samson et al., 1985a,b; Powers et al., 1984b; Gibbs et al., 1985). Gibbs et al. (1984) reported additionally, that in base-line studies of ICA occlusion patients, high OEF values were found only if the CBF to cerebral blood volume ratio fell below a critical value considered to reflect in-directly the lower threshold of autoregulation. Finally, in a study of

the effects of intravenous angiotensin II induced arterial hypertension
in 10 patients with ICA occlusion, the brain areas exhibiting MP at
baseline showed a statistically significant improvement of the
asymmetries in both CBF and OEF (Samson et al., in preparation), which
mimicked the effects of EC-IC bypass. This observation definitely
demonstrated the perfusion pressure dependency of the CBF in brain
regions with chronic MP.

In a group of 51 patients with ICA occlusion consecutively studied
at Orsay, high absolute values of OEF (> 0.60) were found in 12 % of the
occluded ICA territories, a finding in line with reports from others
(Gibbs et al., 1984). However, if this abnormality was defined as
significant OEF asymmetry in the individual case, the incidence of MP
rose up to 41 % in these patients. The striking difference between the
results of these two methods of data analysis presumably reflects the
well-known higher sensitivity of asymmetry indices compared to absolute
value measurements for the detection of individual focal functional
alterations; however, more complex and bilateral abnormalities of the
CBF-CMRO$_2$ coupling may also be involved (see part II). Our data
nevertheless indicate that a state of chronic hemodynamic insufficiency
was present in nearly half of our patients.

Furthermore, MP was found in almost every patient (Lassen, 1982;
Feeney and Baron, 1986) with pure ophthalmic collateral pattern at
angiography, confirming the poor hemodynamic efficiency of this pattern
of collateral revascularization (Norrving et al., 1982; Powers et al.,
1986). However, unlike Gibbs et al. (1984) we did not find any
significant relationship between a bilateral extension of ICA occlusion
and high OEF absolute values (see part II); in addition, the frequency
of significant asymmetries of OEF was, in our series, roughly similar in
patients with unilateral and in those with bilateral ICA obstruction
(11/25 and 7/21, respectively).

In about 50 % of the cases, the MP pattern was associated with a
significant, although moderate CMRO$_2$ decrease. This may result from
three different pathophysiological mechanisms, namely underlying
ischemic damage without gross CT scan changes (Lassen, 1982), actual
true ischemia (CMRO$_2$ dependent on CBF), and associated deafferentation
by deactivation (Feeney and Baron, 1986).

The fact that this focal metabolic alteration associated with MP

remained unaltered despite improving the CBF by EC-IC bypass or angiotensin II infusion (Samson et al., 1985a; Powers et al., 1984b; Gibbs et
al., 1985; Samson et al., in preparation) rules out reversible ischemia
as a significant factor in most instances. However, at least in one of
our EC-IC bypass patients with MP (case 9 of Samson et al., 1985a) a
significant focal $CMRO_2$ depression disappeared after EC-IC bypass,
suggesting a situation of true ischemia ("chronic penumbra"?).

Matched decrease in CBF and $CMRO_2$

The second pattern of functional alteration found with a relatively
high frequency (11 of the 51 patients of our series) in an occluded ICA
territory, is the decrease in both CBF and $CMRO_2$ without any change in
the OEF. Such a pattern remains usually unaltered by EC-IC bypass
(Samson et al., 1985a,b; Powers et al., 1984b; Gibbs et al., 1985) and,
in our experience, was not modified by angiotensin II infusion (Samson
et al., in preparation). This agrees with the hypothesis that such a
functional alteration reflects a primary metabolic abnormality related
either to the "deactivation" surrounding an infarct (Feeney and Baron,
1986) or to a selective neuronal loss (Lassen, 1982).

II. Bilateral functional alterations

In a series of 12 patients who underwent EC-IC bypass (Samson et
al., 1985a,b), we found post-operatively a bilateral and widespread
increase of both CBF and $CMRO_2$; these changes were however only found
in the patient group with bilateral cervical arterial obstructive
lesions. Our findings are, therefore, not irreconcilable with those of
Gibbs et al. (1985), who did not find significant post EC-IC bypass
changes in CBF and $CMRO_2$, as they mainly studied patients with
strictly unilateral ICA occlusion.

There is no straight forward explanation of this post-operative
increase in CBF and $CMRO_2$. Hence, it is not the pattern of changes
expected from the reversal of a hemodynamic anomaly, which should
feature an increase of CBF, a decrease of OEF and little or no changes
in $CMRO_2$ (Baron et al., 1981). On the other hand, a spontaneous
improvement of CBF and $CMRO_2$ unrelated to the surgery (e.g., due to
alleviation of diaschisis (Feeney and Baron, 1986) can be envisioned, but
remains finally very unlikely for the following reasons: 1. There

were no changes in CBF and $CMRO_2$ in a group of similar but unoperated patients (Samson et al., 1985a,b). 2. Despite the lack of significant changes in mean OEF in the operated group, there appeared two different patterns of individual changes in the OEF: in some patients, the metabolic improvement was associated with a marked increase of CBF (the OEF remaining constant or decreasing), while in the remaining cases the CBF was unaltered following surgery, but there occurred an increase in the OEF. 3. Finally, the improvement of CBF and $CMRO_2$ occurred essentially in patients with multiple cervical arterial occlusions, i.e., those with presumably the lowest CPP (Spetzler et al., 1983).

The hemodynamic nature of those bilateral CBF and $CMRO_2$ changes has been recently further supported by our findings in angiotensin II induced arterial hypertension (Samson et al., in preparation). In patients with ICA occlusion, we selected prospectively 5 subjects with patent contralateral ICA (group I) and 5 with severe stenosis or occlusion of this vessel (group II). Mean changes in MABP (+ 30 $\pm$ 9 vs + 31 $\pm$ 3 mmHg; NS), $PaCO_2$ (- 1.9 $\pm$ 1.5 vs - 1.4 $\pm$ 1.5 mmHg; NS) and PaO_2 (+ 0.1 $\pm$ 6.4 vs - 3 $\pm$ 6.7 mmHg; NS) were similar in both subgroups. Significant bilateral increases in CBF and $CMRO_2$ were found in group II, while no significant changes were found in roup I (Fig.1).

As was already the case in our EC-IC bypass study (Samson et al., 1985a), the changes in CBF and $CMRO_2$ in group II patients were apparently mismatched on the individual basis, despite the lack of alteration in mean OEF.

In summary, these studies indicated that increases in cerebral perfusion pressure selectively induced a widespread metabolic improvement in patients with multiple cervical arterial obstructions, associated with a less consistent increase in CBF. In addition, the lack of changes in mean OEF apparently masked individual variations of this parameter in opposite direction, suggesting dissociated alterations in CBF and $CMRO_2$. We therefore investigated whether our rather unexpected findings could be explained by differences in base-line CBF, OEF and $CMRO_2$ between strictly unilateral and bilateral ICA occlusion patients. On the basis of angiographic data, we selected from a population of 51 consecutively studied ICA occlusion patients, 25 subjects with strictly unilateral ICA occlusion (group A) and 21 with severe (> 50 % in diameter) stenosis (n=15) or occlusion (n=6) of the contralateral ICA (group B).

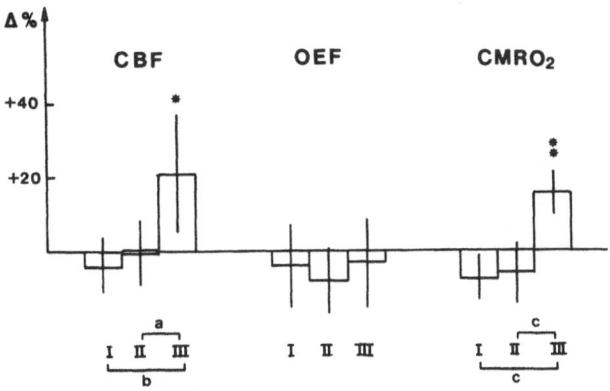

POST. ANGIO II RELATIVE VARIATIONS IN ICA REGIONS

I : PATENT ICA (n=5)

II: UNILATERAL ICA OCCLUSION (n=5)

III: BILATERAL ICA OBSTRUCTION (n=10)

a   p <.05 } with respect to
b   p <.01 } others sub.group.
c   p <.001

*   p <.01 } with respect to 0.
**   p <.001

Fig. 1   Effects of angiotensin II infusion: Results are expressed as the relative variation between pre- and intra-angio-II studies of each paramter (mean + sd) in 3 different groups of ICA territories. (Groups I and II refer to territories of patent and of occluded ICA of patients with strictly unilateral ICA occlusion. Since the physiological variations were very similar in territories of occluded and stenotic ICA of the patients with bilateral ICA obstruction, they were pooled together in group III). A significant increase in both CBF and CMRO2 was found in group III only. CT scan areas were excluded from the data analysis. Statistical comparison of the 3 groups was performed by analysis of variance and the Bonferroni method.

All subjects were studied at least 3 weeks after the last stroke. Clinical status, CT scan finding and number of focal MP areas were similar in both groups. As shown in Fig. 2, the mean $CMRO_2$ and OEF values on each side were significantly lower in group B than in group A patients. In contrast, CBF values were similar in the two

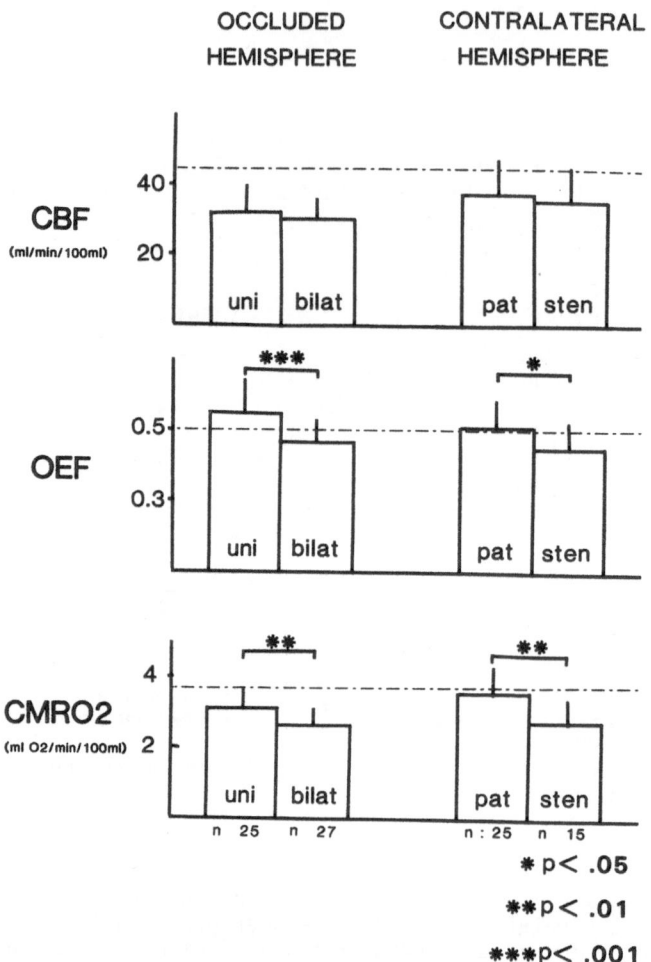

Fig. 2   CBF, OEF and CMRO2 values (mean ± sd) in the ICA
territories of patients with unilateral (group A) or bilateral
(group B) ICA obstruction: Territories of completely occluded ICA
of the patients of group A (UNI) and group B (BILAT) were compared.
A similar comparison was made between territories of patent ICA
(PAT) of group A patients and territories of stenotic ICA (STEN) of
group B patients. (A and B referring to patients with strictly
unilateral and to those with bilateral arterial obstructive
disease, see text for details); CMRO2 and OEF values were
significantly lower on both sides in group B than in group A,
but CBF values were similar.

subgroups, although significantly decreased with respect to controls in both unilaterally and bilaterally occluded ICA territories. These results suggest that a widespread metabolic depression exists in group B patients (Samson et al., 1985b) and that it may be associated with an anomaly of the flow-metabolism coupling mechanisms.

To analyze further this intriguing finding, the individual OEF values were plotted against the corresponding CBF values. As shown in Fig. 3a, the shape of the CBF-OEF relationship was similar the territories of unilaterally occluded, contralateral patent and control ICA. In accordance with the concept of MP, higher OEF values were found at lower CBF values, this pattern being found more often in occluded than in patent or control ICA territories. The metabolic depression present in group B patients is reflected by a global down-shift of the "normal" CBF-OEF relationship (Fig. 3b). This suggests that the metabolic depression on the one hand, and the CBF abnormalities (failure of autoregulation) on the other hand, may be distinct pathophysiological entities, although possibly concomittant in some patients. One consequence of this superimposition of two different types of changes bears on the interpretation of the OEF data in patients with multiple ICA occlusions, which might be much more complex than previously suspected; for example, normal OEF values may be found in areas of moderate MP.

Finally, this hypothesis provides an explanation to the increase in CBF and $CMRO_2$ found either after EC-IC bypass (Samson et al., 1985a) or during angiotensin II perfusion. As shown in Fig. 4, the CBF changes were negligible in 5 patients (preserved autoregulation); in those cases, the OEF base-line values were below the "normal" CBF-OEF relationship, and the sole effect of the increase in CPP was a rise of the OEF. In the remaining 6 cases, there was an increase in CBF (failing autoregulation): the OEF changes were less predictible, probably as a result of the simultaneous improvement in both MP and metabolic depression, altering the OEF in opposite directions.

The bilateral failure of CBF autoregulation presumably results from a major fall of CPP (Gibbs et al., 1984; Spetzler et al., 1983). The unexpected metabolic depression with a paradoxical OEF decrease might be related to a long-term adaptation to the CPP decrease. One possible mechanism for this implicates a primary metabolic adaptation, in some

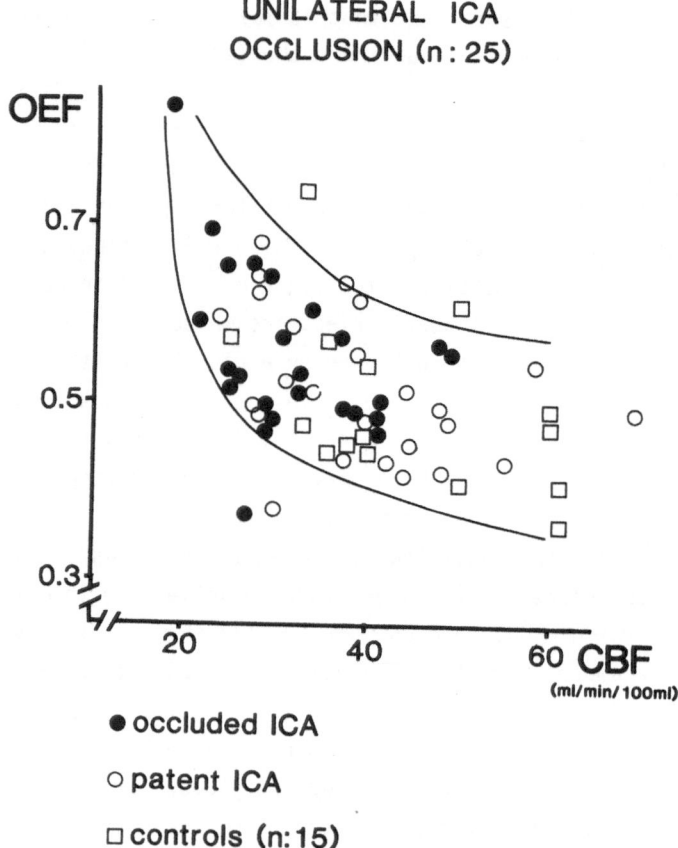

Fig. 3   Relationship between CBF and OEF values in ICA
territories: Fig. 3a: data from patients with unilateral ICA
occlusion (group A) and from age-matached control subjects.
Although the CBF values were generally lower in territories of
occluded than those of patent or control ICA, a consistent CBF-OEF
relationship is found, characterized by an increase of OEF at low
CBF values.

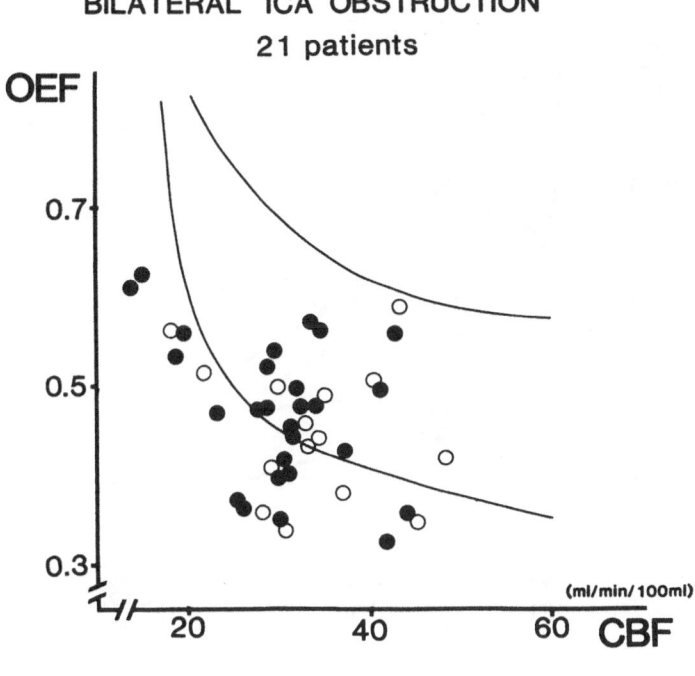

BILATERAL ICA OBSTRUCTION
21 patients

● occluded ICA (n:27)

○ stenotic ICA (n:15)

Fig. 3b   Patients with bilateral ICA obstruction (group B).
The continuous lines show the normal range of the CBF-OEF
relationship; there is a down-shift of this relationship in group
B patients.

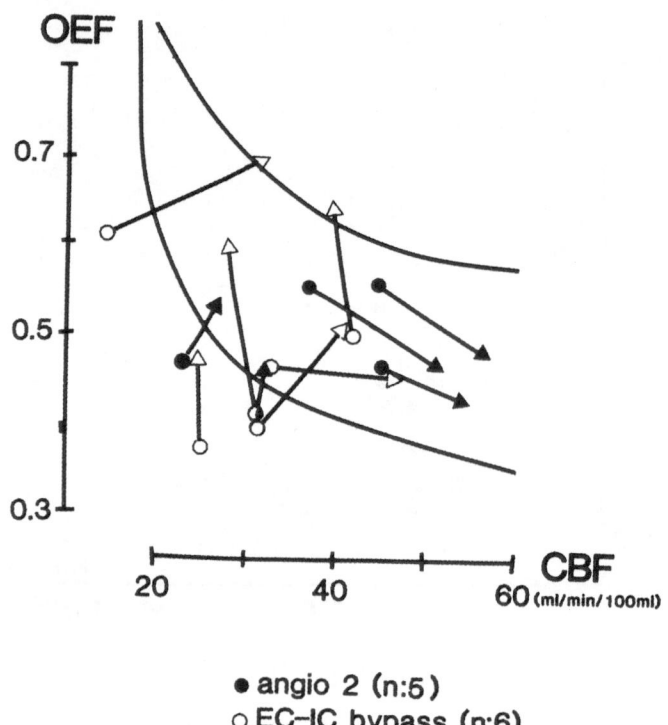

Fig. 4   Changes in CBF and OEF following either EC-IC bypass
or an angiotensin II infusion in patients with bilateral ICA
obstructions: The continuous lines show the "normal" range of the
CBF-OEF relationships. The initial (pre-intervention) values are
shown by circles, and the final (post-intervention) ones by
triangles. See text for further comments.

way similar to the "barbiturate-like" effect of ischemia described in
acute experiments by Astrup (1982), but this would hardly explain the
down-shift of the CBF-OEF relationship. This latter abnormality may,
however, be explained by a state of uneven patchy perfusion (Eklöf et
al., 1972). In this hypothesis, the oxygen delivery would be impeded in
cerebral tissue surrounding unperfused capillaries, a process
potentially resulting in a $CMRO_2$ decrease measured at the spatial
resolution of PET. Additional arguments support this hypothesis: 1. A
similar condition has been suspected to occur in situations of low CPP
with maximal vasodilatation (Eklöf et al., 1972; Dyken et al., 1970;
Barry et al., 1984), likely to occur in patients with bilateral ICA
obstruction (Gibbs et al., 1984). 2. In the cat brain, the number of
cortical perfused channels decreased proportionally to the fall of CPP,
although it was unclear whether CBF autoregulation was always preserved
(Chang et al., 1984). 3. Finally, morphological capillary changes
correlated with the severity of proximal arterial disease (Kishikawa et
al., 1983), have been reported in ischemic retinopathy, and arteriolo-
capillary alterations are a prominent feature of the "granular cortical
atrophy" sometimes found in patients with bilateral ICA occlusion
(Wildi, 1959). Further studies are necessary to investigate this
"microcirculatory" hypothesis, which may be of some practical clinical
importance.

REFERENCES

Astrup, J. 1982. Energy-requiring cell functions in the ischemic brain.
    Their critical supply and possible inhibition in protective
    therapy. J. Neurosurg., 56, 482-497.
Baron, J.C., Bousser, M.G., Rey, A. et al. 1981. Reversal of focal
    "misery-perfusion syndrome" by extra-intracranial arterial bypass
    in hemodynamic cerebral ischemia. A case study with 150 positron
    emission tomography. Stroke, 12, 454-459.
Barry, D.I., Strandgaard, S., Graham, D.I. et al. 1984. Cerebral blood
    flow during dihydralazine-induced hypotension in hypertensive
    rats. Stroke, 15, 102-108.
Chang, B.L., Santillan, G., Bing, R.J. 1984. Red cell velocity and
    autoregulation in the cerebral cortex of the cat. Brain Res., 308,
    15-24.
Dyken, M.L. 1970. Cerebral blood flow, oxygen utilization, and vascular
    reactivity. Neurology, 20, 1127-1132.

Eklöf B., MacMillan, V., Siesjö, B.K. 1972. Cerebral energy state and cerebral venous PO2 in experimental hypotension caused by bleeding. Acta Physiol. Scand., 86, 515-527.

Feeney, D.M., Baron, J.C. 1986. Diaschisis. Stroke, 17, 817-830.

Gibbs, J.M., Wise, R.J.S., Leenders, K.L. et al. 1984. Evaluation of cerebral perfusion reserve in patients with carotid-artery occlusion. Lancet, I, 310-322.

Gibbs, J.M., Wise, R.J.S., Mansfield, A.O. et al. 1985. Regional cerebral blood flow and blood volume before and after EC-Ic bypass surgery and carotid endarterectomy in patients with occlusive carotid disease. J. Cereb. Blood Flow Metabol., 5, Suppl. 1, S19-S20.

Kishikawa, K., Masanobu, U., Asayama, R. 1983. Occlusive thromboaortopathy (Takayasu's disease): cervical arterial stenosis, retinal arterial pressure, retinal microaneurysms and prognosis. Stroke, 14, 730-735.

Lassen, N.A. 1982. Incomplete cerebral infarction - Focal incomplete ischemic tissue necrosis not leading to emollision. Stroke, 13, 522-523.

Norrving, B., Nilsson, B., Risberg, I. 1982. rCBF in patients with carotid occlusion. Stroke, 13, 155-162.

Powers, W.J., Grubb, R.L. Jr., Raichle, M.E. 1984a. Physiological responses to focal cerebral ischemia in humans. Ann. Neurol., 16, 546-552.

Powers, W.J., Martin, W.R.W., Herscovitch, P. et al. 1984b. Extra-cranial-intracranial bypass surgery: Hemodynamic and metabolic effects. Neurology, 34, 1168-1174.

Powers, W.J., Press, A.G., Grubb, R.L. et al. 1986. The hemodynamic effects of carotid stenosis on the cerebral circulation. Stroke, 17, 127.

Samson, Y, Baron, J.C., Bousser, M.G. et al. 1985a. Effects of extra-intracranial arterial bypass on cerebral blood flow and oxygen metabolism in humans. Stroke, 16, 609-616.

Samson, Y., Baron, J.C., Bousser, M.G. 1985. Cerebral hemodynamic and metabolic changes in carotid artery occlusion. A PET study. In "Cerebral Vascular Disease, 5". (Eds. J.S. Meyer, H. Lechner, M. Reivich, E.O. Ott). (Excerpta Medica, Amsterdam, New York, Oxford). pp. 128-135.

Samson, Y., Baron, J.C., Bousser, M.G. et al. 1985b. Extra-intracranial arterial bypass (EIAB) increases CMRO2 in both cerebral hemispheres. J. Cereb. Blood Flow Metabol., 5, Suppl. 1, S17-S18.

Spetzler, R.F., Roski, R.A., Zabramski, J. 1983. Middle cerebral artery perfusion pressure in cerebrovascular occlusive disease. Stroke, 14, 552-555.

Wildi, 1959. Bull. Acad. Suisse Sci. Med., 15, 18-83.

FUNCTIONAL EVALUATION OF EXTRA-INTRACRANIAL ARTERIAL BYPASSES USING PET AND REPEATED BOLUS ADMINISTRATION OF ^{15}O LABELED TRACERS

J.C. Depresseux, J. Lenelle, P. Merlot

Cyclotron Research Center
Liège, Belgium

The extra-intracranial (EC-IC) arterial bypass operations, as performed in patients with stenosis or occlusion of the internal carotid or middle cerebral artery, are to provide extra blood to the brain and to decrease the presumed risk of recurrent cerebral ischemic attacks.

The efficacy of this microsurgial procedure has been evaluated using various approaches:

(a) radiological visualization of the filling of intracranial arteries through the anastomosis, and of the diameter evolution of the feeding artery with time after surgery (Latchaw et al., 1979; Samson and Boone, 1978; Sundt et al., 1976; Yonekawa and Yasargil, 1976);

(b) measuring of the perfusion pressure in vessels below the bypass (Sundt et al., 1976);

(c) studies of regional cerebral blood flow (CBF) and vascular re-activity before and after surgery, using ^{133}Xe methods (Carter et al., 1984; Heilbrun et al., 1975; Schmidek et al., 1971; Thomas et al., 1984) or stable Xe techniques (Yonas et al., 1985);

(d) determination of both CBF and cerebral oxygen uptake rate ($CMRO_2$), using ^{15}O and single photon detection (Grubb et al., 1979) or positron emission tomography (PET) (Baron et al., 1981b; Depresseux and Lenelle, 1986; Samson et al., 1985; Powers et al., 1984);

(e) assessment of the clinical outcome (Chater, 1983; Donaghy, 1976; Gratzl et al., 1976; Guegan et al., 1979; Heilbrun et al., 1975; Reichman, 1974; Yasargil and Yonekawa, 1977) and, more recently, comparison of the outcome of surgically and medically treated patients (EC/IC Bypass Study Group, 1985a; 1985b).

The rationale of such validation studies is provided by two implicit objectives:

(a) deciding on the clinical efficacy of the procedure in comparison with other regimens, (b) extracting more specific indications for the treatment under study.

A review of the literature reveals that these two objectives are interactive because the results of any evaluation of efficacy depend on the predefined criteria for the inclusion of patients in the study. Those criteria effectively define the hypothetical specific indications of the test treatment. Definition of inclusion criteria remains of paramount importance for drawing unambiguous conclusions, but can be open to rediscussion.

It is the purpose of this paper (a) to discuss the present situation of PET studies, in the light of the results of the above international study (EC/IC Bypass Study Group, 1985a, 1985b), and (b) to define our own strategy of evaluation of EC-IC bypasses, using PET.

POTENTIAL ROLE OF PET IN THE EVALUATION OF EC/IC BYPASSES

The effect of an EC/IC bypass and of medical treatment on the clinical outcome of randomized groups of patients with stenosis or occlusion of the carotid or middle cerebral artery was compared in a recently published international cooperative study (EC/IC Bypass Study Group, 1985a, 1985b). That study did not reveal any significant differences in the recurrence rate of ischemic attacks, between surgically and medically treated groups. No difference was found in subgroups of patients with internal carotid occlusion, with internal carotid siphon stenosis, with middle cerebral artery occlusion, with middle cerebral artery stenosis, or with tandem lesions.

Later, controversy arose as to the criteria for selection of patients, statistical power in subgroups, possible exclusion of eligible patients, and non-systematic diagnosis by CT scanning (Ausman and Diaz, 1986; Barnett et al., 1986; Day et al., 1986). Some authors, therefore, maintain that further investigations could be necessary to get a better idea of the indications and effects of the EC-IC bypass procedure.

What is presently the potential of PET methods for documenting that clinical problem, considering recent highlights on the subject? Available PET data on focal cerebral ischemia (Baron et al., 1981b; Depresseux and Lenelle, 1986; Grubb et al., 1979; Samson et al., 1985)

indeed suggest the possibility that subgrouping of patients according
to radiological criteria, as it was done in the cooperative study, may
not be the best approach to identify specific indications for bypass
surgery.

The possible justification for using other inclusion criteria can
be illustrated by considering a model stratifying the tested patient
sample according to deterministic hypotheses. Fig. 1 demonstrates such
an analysis, in which patients are classified in 4 subgroups, according
to their deterministic response to medical or surgical treatment.

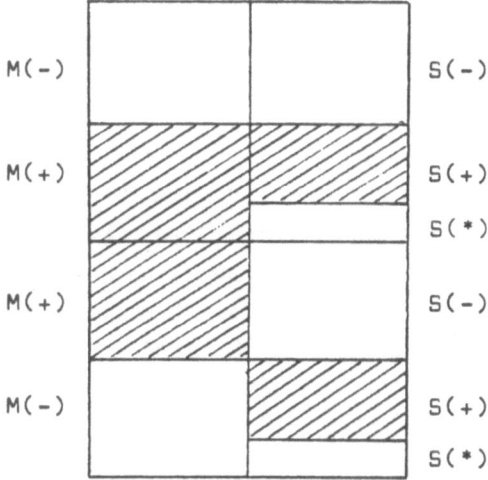

Fig. 1   Illustration of the possible deteministic classes in a
cohort of patients suffering from internal carotid artery and/or
middle cerebral artery occlusion or stenosis. Classes are
defined by the suppressive (+), or the indifferent (-) effect, of
medical (M) or surgical (S) treatment on the recurrence of neurologic ischemic accidents. The side effects of surgery are denoted
by S (*). The model considers the possibility of cases responding
specifically to medical and to surgical treatment, and of cases
with favorable or unfavorable outcome, irrespective of the treatment.

If two treatment groups are properly randomized, and if samples are
sufficiently large, the proportion of successful medical and surgical
treatments, respectively, is given by:

(a) M(+) / N representing correct indications for medical treatment, and (b) (S(+) - S(*)) / N representing correct indications for surgical therapy, including the surgical risk frequency, with N denoting the total sample size.

Results of a randomized comparative study on such a group of patients may thus lead to two possible interpretations, (a) either in terms of testing the null hypothesis of an aleatory response of the globally defined therapeutical groups, or (b) in terms of frequencies in classes of patients with a specific response to the tested therapies. Those two ways of expressing results of a randomized study are fully compatible, but it appears to us that the possible usefulness of the second model is to give support to a search for strategies of patient selection that could define subgroups leading to a more specific definition of therapeutical indications.

In cases of carotid or middle cerebral artery occlusion or severe stenosis, PET allows to define several subgroups with very different patterns of uncoupling between CBF and metabolism (Baron et al., 1981a, 1981b, 1983; Frackowiak, 1985; Gibbs et al., 1984; Lenzi et al., 1981; Samson et al., 1985; Wise et al., 1983), suggesting different therapeutical approaches. Furthermore, some of these subgroups, as studied without randomization, showed a reversal of functional disturbances following EC/IC bypass (Baron et al., 1981b; Depresseux and Lenelle, 1979; Powers et al., 1984; Samson et al. 1985).

They provide arguments maintaining the interest in a randomized trial of medical versus surgical therapy, with patients selected according to clinical + radiological + PET criteria. The possibility of a more specific response in PET-selected subgroups of patients may allow to draw significant conclusions from a relatively small number of patients.

STRATEGY OF REPEATABLE MULTIPARAMETER PET METHODS FOR CLINICAL USE

The combination of PET and ^{15}O-labeled tracers represents a unique possibility for the noninvasive evaluation of local CBF, $CMRO_2$, and extraction fraction of oxygen (CEO_2), in transaxial slices of the brain in man. Various methodological approaches have been published to date, differing in the time profile of the input function, in data collection mode and in operational procedures (Depresseux, 1983;

Depresseux et al., 1983; Frackowiak et al., 1980; Ginsberg et al., 1982; Herscovitch et al., 1983; Huang et al., 1983; Jones et al., 1976; Mintun et al., 1984; Raichle et al., 1983). This variety of methods results from different compromises between the possibilities of data collection and processing on the one side, and optimization of physiological attainments on the other.

From the technical point of view, accuracy and precision of determinations are indeed conditioned by four major sources of noise and/or distortion:

(a) the spatial resolution achieved with PET is such that each local tomographic data is a weighted sum of contributions from different cerebral functional compartments, particularly gray and white matter;

(b) the Poisson distribution of radioactivity countings is propagated through the reconstruction algorithms within the tomographic image contents;

(c) the number of parameters which are computable is limited by the available quantity of information and may be at odds with the complexity of the model, resulting in inaccuracies of data processing:

(d) the permeability of water across the blood-brain barrier is limited (Eichling et al., 1974). It was nevertheless demonstrated that this limitation has negligible bearing on CBF estimates in man, using ^{15}O-labeled radiowater (Raichle et al., 1983).

From the physiological point of view, the main requirements on a clinically useful method can be listed as follows:

(a) repeatability of determinations,

(b) high temporal resolution,

(c) acceptable radiation absorbed dose to the patient,

(d) rapid data processing,

(e) determination of multiple parameters.

In an attempt at meeting those objectives, we designed and validated a method for the concommitant assessment of CBF and $CMRO_2$ from the data recorded after bolus inhalation of $^{15}O_2$ and $C^{15}O_2$, respectively (Depresseux, 1983; Depresseux et al., 1983).

The algorithm was based on data of two time-integrated PET images obtained 30 - 165 and 165 - 300 s after inhalation of the tracer.

Fig. 2 gives the general scheme of the method.
Administration of ^{15}O-labeled CO_2 leads to the formation of radiowater within the pulmonary capillary bed and allows to perform tomograms
of the quantitative distribution of radiowater within the brain. Local
CBF and volume of distribution of radiowater (CWV) are computed for each
tomographic pixel, from local image data and measured concentrations of
the tracer in arterial blood.

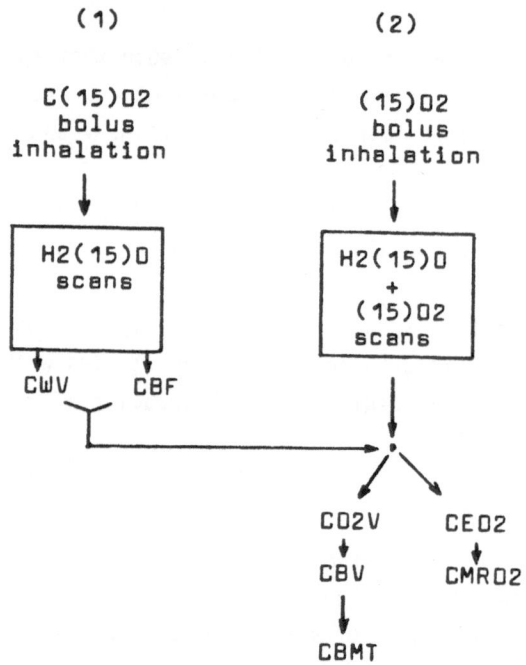

Fig. 2   Organization scheme of our method for concommitant
evaluation of CBF, CMRO2, CEO2, CWV, cerebral blood volume (CBV)
and cerebral blood mean transit time (CBMT), using sequential
PET images obtained after bolus inhalation of 15-O-labeled CO2
and O2. Each PET sequence allows the primary computation of 2 parameters; other ones are computed secondarily.

The administration of ^{15}O-labeled O_2 leads to the distribution
of radio-oxygen to tissues, as a function of local blood flow, and its
local extraction from the blood, with generation of radiowater. Tomograms then represent measures of local radioactivity concentrations
corresponding to the sum of local radio-oxygen, locally produced radiowater, and local recirculating radiowater. Local CEO_2 and CO_2V are

computed for each tomographic pixel, from the local radioactivity data, from the measurements of arterial blood concentrations of radio-oxygen and radiowater, and from previously determined local CBF and CWV.

The method thus allows a pluri-parameter analysis for simultaneous estimates of CBF and $CMRO_2$, taking into account the necessary corrections for local CWV and CO_2V. Computations are straightforward and are compatible with the processing of functional PET images on a pixel-by-pixel basis.

Short-time and repeated determinations of those parameters appear to be particularly suited to the study of pre- and postoperative blood flow, blood volume, and oxygen metabolism in patients, and to the study of effects of compression tests on the anastomosis.

PET STRATEGY FOR ASSESSING THE FUNCTIONAL RESULTS OF BYPASSES

The strategy we are currently using to assess the function of EC/IC bypasses proceeds as follows:

(a) by comparing the circulatory and metabolic parameters immediately before and 2 - 20 weeks after surgery, in correlation with the clinical symptoms and with the radiological criteria of shunt patency;

(b) by performing, after surgery, an additional PET study during 4.5-min compression of the superficial temporal artery feeding the anastomosis.

We present an exemplary observation illustrating the potential of the method: Fig. 3 shows the parametric PET images obtained in a patient suffering from Moya-Moya disease, with bilateral internal carotid artery occlusion and a right EC-IC bypass. CT demonstrated an asymptomatic cerebral infarct in the right prefrontal region. PET images showed a decrease in CBF, with a corresponding mild increase in CEO_2 in the anterior two thirds of the left cerebral hemisphere and in both frontal regions. Decreased CBV in regions with lowered CBF, indicates the absence of recruitment of the perfusion reserve, possibly related to diffuse vascular Moya-Moya lesions. CBF, $CMRO_2$, and CBV were decreased in the infarcted right prefrontal region. Compression of the right superficial temporal artery resulted in an immediate decrease in CBF in a large area of the right cerebral hemisphere.

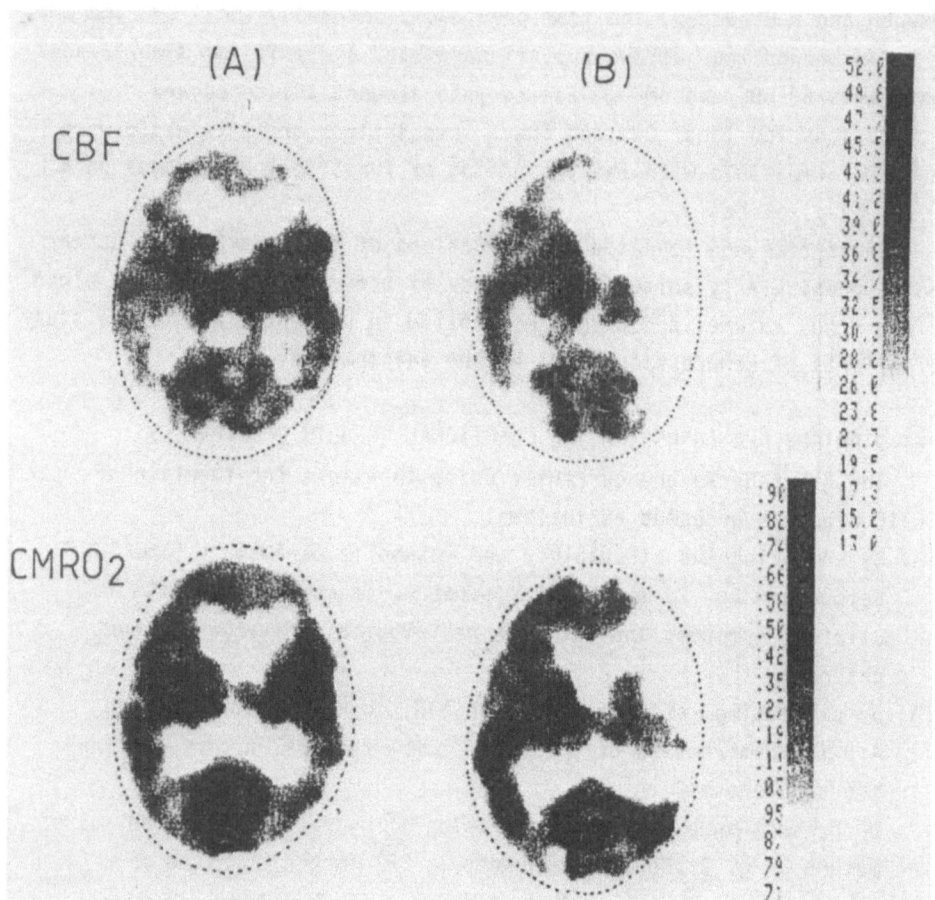

Fig. 3   (first part, continued on next page)

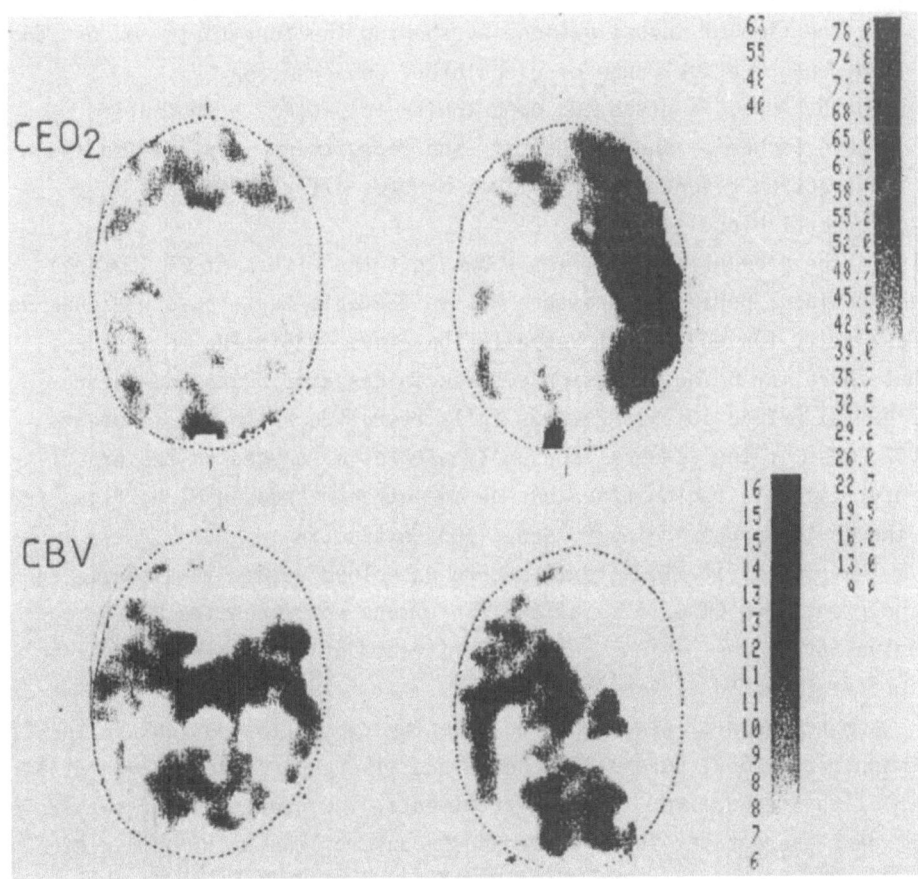

Fig. 3   Parametric PET images of CBF, CMRO2, CBV, and CEO2
obtained by sequential bolus administration of 15-O-labeled CO2
and O2 in a patient with bilateral internal carotid artery
occlusion and a right EC-IC bypass. CT revealed an asymptomatic right prefrontal infarct. Images were obtained before (A)
and during (B) 4.5-min compression of the superficial temporal
artery (with permission from Depresseux and Lenelle, 1986).

This observation illustrates the potential of the method we are systematically utilizing in shunted patients.

(a) It directly demonstrates the hemodynamic effectiveness of the shunt at the time of investigation, by showing the territorial extent and the quantitative range of circulatory compensation.

(b) Furthermore, it gives the opportunity to produce a controlled acute ischemia, and to quantify the recruitment of perfusion and extraction reserves in the first minutes after a decrease in cerebral blood supply.

In the present case, it was shown that the effect of STA compression on local perfusion pressure was so dramatic that there remained no possibility for additional vasodilation, thus confirming the concept that there may be no perfusion reserve in cases of acute and severe ischemia. Extraction reserve was fully recruited, with CEO_2 close to 100%: most of the cerebral consumption rates of oxygen in the experimental ischemic region were thus dependent on decreased blood flow, from a threshold corresponding to about 100% extraction.

The possibility to determine cerebral blood volume in a single run concurrent with $CMRO_2$ also allows for a more comprehensive PET evaluation of the patient before (for treatment indication) and after (for treatment justification) surgery.

A more powerful step could be taken by submitting patients with PET-demonstrated focal cerebral ischemia and misery perfusion (Baron et al., 1981b) to a randomized trial of treatments. The conditions of such an approach are not yet fully agreed on because of the small number of active PET centers and the above mentioned heterogeneity of methods. Cooperation between centers, supported by international programs, could help to tackle such a question.

ACKNOWLEDGEMENTS

The present research was supported by grants no. 1.5.242.86 F and 1.4.647.84 from the Belgian National Fund for Scientific Research.

REFERENCES

Ausman, J.I. and Diaz, F.G. 1986. Critique of the extracranial-intracranial bypass study. Surg. Neurol., 26, 218-221.

Barnett, H.J.M., Fox, A., Hachinski, V., Peerless, S.J., et al. 1986. Further conclusions from the extracranial-intracranial bypass trial. Surg. Neurol., 26, 227-235.

Baron, J.C., Bousser, M.G., Comar, D., et al. 1981a. Noninvasive tomographic study of cerebral blood flow and metabolism in vivo. Eur. Neurol., 20, 273-284.

Baron, J.C., Bousser, M.G., Rey, A., et al. 1981b. Reversal of focal "misery perfusion syndrome" by extra-intracranial arterial bypass in hemodynamic cerebral ischemia. Stroke, 12, 454-459.

Baron, J.C., Rougemont, D., Lebrun-Grandie, P., et al. 1983. Local cerebral blood flow and oxygen consumption in evolving irreversible ischemic infarction. "In Positron Emission Tomography of the Brain" (Eds. W.-D. Heiss and M.E. Phelps). (Springer-Verlag, Berlin). pp. 120-125.

Carter, L.P., Crowell, R.M., Sonntag, V.K.H., et al., 1984. Cortical blood flow during extracranial-intracranial bypass surgery. Stroke, 15, 836-839.

Chater, N. 1983. Neurosurgical extracranial-intracranial bypass for stroke with 400 cases. Neurol. Res., 23, 287-309.

Day, A.L., Rhoton, A.L. and Little, J.R. 1986. The extracranial-intracranial study. Surg. Neurol., 26, 222-226.

Depresseux, J.C. 1983. A method for the local evaluation of the volume of rapidly exchangeable water in the human brain. In "Positron Emission Tomography of the Brain" (Eds. W.-D. Heiss and M.E. Phelps). (Springer-Verlag, Berlin). pp. 95-102.

Depresseux, J.C., Cheslet, J.P. and Franck, G. 1983. An original method for the concommitant tomographic assessment of cerebral blood flow, oxygen extraction rate and exchangeable water volume in man. J. Cereb. Blood Flow Metab., 3, (Suppl. 1), 152-153.

Depresseux, J.C. and Lenelle, J. 1986. Apport de la tomographie d'émission positonique dans l'évaluation des anatomoses extra-intracraniennes. Circ. Met. Cerv., sous press.

Donaghy, P. 1976. Evaluation of extra-intracranial blood flow diversion. In "Microsurgical Anastomoses for Cerebral Ischemia" (Ed. G.M. Austin). (Thomas, Springfield). pp. 256-274.

EC/IC Bypass Study Group. 1985a. The international cooperative study of extracranial-intracranial arterial anastomosis: methodology and entry characteristics. Stroke, 16, 397-406.

EC/IC Bypass Study Group. 1985b. Failure of extracranial-intracranial bypass to reduce the risk of ischemic stroke. Results of an international randomized trial. New Engl. J. Med., 313, 1191-1200.

Eichling, J.O., Raichle, M.E., Grubb, R.L., et al. 1974. Evidence of the limitations of water as a freely diffusible tracer in the brain of the Rhesus monkey. Circ. Res., 35, 358-364.

Frackowiak, R.S.J. 1985. Pathophysiology of human cerebral ischemia: studies with positron tomography and 15-oxygen. In "Brain Imaging and Brain Function" (Ed. L. Sokoloff). (Raven Press, New York). pp. 139-161.

Frackowiak, R.S.J., Lenzi, G.L., Jones, T., et al. 1980. Quantitative measurement of regional cerebral blood flow and oxygen metabolism in man, using 15-O and positron emission tomography: theory, procedure and normal values. J. Comput. Assist. Tomogr., 4, 727-731.

Gibbs, J.M., Wise, R., Leenders, K., et al. 1984. Evaluation of cerebral perfusion reserve in patients with carotid artery occlusion. Lancet, 1, 310-314.

Ginsberg, M.D., Lockwood, A.H. and Busto, R. 1982. A simplified in vivo autoradiographic strategy for the determination of regional cerebral blood flow by positron emission tomography: theoretical considerations and validation studies in the rat. J. Cereb. Blood Flow Metab., 2, 89-98.

Gratzl, O., Schmidek, P., Spetzler, R., et al. 1976. Clinical experience with extra-intracranial arterial anastomosis in 65 cases. J. Neurosurg., 44, 313-324.

Grubb, R.L., Ratcheson, R.A., Raichle, M.E., et al. 1979. Regional cerebral blood flow and oxygen utilization in superficial temporal-middle cerebral artery anastomosis patients. J. Neurosurg., 50, 733-741.

Guegan, R., Deruty, R., Reg, A., et al. 1979. EICA in transient ischemic attacks and neurological deficits. Acta Neurochir., 28, (Suppl.), 302-305.

Heilbrun, M.P., Reichman, O.H., Anderson, R.E., et al. 1975. Regional cerebral blood flow studies following superficial temporal-middle cerebral artery anastomosis. J. Neurosurg., 43, 706-716.

Herscovitch, P., Markham, J. and Raichle, M.E. 1983. Brain blood flow measurement with intravenous H-2 15-O. I. Theory and error analysis. J. Nucl. Med., 24, 782-789.

Huang, S.C., Carson, R.E., Hoffman, E.J., et al. 1983. Quantitative measurement of local cerebral blood flow in humans by positron computed tomography and 15-O water. J. Cereb. Blood Flow Metab., 3, 141-153.

Jones, T., Chesler, D.A. and Ter-Pogossian, M.M. 1976. The continuous inhalation of oxygen-15 for assessing regional oxygen extraction in the brain of man. Br. J. Radiol., 49, 339-343.

Latchaw, R.E., Ausman, J.I and Lee, M.C. 1979. Superficial temporal-middle cerebral artery bypass: a detailed analysis of multiple pre- and postoperative angiograms in 40 consecutive patients. J. Neurosurg., 51, 455-465.

Lenzi, G.L., Frackowiak, R.S.J., Jones, T., et al. 1981. CMRO-2 and CBF by the oxygen-15 inhalation technique: results in normal volunteers and cerebrovascular patients. Eur. Neurol., 20, 285-290.

Mintun, M.A., Raichle, M.E., Martin, W.R.W., et al. 1984. Brain oxygen utilization measured wiht 0-15 radiotracers and positron emission tomography. J. Nucl. Med., 25, 177-187.

Powers, W.J., Martin, W.R., Herscovitch, P., et al. 1984. Extracranial-intracranial bypass surgery: hemodynamic and metabolic effects. Neurology, 34, 1168-1174.

Raichle, M.E., Martin, W.R.W., Herscovitch, P., et al. 1983. Brain blood flow measured with intravenous H-2 (15-O). II. Implementation and validation. J. Nucl. Med., 24, 790-798.

Reichman, O.H. 1974. Neurosurgical microsurgical anastomosis for cerebral ischemia: five years' experience. In "Cerebrovascular Disease" (Ed. P. Scheinberg). (Raven Press, New York). pp. 311-330.

Samson, D.S. and Boone, S. 1978. (EC-IC) arterial bypass: past performance and current concepts. Neurosurg., 3, 79-86.

Samson, Y., Baron, J.C., Bousser, M.G., et al. 1985. Conséquences hémo-
   dynamiques et métaboliques régionales de l'anastomose temporo-
   sylvienne. Etude de 15 patients par tomographie par émission de
   positons. Neurochir., 31, 31-36.
Schmidek, P., Steinhoff, H. and Gratzl, O. 1971. rCBF measurements in
   patients treated for cerebral ischemia by extra-intracranial
   vascular anastomosis. Eur. Neurol., 6, 364-368.
Sundt, T.M., Siekert, R.G., Sharbrough, R.W., et al. 1976. Bypass
   surgery for vascular disease of the carotid system. Mayo Clin.
   Proc., 50, 677-692.
Thomas, M., Hennerici, M. and Marshall, J. 1984. Cerebral blood flow
   after carotid occlusion and extracranial-intracranial bypass.
   J. Neurol., Neurosurg., Psychiat., 47, 148-152.
Wise, R.J.S., Bernardi, S., Frackowiak, R.S.J., et al. 1983. Serial
   observations of the pathophysiology of acute stroke. The
   transition from ischaemia to infarction as reflected in regional
   oxygen extraction. Brain, 106, 197-222.
Yasargil, M.G. and Yonekawa, Y. 1977. Results of microsurgical extra-
   intracranial arterial bypass in the treatment of cerebral
   ischemia. Neurosurg., 1, 22-24.
Yonas, H., Gur, D., Good, B.C., et al. 1985. Stable Xenon CT blood flow
   mapping for evaluation of patients with extracranial-intracranial
   bypass surgery. J. Neurosurg., 62, 324-333.
Yonekawa, Y. and Yasargil, M.G. 1976. Extra-intracranial arterial
   anastomosis: clinical and technical aspects. Results. Adv. and
   Techn. Standards in Neurosurg., 3, 47-78.

POSITRON EMISSION TOMOGRAPHY IN CEREBROVASCULAR DISORDERS:
RESULTS AND PERSPECTIVES

G.L. Lenzi, F. Fazio, C. Fieschi
Clinica Neurologica, Dept. of Neurol. Sciences, Rome, Italy

A technique is helpful to the clinician when it helps to explain the clinical presentation and/or when it helps to predict the future course, and/or when it correctly channels a treatment. Neuroimaging techniques are, in this respect, a classical example. The best known technique, the CT scan, is in fact relevant for the identification, for the management and for the follow-up of many organic brain syndromes, from tumors to hydrocephalus to cerebrovascular disorders. However, the CT scan is useless for explaining widespread neuropsychiatric disorders such as depression, anxiousness, psychosis. These disorders in fact belong to the "functional" sphere and not to the "organic" brain syndromes in the present context of these definitions.

Furthermore, CT scan, and possibly also the more recent MRI, cannot give information on aspects other than those linked to tissue's density, that is percent content in water.

However, the behavior of some basic functional aspects of cerebral tissue appears fundamental in predicting the clinical course and final prognosis of a disease, in particular for cerebrovascular disorders.

Other neuroimaging techniques, directed more toward the representation of basic functional aspects of the brain, are thus potentially useful for clinicians in the study of CVD. These techniques are positron emission tomography (PET), and single photon emission computerized tomography (SPECT). Both represent main branches of the emission computerized tomography general approach.

The main aim of the present short review is the analysis of the results obtained to date with PET, focussing in particular on the revenue offered to neurologists as real advantages in the management of cerebrovascular patients, and following through from the analysis of the results to bring into focus the perspectives and limits of this technique.

CLINICAL RESULTS OF PET IN CVD

The major accomplishment, so far, of PET in the field of CVD has been to acquire a greater knowledge of the mechanisms underlying the pathophysiology of human cerebral ischemia. In particular, the simultaneous measurement of CBF, CMRO2, OER, and CBV obtained in many PET centers, have led to a better understanding of this extremely relevant clinical entity. In fact treatment of cerebral ischemia is being directed more and more towards the very first hours and it requires knowledge of the time-course of the transition between a potentially recoverable ischemia and completed infarction. Also preventive treatment of patients "at risk" needs a more thorough assessment and greater consideration of hemodynamic conditions in order to recognize the correct sub-population that could truly benefit from a particular therapy; a therapy which might otherwise appear to be useless if applied to an unselected sub-population.

In pathophysiological terms, cerebral ischemia is a condition in which cerebral energy metabolism becomes impaired due to inadequate blood supply. In physiological conditions, the local CBF is metabolism dependent: rCBF = f(rCMRO2). In ischemia there is a reversal and the metabolism becomes flow rate dependent. In normal conditions a considerable excess of energy substrates is delivered to the brain: the oxygen is 2-3 times and the glucose is 7 times the normal requirement of the nervous tissue per minute. The glucose is actively transported from blood to brain, while the oxygen diffuses passively into the tissue. Active neurons burn more substrates than the silent ones and the close relationship between metabolism and flow leads to a physiological increase in rCBF in the active regions. This regional coupling is expressed by the fractional extraction of oxygen (OER).

It follows that by increasing extraction a twofold increase in metabolic activity (or vice-versa a comparable decrease in blood supply) can be accomodated. Thus, tissue hypoperfusion does not in itself necessarily imply ischemia and tissue hypoxia may coexist with normal or also increased metabolic activity.

In fact, CBF and CMRO2 are linearly related, but the angular coefficient of their linear relationship may change a great deal. One classical example is the effect of hyperventilation, which greatly increases this angular coefficient (that is the OER).

Only when the hypoperfusion cannot be compensated for and therefore local metabolism is affected, is there a true ischemia. In this sense, the situation of "compensated hypoperfusion" is one at risk of hemodynamic unbalance: the "critical perfusion" situation.

The recognition and understanding of this situation represent one of the major achievements of PET in pathophysiology. However, we must remember that a fundamental role appears to be played by the changes in the peripheral resistance of the cerebral vascular tree. The measurements of the cerebral blood volume (CBV) have shown how the main mechanism of autoregulation acts through increase or decrease of CBV in order to maintain CBF constant. A rise in systemic blood pressure results in a vasoconstriction and an increase in peripheral resistance. Thus, the decrease in CBV is the counterpart of the stability of CBF. Vice-versa, as the systemic blood pressure falls, CBV increases and CBF again remains constant. Many studies have been performed to assess the relative frequency of patients with critical perfusion in respect to clinical presentation of RIA or to the presence of an occlusion of an internal carotid artery. The poor selection of the patient population has however brought about a wide variability in the results.

In general, when the patient presents with a normal CT scan and without large vessel disease, the PET and SPECT landscapes are normal. But many cases with clinical RIA in fact showed a CT scan hypodensity and/or had a significant pathology of the large neck vessels. Thus, a wide variety of changes in rCBF, rCMRO2 and rOER have been reported. In general, the long dismissed concept of hemodynamic (as opposed to embolic) focal ischemia has received some support from PET studies after the first full report of "reversal of focal misery-perfusion syndrome" by extra-intracranial arterial bypass in hemodynamic cerebral ischemia in the patient studied by Baron et al. (1981).

Combined studies of the oxygen metabolism and of the glucose metabolism in this type of patient (that is, with TIA and carotid occlusion) have shown that in general CMRGlu is better preserved than CMRO2 in the affected hemisphere, "suggesting enhanced anaerobic glycolysis triggered by long-standing tissue hypoxia" (Baron et al., 1984).

In the larger series of patients studied by Gibbs et al. (1984) (seven patients) and by Powers et al. (1985) (twenty-four patients), the

evaluation of cerebral blood volume (CBV) has provided further
information on the consequences of ICA occlusion. The "critical" or
"misery" perfusion is accompanied by an increase in rCBV, indicating an
impaired autoregulation and a maximal vasodilation of resistance vessels
distal to the occluded ICA. However, rCBV may be increased in the
affected territory without any detectable change in CBF and OER. In the
seven patients selected by Powers et al. (1984) because of normal CT
scan and impaired CBF, concomitant to a decrease of rCBF to the
symptomatic hemisphere, there was a slight decrease in rCMRO2 and an
increase in rCBV and rOER. Meaning that the ischemic hemispheres showed
loss of the normal coupling between flow and metabolism, rCMRO2 was
maintained by an increase in rOER, with progressively higher extraction
needed as flow decreased. In this series "the greatest declines in rCBF
occurred in those patients with the least evidence of vasodilation,
suggesting that autoregulatory capacity may vary from individual to
individual" (Powers et al., 1984). This is in contrast with Gibbs et al.
(1984) who reported an increase of rOER only in those five patients with
the lowest rCBF/rCBV ratio, that is with the largest increases in rCBV.
However, this observation was made on a mixed TIA-stroke population.

The general meaning is that PET may help to identify those stroke-
prone patients who are at an increased risk of stroke on a low-flow
basis by demonstrating focal regions of diminished cerebral perfusion.

The data presented by the St. Louis group have helped to establish
the thresholds for normal functioning of the brain. The minimum rCBF and
rCMRO2 levels observed in viable brain tissue were 15 and 1.3 mls/100
g/min respectively (Powers et al., 1985). However, rCBF values showed
high variability, while rCMRO2 data was more consistent with the final
outcome. Below these values there is irreversible infarction.

In addition to these data which point towards the identification of
a hemodynamic unbalance, a parallel reduction in flow and metabolism,
with normal OER has been reported in the cortical territory distal to
an ICA or MCA occlusion (Grubb et al., 1979; Baron et al., 1981;
Sgouropoulos et al., 1985). This condition of metabolic depression could
be due either to neuronal loss, or to functional deactivation or to
both, affecting these cortical areas. The possible reversibility of this
metabolic depression after an EC-IC by-pass (Samson et al., 1985) is not
consistent with those two explanations, but its precise mechanism still

remains obscure.

No further comment will be made on these aspects of metabolic and functional depression, that is on the "diaschisis". However, it should be pointed out that in our opinion demonstration of functional inactivation is one of the most fascinating aspects of the neuroimaging techniques and their utilization for clinical purposes appears very promising. Unfortunately more SPECT than PET studies have been performed so far in this field.

The number of PET studies performed in stroke is not much larger than that performed in TIAs:

Our review of the literature includes 10 patients studied during the first 24 hours, 9 studied during the 2nd day, 14 during the 3rd day and 11 during the 4th day. Apart from the apparently scanty amount of data, the results have brought an understanding of events taking place in acute cerebral ischemia. The role of CBF, apart from initiating a cascade of events has been reduced to the point where Ackerman has labelled CBF and its modifications as an "epiphenomenon". In fact, it is well recognized that there is a wide variability of rCBF after stroke both with or without carotid occlusion.

PET studies have indicated that in the very early phase of cerebral ischemia, cerebral tissue in and around the area of depressed flow exhibits an increased oxygen extraction. This indicates that at the onset of a major reduction of CBF, trespassing the threshold of 15 mls/100 g/min for a period of time lasting probably well over a few minutes, mitochondrial function remains intact, resulting in a maximal extraction of oxygen from the residual trickle of arterial blood. And as previously stated, the metabolism becomes flow-dependent and flow-limited.

In the early hours after an ischemic stroke, practically all the patients show a marked focal elevation of oxygen extraction (Wise et al., 1983). Within the following hours, rOER tends to fall, indicating that the balance between oxygen supply and demand is tilting in favor of the former. That is, the tissue becomes hyperemic relative to its underlying metabolic demands, whatever the absolute level of blood flow. The frequent fall in rOER below the normal value may simply imply reperfusion of the infarcted tissue or indicate a further progressive decline in the tissue's metabolism, perhaps because of delayed cell death following a critical degree or duration of ischemia. In addition,

OER per se is not a reliable predictor of tissue viability. It is the combination of rOER and rCMRO2 evaluations which is highly predictive: a low rOER together with a low rCMRO2 indicates irreversible infarction.

A regional pattern of differential tissue vulnerability becomes apparent in the first hours: cortical regions supplied by the occluded arterial branch show a very high OER, whereas deep regions (basal grey and subcortical white matter) show an early decrease in OER. Wise et al. (1983) have considered this finding as indicative of an early change from ischemia to infarction in the deep tissue, probably related to the anatomy of the microvasculature (Plets, 1981). The early irreversible changes occurring in deep cerebral structures may limit the potential clinical benefit derived from maintenance of cortical function. Therapy has to be administered in a very short time interval: the therapeutical window. However, together with the experimental data, PET studies have shown that this window is definitely larger than the few minutes reported in classical text-books. Further studies, performed with stroke units, working in close proximity to a fast PET camera, may be crucial in order to fully clarify this point. The final picture of a low OER and a low CMRO2 defines established infarction.

During this period, rCMRGlu is not as depressed as the oxygen metabolism. Within the infarct, regional oxygen consumption and glucose metabolism are significantly correlated, with a ratio of two moles of oxygen per mole of glucose (1/3 that of normal tissue). This finding has led Wise et al. (1983) to suggest that the metabolizing tissue of a recent cerebral infarct utilizes anaerobic glycolysis. This (relatively) increased glucose consumption could be due to the migration of phagocytic cells in the lesion (Pozzilli et al., 1985). Kushner et al. (1986) have observed some consistent relationship between clinical outcome and the severity of the metabolic abnormality at presentation. These observations are derived from 36 studies in acute or subacute strokes, 1/3rd of which were studied within 3 days from the onset of symptoms and 6 within 2 days.

However, the interpretation is difficult due to the problems involved in the direct application of the Sokoloff model to damaged tissue. Baron et al. (1985) describe an increase of the ratio CMRO2/ CMGlu outside the area of maximal tissue damage (as judged by CT scan

data). Possibly other substrates, such as ketone bodies and aminoacids, are oxidized for energy production in the surviving tissue
surrounding a recent infarct.

In chronic infarction, PET measurements show that blood flow and
oxidative metabolism are reduced in and around the lesion, while the
coupling between the two reverts to the balance found in normal cerebral
tissue. Studies of chronic multi-infarct dementia patients have shown
focal reductions in cerebral oxygen and glucose utilization, which have
a normal coupling to tissue blood flow. However, the findings indicating
a coupled decrease of CBF and metabolism in otherwise unimpaired
cerebral regions may also be due to the occurrence of disconnection
effects (diaschisis).

Frackowiak et al. (1981) have observed no significant elevation of
the OER in mild or severe dementia of the vascular type, thus supporting
the hypothesis of Hachinski et al. (1974) that chronic global cerebral
ischemia is not a major pathogenetic mechanism in dementia. Further
evidence that flow meets regional tissue metabolism demands comes from
the PET study on the effect of a vasodilator drug in MID patients
(Gibbs, 1985). Measurements performed in these patients after six months
of treatment have failed to show any changes in blood flow and/or oxygen
extraction.

Taking into consideration all the data summarized here, just what
are the perspectives and limits of PET in the field of cerebrovascular
disorders? What is its outcome for CVD management? Are the results more
important for physiologists or may they also have meaning for
clinicians?

One must remember that neuroimaging modalities have two faces. The
"qualitative" face is appealing but it does not fully answer the
quantitative questions raised by scientific medicine in the field of
pathophysiology. The "quantitative" face, on the other hand, should not
be imbellished by the niceties of the color images which can hide the
problems still present that hinder their correct interpretation.

In spite of these limitations, the pathophysiological information
obtained by PET is highly relevant. This is especially true in critical
situations where the tissue morphology is intact, in spite of radical
changes in hemodynamic reserve and/or energy metabolism.

The area where the largest gains are expected is in the selecting of patients for specific therapeutical protocols and in monitoring in therapeutical efficacy "real time".

The major problems in this direction are two-fold: one is the limited access of acute cerebrovascular patients to PET facilities. These facilities are, in fact, seldom "clinically" oriented to acute neurological problems. A second aspect is not so much a limitation of the technologies on hand but rather the limited amount of therapeutical proposals available so far in the acute phase of cerebral ischemia. This is a clinical pharmacological "black-spot" that optimistically will be deleted by new pathophysiological and experimental knowledge.

Improved technologies, more specific development of radio-pharmaceuticals and of kinetic models with which to study metabolic aspects of functional relevance, but above all, a closer collaboration with clinical centers and an active participation of clinicians in these studies, are the basis for some cautious optimism that this short review hopes to have inspired.

REFERENCES

Baron, J.C., Bousser, M.G., Rey, A. et al. 1981. Reversal of focal "misery-perfusion syndrome" by extra-intracranial arterial bypass in hemodynamic cerebral ischemia. Stroke, 12, 454-459.

Baron, J.C., Rougemont, D., Soussaline, F. et al. 1984. Local inter-relationships of cerebral oxygen consumption and glucose utilization in normal subjects and in ischemic stroke patients: a positron tomography study. J. Cereb. Blood Flow Metabol., 4, 140-149.

Baron, J.C., Rougemont, D., Samson, Y. et al. 1985. Local interrela-tionships of cerebral oxygen consumption and glucose utilization in normals and in ischemic stroke patients. In "The Metabolism of the Human Brain Studied with Positron Emission Tomography". (Eds. T. Greitz et al.). (Raven Press, New York). pp 377-386.

Frackowiak, R.S.J., Pozzilli, C., Legg, N.J. et al. 1981. Regional cerebral oxygen supply and utilization in dementia: a clinical and physiological study with oxygen-15 and positron tomography. Brain, 104, 753-778.

Gibbs, J.M. 1985. Cerebral blood flow and metabolism in dementia, with reference to the effects of pharmacological intervention. In "Proceedings of British Association of Psychopharmacology Meeting". (Ed. M. Trimble). (Pergamon, Oxford).

Gibbs, J.M., Wise, R.J.S., Leenders, K.L. et al. 1984. Evaluation of cerebral perfusion reserve in patients with carotid artery occlusion. Lancet, I, 310-314.

Grubb, R.L., Ratcheson, R.A., Raichle, M.E. et al. 1979. Regional
    cerebral blood flow and oxygen utilization in superficial temporal
    middle cerebral artery anastomosis patients: an exploratory
    definition of clinical problems. J. Neurosurg., 50, 733-741.
Hachinski, V.D., Lassen, N.A., Marshall, J. 1974. Multi-infarct
    dementia. A cause of mental deterioration in the elderly. Lancet,
    II, 207-209.
Kushner, M., Reivich, M., Fieschi, C. et al. 1986. Focal and remote
    effects on local cerebral glucose metabolism of acute ischemic
    infarction in man. In "Acute Brain Ischemia Medical and Surgical
    Therapy". (Raven Press, New York). pp. 89-95.
Plets, C. 1981. Macroscopic and microscopic anatomy of cerebral
    circulation. In "Cerebral Blood Flow: Basic Knowledge and Clinical
    Implications". (Ed. J.M. Minderhound). (Excerpta Medica,
    Amsterdam). pp. 1-19.
Powers, W.J., Martin, W.R.W., Herscovitch, P. et al. 1984. Extracranial-
    intracranial bypass surgery: hemodynamic and metabolic effects.
    Neurology, 34, 1168-1174.
Powers, W.J., Grubb, R.L., Darriet, D. et al. 1985. Cerebral blood flow
    and cerebral metabolic rate of oxygen requirements for cerebral
    function and viability in humans. J. Cereb. Blood Flow Metabol., 5,
    600-608.
Pozzilli, C., Lenzi, G.L., Argentino, C. et al. 1985. Imaging of
    leukocytic infiltration in human cerebral infarcts. Stroke, 16,
    251-255.
Samson, J., Baron, J.C., Bousser, M.G. et al. 1985. Effects of extra-
    intracranial arterial bypass on cerebral blood flow and oxygen
    metabolism in humans. Stroke, 16, 600-616.
Sgouropoulos, P., Baron, J.C., Samson, Y. et al. 1985. Stenoses serrees
    et occlusions persistantes de l'artere cerebrale myoenne:
    consequences hemodynamiques et metaboliques: estudies par
    tomographie a positron. Rev. Neurol., 141, 698-705.
Wise, R.J.S., Bernardi, S., Frackowiak, R.S.J. et al. 1983. Serial
    observations on the pathophysiology of acute stroke. Brain, 106,
    197-222.

B R A I N

Movement Disorders

CHANGES OF CEREBRAL GLUCOSE METABOLISM IN MOVEMENT DISORDERS

F.J. Schuier

Dept. of Neurology, University Hospital
University of Düsseldorf, FRG

This is a short summary of the literature on local cerebral glucose metabolism in movement disorders as studied with PET and the ^{18}F-fluorodeoxyglucose technique. For a comprehensive review of PET findings in movement disorders, including changes in flow, oxygen and glucose metabolism, as well as neurotransmitter changes, the reader is referred to a recently published monograph (Leenders, 1986).

PARKINSON'S DISEASE

A global depression of glucose metabolism in all brain structures, related to the severity of bradykinesia and accompanying dementia, has been described by several authors (Heiss et al., 1985; Kuhl et al., 1984a, 1984b; Martin et al., 1984a). There seemed to be no focal changes in the basal ganglia of the more advanced cases reported by Kuhl and associates (Kuhl et al., 1984a, 1984b). In acute stages of the disease and in hemiparkinsonian cases, hypermetabolism was found in the basal ganglia contralateral to the affected limbs (Martin et al., 1984a). Early glucose hypermetabolism is accompanied by hyperperfusion (Perlmutter and Raichle 1985; Raichle et al., 1984; Wolfson et al., 1985) and oxygen hypermetabolism (Wolfson et al., 1985) in the pallidum area of the contralateral basal ganglia. The occurence and degree of asymmetry may depend on the time course, severity, and nature of symptoms (Leenders, 1986).

Animal models of Parkinson's disease (PD) did not yield unequivocal results. Hypermetabolism in the basal ganglia was found after acute lesions of the substantia nigra or after MPTP treatment by some authors (Wooten and Collins 1981), but hypometabolism by others (Porrino et al., 1985; Schwartz et al., 1976).

A regional decrease in parietal cortex glucose utilization with progressing disease, described by Kuhl and associates (Kuhl et al., 1984a), contrasts with observations of a focal flow decrease in the frontal mesocortex (Perlmutter and Raichle, 1985).

There is general agreement on the lack of any effect of medication on glucose utilization (Rougemont et al., 1983, 1984), supported by no effect on oxygen metabolism (Leenders et al., 1985) and no correlation of regional glucose metabolism with the effectiveness of treatment (Fig. 1).

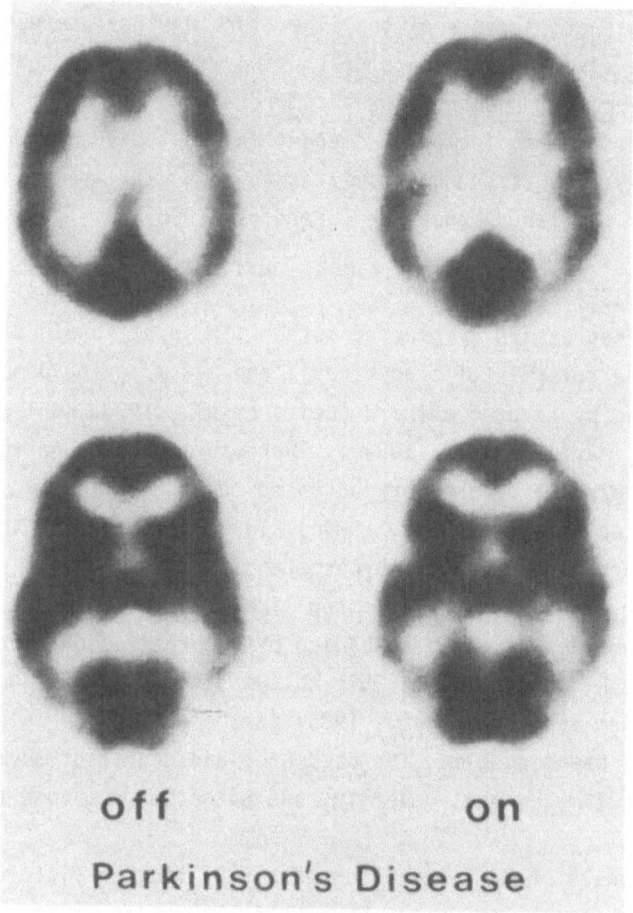

Fig. 1   No difference in cerebral glucose metabolism between on and off state in one PD patient (from Kuhl et al., 1984a, with permission).

No effect of efficacious drug therapy on glucose metabolism is supported by earlier findings of unchanged regional gray matter blood flow after treatment (Melamed et al., 1978). This again is in contrast with observations of L-Dopa mediated increases in glucose metabolism of the whole brain, but particularly in the substantia nigra and striatum, after MPTP lesions in the monkey (Porrino et al., 1985). L-Dopa also seems to increase blood flow by a direct effect on the cerebral vasculature (Leenders et al., 1985).

HUNTINGTON'S DISEASE

Conflicting results on glucose metabolism in Huntington's disease (HD) were obtained by several groups (Heiss et al., 1985; Kuhl et al., 1982, 1985; Martin et al., 1984b, Young et al., 1986). Significant loss of caudate metabolism is correlated with the severity of functional impairment (Mazziotta et al., 1985). It is more sensitive to the clinical symptoms than the atrophy seen on CT (Fig. 2).

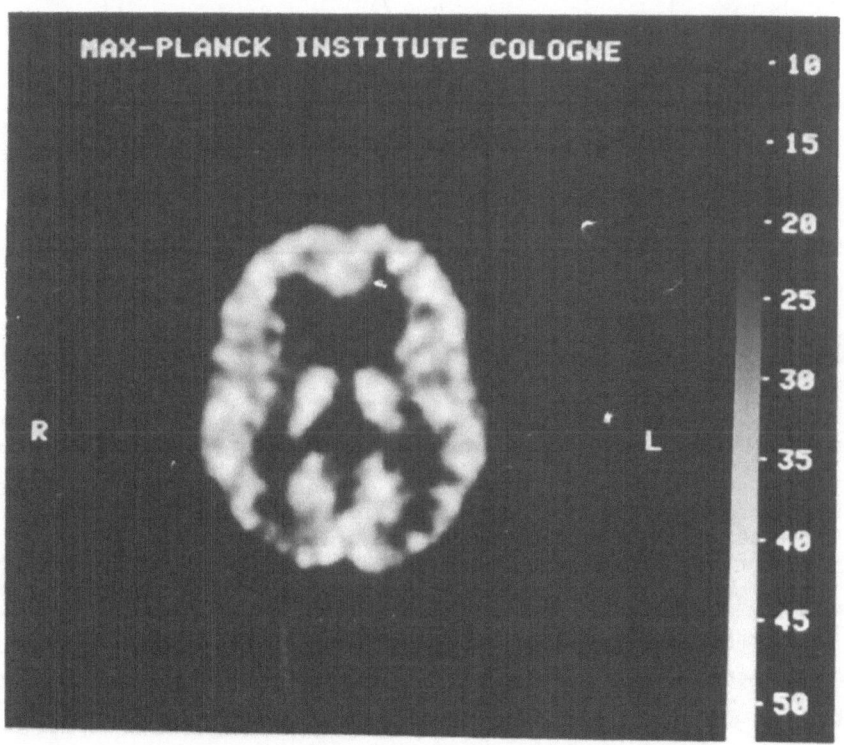

Fig. 2   Loss of striatal glucose metabolism in a patient with severe HD.

Caudate hypometabolism is already apparent in about 50% of persons
at risk and may be a predictor of the disease (Fig. 3).

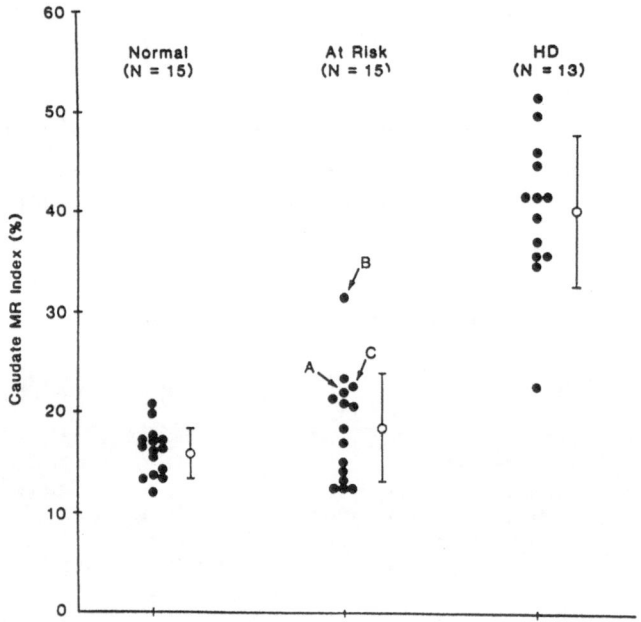

Fig. 3   Huntington's disease. Correlation between caudate glucose
hypometabolism and stage of the disease. Two subjects at risk, with
decreased caudate metabolism (arrows), later developed clinical
signs of the disease (from Kuhl et al., 1985; with permission)

In contrast with the cortical hypometabolism in PD related to
dementia, even in advanced dementia no cortical hypometabolism was found
in HD (Kuhl et al., 1984; 1985; Young et al., 1986). The absence of
cortical changes supports the concept of a subcortical type of dementia

in HD (Albert, 1978). However, corresponding with an initially observed non-significantly decreased fronto-parietal metabolic ratio (Kuhl et al., 1982), recent studies with longer follow-up do suggest focal frontal and cingulate glucose hypometabolism with advancing dementia Mazziotta et al., 1985).

WILSON'S DISEASE

A general decrease in glucose utilization, without any change of regional distribution, was found in 4 patients with Wilson's disease (WD); this metabolic depression seemed to be roughly correlated with the severity of symptoms (Hawkins et al., 1983).

TORSION DYSTONIA

No focal abnormalities of glucose utilization were found in spasmodic torticollis by Stoessl and colleagues (1986), while Martin (1985) described putaminal asymmetry unrelated to the side of head turning.

In hemidystonia consequent to birth injury, we found significant hypometabolism in the contralateral striatum, without corresponding abnormality on CT (Fig. 4). This finding is in agreement with case of posttraumatic hemidystonia reported by Perlmutter and Raichle (1984), where oxygen hypometabolism with hyperperfusion and hypervolemia of the contralateral basal ganglia could be demonstrated.

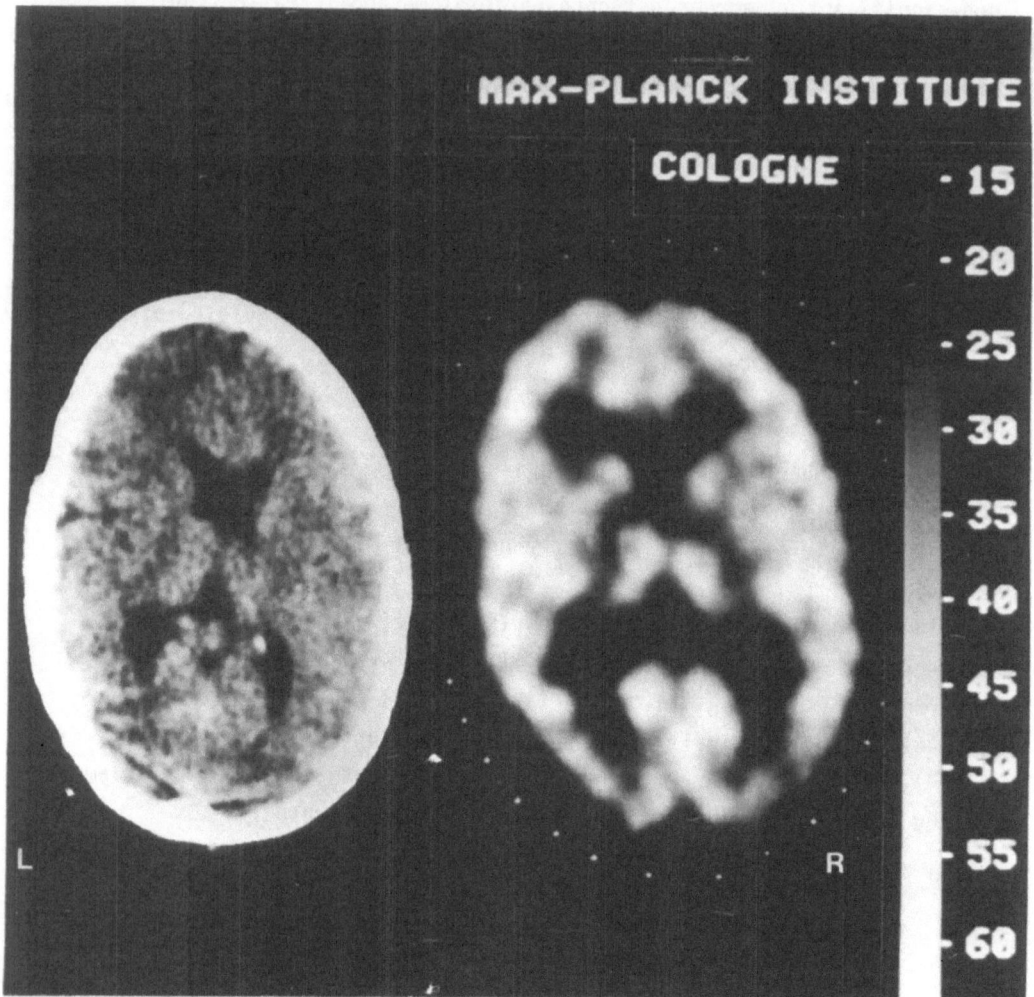

Fig. 4   No morphological defect on CT (left image) in a 20-year-old patient with severe left-sided hemidystonia. FDG-PET (right image) shows contralateral basal ganglia hypometabolism.

REFERENCES

Albert, M.L. 1978. Alzheimer's disease: Senile dementia and related
    disorders. In "Aging", Vol. 7.(Eds. R. Katzman, R.D. Terry and
    K.L. Bick). (Raven Press, New York). pp. 173-180.
Hawkins, R.A., Phelps, M.E., Mazziotta, J.C., et al. 1983. A study of
    Wilson's disease with 18-F FDG and positron tomography. J. Cereb.
    Blood Flow Metab., 3 (Suppl. 1), 498-499.
Heiss, W.-D., Beil, C., Herholz, K., et al. (Eds.) 1985. Atlas of
    Positron Emission Tomography of the Brain. (Springer Verlag,
    Berlin-Heidelberg-New York).
Kuhl, D.E., Markham, C.H., Metter, E.J., et al. 1985. Local cerebral
    glucose utilization in symptomatic and presymptomatic Huntington's
    disease. In "Brain Imaging and Brain Function". (Ed. L. Sokoloff).
    (Raven Press, New York). pp. 199-209
Kuhl, D.E., Metter, E.J. and Riege, W.H. 1984a. Patterns of local
    cerebral glucose utilization determined in Parkinson's disease
    by the 18-F-Fluorodeoxyglucose method. Ann. Neurol., 15, 419-424.
Kuhl, D.E., Metter, E.J., Riege, W.H., et al. 1984b. Patterns of
    cerebral glucose utilization in Parkinson's disease and Hunting-
    ton's disease. Ann. Neurol., 15, (Suppl. 1), 119-125.
Kuhl, D.E., Phelps, M.E., Markham, C.H., et al. 1982. Cerebral metab-
    olism and atrophy in Huntington's disease determined by 18-FDG
    and computed tomographic scan. Ann. Neurol., 12, 425-434.
Leenders, K.L. (Ed.) 1986. Movement disorders: A study with positron
    emission tomography. (Thesis, Rodopi Press, Amsterdam).
Leenders, K., Wolfson, L., Gibbs, J., et al. 1985. Regional cerebral
    blood flow and oxygen metabolism in Parkinson's disease and their
    response to L-Dopa. J. Cereb. Blood Flow Metab., 5, (Suppl. 1),
    488-489.
Martin, W.R.W. 1985. Positron emission tomography in movement dis-
    orders. Can. J. Neurol. Sci., 12, 6-10.
Martin, W.R.W., Beckman, J.H., Calne, C.B., et al. 1984a. Cerebral
    glucose metabolism in Parkinson's disease. Can. J. Neurol. Sci.,
    11, 169-173.
Martin, W.R.W., Hayden, M.R., Suchowersky, O., et al. 1984b. Striatal
    metabolism in Huntington's disease and benign hereditary chorea.
    Ann. Neurol., 16, 126.
Mazziotta, J.C., Wapensky, J., Phelps, M.E., et al. 1985. Cerebral
    glucose utilization and blood flow in Huntington's disease:
    symptomatic and at-risk subjects. J. Cereb. Blood Flow Metab.,
    5, (Suppl. 1), 25-26.
Melamed, E., Lavy, S., Cooper, G., et al. 1978. Regional cerebral blood
    flow in Parkinsonism. Measurement before and after Levodopa.
    J. Neurol. Sci., 38, 391-397.
Perlmutter, J.S. and Raichle, M.E. 1985. Reduced blood flow in the
    frontal mesocortex in Parkinsonian patients. J. Cereb. Blood Flow
    Metab., 5, (Suppl. 1), 171-172.
Perlmutter, J.S. and Raichle, M.E. 1984. Pure hemidystonia with basal
    ganglion abnormalities in positron emission tomography. Ann.
    Neurol., 15, 228-233.
Porrino, L.J., Burns, R.S., Crane, A.M., et al. 1985. Measurement of
    local cerebral glucose metabolism in a primate model of Parkin-
    sonism. J. Cereb. Blood Flow Metab., 5, (Suppl. 1), 167-168.

Raichle, M.E., Perlmutter, J.S. and Fox, P.T. 1984. Parkinson's
    disease: metabolic and pharmacological approaches with positron
    emission tomography. Ann. Neurol., 15, (Suppl. 1), 131-132.
Rougemont, D., Baron, J.C., Collard, P., et al. 1983. Local cerebral
    metabolic rate of glucose (lCMRGlc) in treated and untreated
    patients with Parkinson's disease. J. Cereb. Blood Flow Metab.,
    3, (Suppl. 1), 504-505.
Rougemont, D., Baron, J.C, Collard, P., et al. 1984. Local cerebral
    glucose utilisation in treated and untreated patients with Parkin-
    son's disease. J. Neurol., Neurosurg., Psychiat., 47, 824-830.
Schwartz, W.J., Sharp, F.R., Gunn, R.H., et al. 1976. Lesions of as-
    cending dopaminergic pathways decrease forebrain glucose uptake.
    Nature, 261, 155-157.
Stoessl, A.J., Martin, W.R.W., Clark, C., et al. 1986. PET studies of
    cerebral glucose metabolism in idiopathic torticollis. Neurology,
    36, 653-657.
Wolfson, L.I., Leenders, K.L., Brown, L.L., et al. 1985. Alterations of
    regional cerebral blood flow and oxygen metabolism in Parkinson's
    disease. Neurology, 35, 1399-1405.
Wooten, G.F. and Collins, R.C. 1981. Metabolic effects of unilateral
    lesions of the substantia nigra. J. Neurosci., 1, 285-291.
Young, A.B., Penney, J.B., Starosta-Rubinstein, S., et al. 1986. PET
    scan investigations of Huntington's disease: cerebral metabolic
    correlates of neurological features and functional decline.
    Ann. Neurol., 20, 296-303.

PROGRESSIVE SUPRANUCLEAR PALSY STUDIED BY PET

B. Mazière[1], J.C. Baron[1,2], C. Loc'h[1],
H. Cambon[1,2], Y. Agid[3]

[1]Service Hospitalier Frédéric Joliot, CEA,
Dept. de Biologie, Orsay, France
[2]Clinique des Maladies du Système Nerveux,
Hopital La Salpétrière, Paris, France
[3]Clinique de Neurologie et de Neuropsychologie,
Hopital La Salpétrière, Paris, France

Among the movement disorders progressive supranuclear palsy (PSP) is a degenerative neurological disease characterized by a loss of voluntary control of vertical gaze, dysarthria, diffuse body rigidity with dystonic extension of the neck and dementia (Steele, 1975).

In post-mortem investigations it was observed that the number of dopamine receptors in the striatum of patients with PSP was reduced by almost 50 % compared to controls (Bokobza et al., 1984). Recent developments in positron emission tomography (PET) have shown that, using appropriate ligands, it was possible to investigate in vivo the distribution of specific binding sites in humans (Phelps and Mazziotta, 1985). The method has been applied to muscarinic receptors in myocardium (Syrota et al., 1984) and to benzodiazpine (Samson et al., 1985), serotonin (Baron et al., 1985a), opiate (Frost et al., 1985) and dopamine (Wagner et al., 1983; Baron et al., 1985b; Leenders et al., 1984; Mazière et al., 1985; Farde et al., 1985; Crawley et al., 1983) receptors in brain, and has consistently shown preferential accumulation of the labeled tracer in regions expected from in vivo binding assays to have the highest receptor density.

A major advantage of PET over post-mortem studies is that it provides insight into receptor changes at various stages of the illness, as well as pharmacological modifications of such changes.

In order to try to determine at what stage of the disease and to what extent the impairments of the central dopaminergic functions can be matched with regional modifications of the dopaminergic D2 receptors, 7 patients with PSP were studied by PET using [76]Br-bromospiperone as specific ligand.

PATIENTS

The patient group included 3 women and 4 men (mean age 66.4 $\pm$ 6 years) suspected on clinical grounds of progressive supranuclear palsy (Table 1). They all complained of falls, and were found to have intellectual disability suggesting sub-cortical dementia. In addition, none of them responded favourably to DA agonists. All were off medication for at least 3 days before study.

Seven sex- and age-matched control subjects (mean age 67.2 $\pm$ 7.5 years) were consecutively selected from a larger control series. None of them was on medication known to interfere with DA receptors.

MATERIALS AND METHODS

1. Preparation of the labeled radiopharmaceutical

^{76}Br was prepared by irradiating an arsenic target with a beam of 30 MeV helium-3 ions. The target was dissolved in an acidic medium and after oxidation the radioactive bromide was distilled and trapped as bromide in diluted ammonia which was then taken to dryness. ^{76}Br$_2$, generated in situ by an H_2O_2-acetic acid mixture, was allowed to react for 10 min with an excess of spiperone by means of an electro-philic substitution reaction. The radioactive bromo compound, separated from the cold precursor by high-performance liquid chromatography, was dissolved in dilute acetic acid. The solution was sterilized by filtration through a Millipore membrane and brought to isotonicity using diluted NaOH (final pH 4).

2. PET studies

PET scans were performed by means of a time-of-flight tomograph (Soussaline et al., 1984) which allows simultaneous acquisition of 7 slice images, 12 mm thick on average. The undetected space between slices is 3 mm. By means of bony landmarks and laser beams, the subject was carefully positioned so that the lowest slice, 1 cm above and parallel to the orbito-meatal (OM) plane, included the cerebellar hemispheres and the third slice (OM + 4 cm) the basal ganglia. After collection of transmission scan data via an external ^{68}Ge source for subsequent correction of radiation attenuation effects, 1 mCi (37 MBq) of ^{76}Br-bromospiperone in isotonic acetate solution was injected in a brachial vein of the subject.

TABLE 1 : Patients' clinical data

PATIENT AGE/SEX	DISEASE DURATION (yrs)	VERTICAL GAZE PALSY	AXIAL HYPERTONIA[a]	BRADYKINESIA[a]	FUNCTIONAL DISABILITY[a]	"FRONTAL" DEMENTIA[a]	C.T. SCAN	RESPONSE TO DA AGONIST[b]
1/62/M	7	Present	+++	+++	+++	+++	Mild hydrocephalus	-
2/66/M	10	Present	++	++	++	++	Normal	-
3/62/F	2	Present	+	+	+	+/-	Normal	+
4/72/M	1	Present	++	+	+	++	Mild cortical atrophy	+
5/74/F	6	Present	+	++	++	+	Mild cortical atrophy	-
6/71/M	2	Present	++	++	++	++	Moderate hydrocephalus	-
7/58/F	3	Present	++	++	++	++	Normal	-

a : Alteration mild (+), moderate (++), severe (+++) or questionable ($\pm$).

b : DA = dopaminergic ; response negative (-) or questionable ($\pm$).

For the initial kinetic distribution study, eight 30 to 60 min scans (accumulating a total of 300 000 counts typically for each brain level) were performed starting at the end of the injection and continuing for 26 h.

Venous blood samples were collected 15 min before the end of each scan and their radioactivity content assayed by means of a sodium iodide well counter.

3. Data analysis

On the 4.5 hr images, the striatum and the cerebellum were clearly visible in each case. Two methods were used to analyze the data as objectively as possible. One method used computer-controlled delineation of percentage isocontour, yielding irregular regions of interest for cerebellum and for striatum. The other method used circular regions of interest covering each cerebellar hemisphere (area 12 cm², positioned using a standard procedure) and each striatal area (area 3 cm²). For each study, a mean (average of right and left values) striatal and a mean cerebellar value was obtained, expressed in percentage of the injected dose per ml brain (corrected for ^{76}Br decay); the value of the striatum/cerebellum ratio was then calculated. The data from PSP patients were compared to control values using Student's t test.

RESULTS

In cerebellum, the mean tracer concentration at t = 4.5 hr, expressed in % of injected dose per liter brain, was 1.28 ($\pm$ 0.32) and 1.47 ($\pm$ 0.41) in controls and PSP patients, respectively (no significant difference). Likewise, the corresponding values in striatum were not significantly different in controls and PSP patients (2.27 $\pm$ 0.45 and 1.94 $\pm$ 0.61, respectively).

In controls, the individual striatum/cerebellum radioactivity concentration ratios ranged from 1.45 in a 79 yr old lady to 1.95 in a 59 yr old man, with a mean value of 1.74 ($\pm$ 0.17). In PSP patients, it ranged from 0.90 to 1.57, with a mean of 1.32 ($\pm$ 0.23). The difference between PSP and controls is highly significant (t = 3.955, df = 12, p < 0.02) (Table 2).

TABLE 2

Number	Sex	Age (yrs)	CONTROLS Striatum/cerebellum ratio	Number	Sex	Age (yrs)	PSP PATIENTS Striatum/cerebellum ratio
1	M	59	1.95	1	M	62	1.29
2	M	67	1.75	2	M	66	1.42
3	F	63	1.63	3	F	62	1.46
4	M	72	1.73	4	M	72	0.90
5	F	79	1.45	5	F	74	1.18
6	M	72	1.85	6	M	71	1.43
7	F	59	1.85	7	F	58	1.57
Mean $\pm$ 1 SD		67.2 ($\pm$ 7.5)	1.74 ($\pm$ 0.17)			66.4 ($\pm$ 6.1)	1.32 ($\pm$ 0.23)*

* $p < 0.02$ with respect to controls

DISCUSSION

The potent neuroleptic spiperone binds with high affinity to the D2 class of dopaminergic (DA) receptors. Bromospiperone retains the binding characteristics of spiperone (Huang et al., 1980), and has been shown to accumulate specifically in the striatum of baboons and humans in vivo (Mazière et al., 1984).

We chose to label spiperone with ^{76}Br because of its high specific radioactivity and long physical half-life (16.2 hrs) allowing late imaging and, hence, more stable conditions. Extensive studies in rats and baboons have demonstrated displaceable and saturable binding of bromospiperone to striatal DA receptors in vivo (Mazière et al., 1984; Kulmala et al., 1981; Owen et al., 1983). In control human subjects, ^{76}Br-bromospiperone slowly accumulated in striatum, leading to a striatum/cerebellum concentration ratio of 2.2 at 4.5 hr after injection in young subjects (Mazière et al., 1985), a value which included the partial volume effects (Mazziotta et al., 1981). In subjects loaded with cold neuroleptics, this ratio was reduced to 1.2, another argument indicating specific binding to striatal DA receptors in humans in vivo (Mazière et al., 1985). A major factor in the reliability of the method is the very small injected drug amount, theoretically resulting in 0.5-2 % occupation of the dopaminergic receptors in human striatum (Mazière et al., 1985; Ruberg et al., 1984).

We found a significant decrease ($p > 0.002$) in the mean striatum/cerebellum ratio of PSP patients as compared to controls (Table 2).

The physiological meaning of the striatum/cerebellum ratio has been investigated by compartmental modeling of the kinetics of DA antagonists in brain in vivo (Mintun et al., 1984; Friedman et al., 1984). These studies suggest that this ratio depends essentially on the receptor-ligand interaction (i.e., affinity constant and receptor density), and less so on a number of other parameters as accessibility to the receptors (i.e., blood tracer concentration, blood flow, and penetration through the blood-brain barrier), competition with the endogeneous (agonist) ligand, and non-specific binding. We used the striatum/cerebellum ratio as a reasonably accurate and easily measurable index of specific binding, provided it was measured at post-injection intervals long enough to reach essentially stable tracer concentration in brain and in blood (Wong et al., 1984). The non-specific components of this ratio (accessibility to the receptor sites and non-specific binding) likely played no part in the decrease observed in PSP patients. Hence, the blood ^{76}Br concentration at scanning time was identical in PSP patients and controls (0.49 $\pm$ 0.16 and 0.48 $\pm$ 0.10 % injected dose/liter, respectively), and the early (t = 15 min) ^{76}Br uptake in cerebellum was similar in PSP patients (n = 2) and controls (n = 4), suggesting equal accessibility of the ligand to the receptors. Also the tracer uptake at t = 4.5 hrs in cerebellum was similar in PSP and controls indicating comparable non-specific binding. Finally, dopamine levels should be markedly depressed in the striatum of PSP patients (Bokobza et al., 1984), theoretically allowing increased, not decreased, bromospiperone binding (Friedman et al., 1984). These considerations strongly suggest that the reduced striatum/cerebellum ratio reflected decreased specific binding compared to controls.

A decrease in specific binding of bromospiperone to striatal DA receptors can result from decreased affinity or decreased receptor density, or both. Since affinity is rarely affected by disease (as is true also of ^{3}H-spiperone in PSP brain post-mortem, Bokobza et al., 1984), decreased receptor density presumably explains our results. If the difference in bromospiperone uptake between striatum and cerebellum is taken to represent specific binding (Laduron et al., 1978), the age-adjusted loss of striatal receptor sites amounts to 60 %; this value is close to the figure of 45 % found in the striatum of 9 PSP patients post-mortem (Ruberg et al., 1985). Since bromospiperone has affinity for both the D2 dopaminergic and the serotoninergic (5 HT$_2$) receptors (Stoof, 1983), these results may imply loss of D2 or 5 HT$_2$ sites, or both. However, the fraction of ligand bound to 5 HT$_2$ receptors in striatum is probably less than 20 % of total specific binding (Wagner et al., 1983; Ruberg et al., 1984), indicating that the observed decrease in binding capacity essentially represents loss of D2 receptor sites. Post-mortem binding studies recently documented a mean decrease of 45 % in striatal D2 receptor density in PSP (Ruberg et al., 1985). The present study confirms these data and extends them by showing this loss to occur during life not only in advanced, but also in early stages of the disease.

This study demonstrates that alterations in brain receptor density as a result of degenerative disease can be detected _in vivo_ using PET.

REFERENCES

Baron, J.C., Samson, Y., Crouzel, C. et al. 1985b. Pharmacologic studies in man with PET: an investigation using 11C-labeled ketanserin, a 5-HT2 receptor antagonist. In "Cerebral Blood Flow and Metabolism Measurement". (Eds. A. Hartmann, S. Hoyer). (Springer, Berlin, Heidelberg, New York). pp. 473-480.

Baron, J.C., Comar, D., Zarifian, E. et al. 1985a. Dopaminergic receptor sites in human brain: positron emission tomography. Neurology, 35, 1624.

Bokobza, B., Ruberg, M., Scatton, B. et al. 1984. 3H-spiperone binding, dopamine and HVA concentrations in Parkinson's disease and supranuclear palsy. Eur. J. Pharmacol., 99, 167-175.

Crawley, J.C.W., Smith, T., Veall, N. et al. 1983. Dopamine receptors displayed in human living brain with 77Br-p-bromospiperone. Lancet, II, 975.

Farde, L., Ehrin, E., Eriksson, L. et al. 1985. 11C-labeled dopamine-2-receptor antagonists as tools for quantitative studies or dopamine receptors in the human brain. In "Brain 85", 16-20 June 1985, Ronneby, Sweden, pp. 205.

Friedman, A.M., Dejesus, O.T., Revenaugh, B.A. et al. 1984. Measurements in vivo of parameters of the dopamine system. Ann. Neurol., 15, (Suppl.), 566-576.

Frost, J.J., Wagner, H.N., Dannals, R.F. et al. 1985. Imaging opiate receptors in the human brain by positron tomography. J. Comput. Assist. Tomogr., 9, 231-236.

Huang, C.C., Friedman, A.M., So, R. et al. 1980. Synthesis and biological evaluation of p-bromospiperone as potential neuroleptic drug. J. Pharm. Sci., 69, 984-986.

Kulmala, H.K., Huang, C.C., Dinerstein, R.J. et al. 1981. Specific in vivo binding of 77-Br-p-bromospiroperidol in rat brain: a potential tool for gamma ray imaging. Life Sci., 28, 1911-1916.

Laduron, P.M., Janssen, P.F.M., Leysen, J.E. 1978. Spiperone, a ligand of choice for neuroleptic receptors. 2. Regional distribution and in vivo displacement by neuroleptic drugs. Biochem. Pharmacol., 27, 371-321.

Leenders, K.L., Herold, S., Brooks, D.J. et al. 1984. Pre-synaptic and post-synaptic dopaminergic systems in human brain. Lancet, II, 110-111.

Mazière, B., Loc'h, C., Hantraye, P. et al. 1984. 76-Br-bromospiperidol: a new tool for quantitative in vivo imaging of neuroleptic receptors. Life Sci., 35, 1349-1356.

Mazière, B., Loc'h, C., Baron, J.C. et al. 1985. In vivo quantitative imaging of dopamine receptors in human brain using positron tomography and 76Br-bromospiperone. Eur. J. Pharmacol., 114, 267-272.

Mazziotta, J.C., Phelps, M.E., Miller, J. et al. 1981. Tomographic mapping of human cerebral metabolism: normal unstimulated state. Neurology, 31, 503-516.

Mintun, M.A., Raichle, M.E., Kilbourn, M.R. et al. 1984. A quantitative model for the in vivo assessment of drug binding sites with positron emission tomography. Ann. Neurol., 15, 217-227.

Owen, F., Poulter, M., Marshall, R.D. et al. 1983. 77Br-
    p-bromospiperone: a ligand for in vivo labelling of dopamine
    receptors. Life Sci., 3, 765-768.
Phelps, M.E., Mazziotta, J.C. 1985. Positron emission tomography: human
    brain function and biochemistry. Science, 228, 799-809.
Ruberg, M., Bokobza, B., Javoy-Agid, F. et al. 1984. 3H-spiperone
    binding in the nigrostriatal system in human brain. Eur. J.
    Pharmacol., 99, 159-165.
Ruberg, M., Javoy-Agid, F., Hirsch, E. et al. 1985. Aminergic,
    cholinergic, and gabaergic systems in the brain of patients with
    progressive supranuclear palsy. Ann. Neurol., 18, 523-529.
Samson, Y., Hantraye, P., Baron, J.C. et al. 1985. Kinetics and
    displacement of 11C-RO 15-1788, a benzodiazepine antagonist,
    studied in human brain in vivo by positron tomography. Eur. J.
    Pharmacol., 110, 247-251.
Soussaline, F., Campagnolo, R., Verrey, B. et al. 1984. Physical
    characterization of a time-of-flight positron emission tomography
    system for wholebody quantitative studies. J. Nucl. Med., 25, P46.
Steele, J.C. 1975. Progressive supranuclear palsy. In "Handbook of
    Neurology", Vol. 22. (Eds. Vinken, Bruyn). (Elsevier Publ. Comp.).
    pp. 217-229.
Stoof, J.C. 1983. Dopamine receptors in the neostriatum: Biochemical
    and physiological studies. In "Dopamine Receptors". (Eds. C.
    Kaiser, J.W. Kebabian). (A.C.S. Symposium Series, Vol. 224). pp.
    117-145.
Syrota, A., Paillotin, G., Davy, J.M. et al. 1984. Kinetics of in vivo
    binding of antagonist to muscarinic cholinergic receptor in the
    human heart studied by positron emission tomography. Life Sci.,
    35, 837-845.
Wagner, H.N., Burns, H.D., Dannals, R.F. et al. 1983. Imaging dopamine
    receptors in the human brain by positron tomography. Science, 221,
    1264-1266.
Wong, D.F., Wagner, H.N., Dannals, R.F. et al. 1984. Effects of age on
    dopamine and serotonin receptors measured by positron tomography
    in the living human brain. Science, 1393-1396.

CENTRAL DOPAMINERGIC MECHANISMS IN MONKEY AND MAN STUDIED BY POSITRON EMISSION TOMOGRAPHY

S.-M. Aquilonius, P. Hartvig, K.L. Leenders, H. Lundqvist
B. Langström, J. Tedroff

Dept. of Neurology, Organic Chemistry,
The Hospital Pharmacy and Gustaf Werner Institute
Uppsala University
Uppsala, Sweden

Positron emission tomography (PET) represents a new methodology of high research potential in clinical neuropharmacology. It must be realised, however, that an effective utilization of the PET technique requires an interplay with the other approaches available in this area of research. Further, before introducing new applications of PET to man, preclinical studies in larger animals, particularly monkeys, is often a prerequisite.

The present brief overview describes the introduction of a battery of ^{11}C-labelled tracers to evaluate in vivo different aspects of central dopaminergic mechanisms, i.e. density of terminals, concentration of degrading enzymes and density of postsynaptic receptor sites.

MATERIALS AND METHODS

Synthesis

[11]C-labelled carbon dioxide was produced by the Tandem accelerator at the University of Uppsala by bombardment of a nitrogen target with a 10 MeV proton beam. The ^{11}C-carbon dioxide was trapped in molecular sieves and converted to ^{11}C-methyl iodide. ^{11}C-labelled nomifensine, L-deprenyl, D-deprenyl and raclopride respectively were produced by a N-methylation procedure as described in principle elsewhere (Langström, 1980).

Chemical and radiochemical purity was established by liquid chromatography whereafter solutions for injection were passed through a 0.22 µ sterile filter.

Volunteers and patients

The healthy volunteers had no history of neuropsychiatric disease - the older group was recruited from an organization of teetotallers. In the patients, the diagnosis of Parkinson's disease was settled by two experienced neurologists who characterized symptomatology and graded severity. Computerized tomography (CT) was performed before PET, the humans wearing individually prepared plastic helmets in order to transfer positioning by means of a fixation system.

Monkeys

Adult Rhesus monkeys (Macaca Mulatta from the Primate Laboratory of Reproductive Research, Uppsala University) of 6 - 9 kg body weight and of known age were studied. In one monkey a unilateral lesion of the nigrostriatal dopaminergic neurons was performed using an infusion of 0.2 mg/kg of 1-methyl-4-phenyl-1,2,3,6-tetrahydropyridine (MPTP) into an internal carotid artery according to the method of Bankiewicz and collaborators (1986).

Before PET, anaesthesia was induced with 100 mg ketamine (Ketalar^R, Parke-Davis) which was repeated as required. The monkeys were laying on a stretcher equipped with a head-holder during imaging.

PET-system

A PC 384-3B positron emission tomograph (Scanditronix, Uppsala, Sweden) was used, equipped with two detector rings, allowing imaging of three consecutive transaxial 14 mm sections. Thus, the slices covered the whole monkey brain while in humans the position was usually chosen so that the upper section included the basal ganglia and the lowest the cerebellum.

Data acquisition was started after intravenous injection of the ^{11}C-labelled tracer (80 - 150 MBq). The amount of radiotracer injected was usually in the interval 20 - 60 µg.

In some experiments brain uptake was studied after large i.v. doses of unlabelled drug or after pharmacological pertubations with pre- or postsynaptically active compounds (mazindol, desipramine, spiperone) as exemplified below.

After data acquisition regions of interest (ROI) were selected manually using a cursor. The time-dependent radioactivity was determined for striata, cortex, thalamus (humans), cerebellum and "back of the brain" (monkey). Brain uptake was expressed as normalized activity, i.e. the ratio of counts per minute (cpm) in the ROI per ml tissue to cpm of the injected ^{11}C-labelled compound per g body weight. The ROI data were transferred to a desk computer (Apple McIntosh, Apple Corp., USA) for further calculations and graphical representations.

RESULTS AND DISCUSSION
[11]C-nomifensine

It is known from in vitro studies using brain homogenates as well as autoradiographic techniques that ^{3}H-nomifensine binds to dopaminergic re-uptake sites with high affinity and specificity. However, ^{3}H-nomi-fensine also binds to noradrenaline re-uptake sites (see Hunt et al., 1974). Consequently, our basic idea was that ^{11}C-labelled nomifensine could be applied as a tracer to measure the density of monoamine nerve terminals in man using PET.

A typical experiment demonstrating the uptake of radioactivity in the brain of a monkey following an i.v. tracer amount of ^{11}C-labelled nomifensine is shown in Fig. 1. The highest uptake was found within the striatal regions whereas "non-dopaminergic" regions such as the "back brain" ROI (comprising the posterior one third of the section) showed lower radioactivities. The experiment was repeated after 0.3 mg/kg of mazindol (Fig. 1), another active blocker of dopamine re-uptake (Javitch et al., 1983). This resulted in a similar uptake within the two aforementioned regions. Equally, after pretreatment of the monkey with 2 - 6 mg/kg of nomifensine the difference between striatal and backbrain uptake disappeared. In contrast, neither desipramine (preferentially blocking noradrenaline re-uptake) nor spiperone (blocking postsynaptic sites) did diminish the relative difference between striatal and backbrain uptake. Taken together, these experimental results indicate that the difference between striatal and backbrain uptake of ^{11}C-nomifensine in the monkey is related to specific dopaminergic re-uptake binding sites. Proof of this was obtained by studying sequentially the monkey with unilateral MPTP-lesion of the nigro-striatal dopamine neurons. No striatal side to side differences in ^{11}C-nomifensine uptake were found before or two days after the lesion. However, the next investigation performed nine days after lesion demonstrated a complete disappearance of specific ^{11}C-labelled nomifensine binding on the lesioned side.

114

11C-Nomifensine monkey before(1) and after(2) mazindol

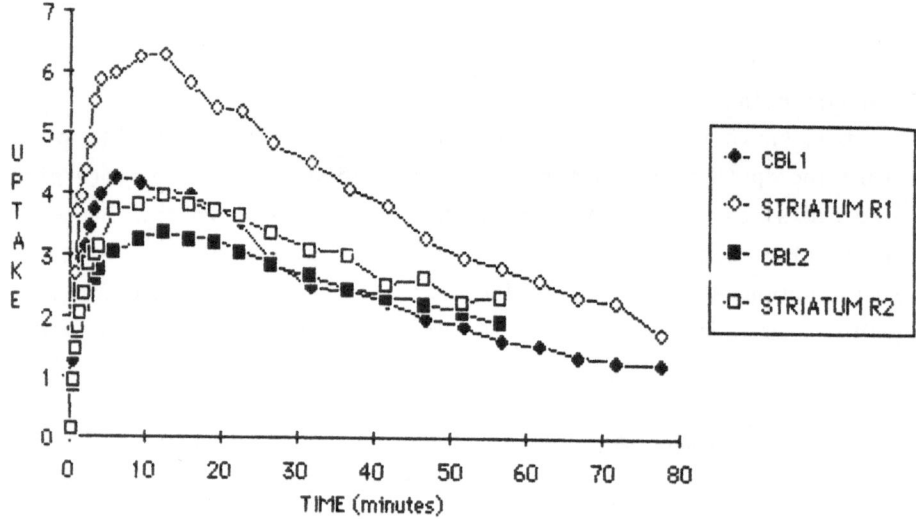

Fig. 1   Time-course of radioactivity in the rhesus monkey brain
after i.v. administration of a tracer dose of 11-C-nomifensine.
Striatum R1 and R2, respectively, refer to the right striatal
region before and after pretreatment with 0.3 mg/kg of mazindol.
CB1 refers to a region in the posterior part of the brain containing the cerebellum.

To date, human PET studies with ^{11}C-nomifensine have been performed
in one healthy volunteer and in one patient suffering from Parkinson's
disease for about five years. The maximal ratio between striatal and cerebellar uptake of radioactivity was 2.3 in the healthy subject and 1.2
in the parkinsonian patient.

In conclusion, PET and ^{11}C-nomifensine enables measurement of the
density of striatal dopaminergic nerve terminals in man in vivo. The
present results have been obtained using racemic ^{11}C-nomifensine.
Further refinement of the technique is likely to be achieved when the
[11]C-labelled active enantiomer becomes available.

^{11}C-deprenyl

It is known that the active L-enantiomer of deprenyl binds irrever-
sibly to monoamine oxidase of the B-type (MAO-B). The affinity of the D-
enantiomer for the enzyme is about 25 times less (see Robinson, 1985).
Consequently, the difference in uptake between the two enantiomers within a specified region of the brain would be proportional to the local
MAO-B concentration. This basic idea has recently been introduced using
PET (Fowler et al., 1986) by labelling both enantiomers separately with
^{11}C. The difference in brain uptake between ^{11}C-L and ^{11}C-D-deprenyl
has now been demonstrated using PET in both monkey and man.
The L-enantiomer is rapidly taken up by the brain tissue and trapped as
illustrated in a healthy volunteer (Fig. 2).

The D-enantiomer, on the other hand, has a similar initial uptake,
but is then quickly eliminated from the brain. In addition, a repeat
study of the same healthy volunteer, one day after oral administration
of 15 mg deprenyl, demonstrated blocked trapping of the ^{11}C-L-deprenyl,
which then followed the same pattern of elimination as ^{11}C-D-de-
prenyl.

To date two young and two elderly healthy volunteers and two parkinsonian patients have been studied in our laboratory using this technique. The difference in uptake between ^{11}C-L- and ^{11}C-D-enantiomers
increased with age. This is in line with the increase with age of cerebral MAO-B concentration in man as found in post-mortem studies
(Fowler et al., 1980). The uptake values in the two parkinsonian patients did not differ from the control values when allowing for age.

In conclusion these tracers enable the assessment of MAO-B concentration in brain in man in vivo. The use of two enantiomers of a suicide
enzyme inhibitor is a new general principle in PET tracer studies.

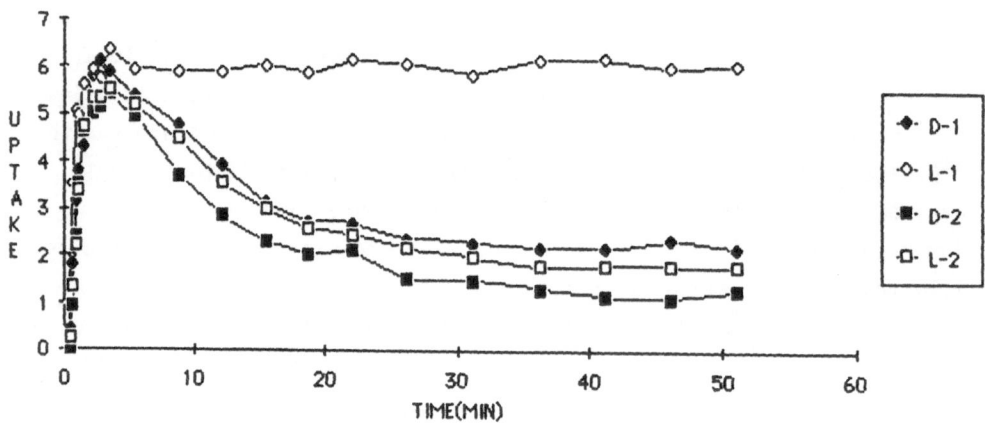

(11C)-DEPRENYL UPTAKE IN A HEALTHY VOLUNTEER (FRONTAL CORTEX)

Fig. 2   Brain radioactivity in a healthy volunteer following tracer doses of 11-C-D- and L-deprenyl. The curves D-2 and L-2 were obtained 24 hours following an oral dose of 15 mg deprenyl.

^{11}C-raclopride

^{11}C-raclopride binds specifically to dopamine (D_2) receptor sites (Köhler et al., 1985). Lately this tracer has been applied in human PET studies (Farde et al., 1986).

In our laboratory sequential administration of ^{11}C-raclopride was performed in a monkey before and after unilateral MPTP lesion. Already two days after the lesion (when ^{11}C-nomifensine uptake was still unchanged) ^{11}C-raclopride radioactivity had increased in the striatum of the lesioned side. This was still present but less pronounced after 9 days. These findings suggest that diminished pre-synaptic dopaminergic function may result in an increase in post-synaptic dopamine D_2 receptor concentration. It will be important to repeat the ^{11}C-raclopride study after a longer period of nigro-striatal dopaminergic degeneration.

The conclusion from PET-studies performed in patients with Parkinson's disease, who have diminished intrastriatal dopaminergic stimulation on a chronic basis, is that striatal dopaminergic receptor concentration is essentially unaltered (see Leenders, 1986; Hägglund et al., 1986).

GENERAL CONCLUSION

1. Preclinical PET-studies in monkeys are of great value in the process of evaluating new ^{11}C-labelled tracer-drugs.

2. For the dopamine system PET-techniques have been worked out for the assessment of the density of terminals and receptors as well as for the determination of brain MAO-B activity. These techniques will enabele a multifactorial characterization of brain neurotransmitter dysfunction in disorders such as Parkinson's disease.

ACKNOWLEDGEMENT

The investigations are supported by the Swedish Medical Research Council, by the Swedish Natural Science Research Council and by Pharmacia AB, Uppsala, Sweden

REFERENCES

Bankiewicz, K.S., Oldfield, E.H, Chiueh, C.C., et al. 1986. Hemi-parkinsonism in monkeys after unilateral internal carotid artery infusion of 1-methyl-4-phenyl-1,2,3,6-tetrahydropyridine (MPTP). Life Sci., 39, 7-16.

Farde, L., Hall, H., Ehrin, E., et al. 1986. Quantitative analysis of D2 dopamine receptor binding in the living human brain by PET. Science, 231, 258-261.

Fowler, J.S., MacGregor, R.R., Wolf, A.P., et al. 1986. Regional distribution of monoamine oxidase A and B in human brain using 11-C-suicide inhibitors and positron emission tomography. Submitted to Science.

Fowler, C.J., Wiberg, A., Oreland, L., et al. 1980. The effect of age on the activity and molecular properties of human brain monoamine oxidase. J. Neural. Transm., 49, 1-20.

Hunt, P., Kannengiesser, M.H. and Raynaud, J.P. 1974. Nomifensine: a potent new inhibitor of dopamine uptake into synaptosomes from rat brain corpus striatum. J. Pharmac., 26, 370-371.

Hägglund, J., Aquilonius, S.-M., Eckernäs, S.-A., et al. 1986. Dopamine receptor properties in Parkinson's disease and Huntington's chorea evaluated by positron emission tomography using 11-C-N-methyl-spiperone. Acta Neurol. Scand., in press.

Javitch, J.A., Blaustein, R.O. and Snyder, S.H. 1983. 3-H-mazindol binding associated with neuronal dopamine uptake sites in corpus striatum membranes. Eur. J. Pharmacol., 90, 461-462.

Köhler, C., Hall, H., Ögren, S.-O., et al. 1985. Specific in vitro and in vivo binding of 3-H-raclopride. A potent substituted benzamide drug with high affinity for dopamine D-2 receptors in the rat brain. Biochem. Pharmacol., 34, 2251-2259.

Langström, B. 1980. On the synthesis of 11-C-compounds. Thesis Acta Universitatis, Upsaliensis, 555, Uppsala.

Leenders, K.L. 1986. Movement disorders: a study with positron emission tomography. Thesis Vrije University, Rodopi, Amsterdam.

Robinson, J.B. 1985. Stereoselectivity and isoenzyme selectivity of monoamine oxidase inhibitors. Enantiomers of amphetamine, N-methyl-amphetamine and deprenyl. Biochem. Pharmacol., 34, 1105-1108.

APPLICATION OF PET IN CLINICAL BRAIN RESEARCH

H.-J. Freund, Neurologische Universitätsklinik, Düsseldorf, FRG

It is a widely held view that PET is a research tool rather than part of clinical routine equipment. In spite of that, this conference is devoted to the clinical efficacy of PET.

From the various fields of application discussed here that for cerebrovascular disease seems to be most advanced, as it was the first where PET was applied. It is now firmly established that amongst the available methods PET is the only one that can provide the information on some parameters of cerebral blood flow and metabolism which are of critical importance for prognosis and therapeutical decisions. Cerebral blood flow and volume in conjunction with oxygen extraction and consumption allow the distinction between various pathological stages such as reduced flow without or with concomitant decrease of oxygen consumption. Oligemia, ischemia, and infarction can be distinguished as well as reversible and irreversible damage. This is of course of major significance for planning therapy. Without knowing these parameters, the clinician has no rational basis for decisions about the indication for extra-intracranial bypass or carotid artery surgery. Future studies on patient selection for surgery may greatly benefit from the information available by PET scanning. The disadvantage of the high coasts of PET examinations may be counterbalanced by the decrease in the number of patients that have to be operated.

It is obvious from the joint study on extra-intracranial bypass surgery as well as from prospective studies on asymptomatic carotid artery disease that the previous criteria used for the indication of such surgical measures are not valid. There is obvious need for better criteria for the selection of patients that may really benefit from such therapeutic procedures. Other diagnostic tools such as CT, MRI or angiography hold little promise in that direction. In my opinion it is only the improvement of ultrasound or endoscopic techniques that can - from the other end - help to improve on the indication for carotid artery surgery by recognizing those stenotic lesions that are emboligenic.

The optimal use of the potential of the PET technology will depend on a careful correlation with the individual determinants for the course of the disease. In addition to the progression of the underlying disease process there are several factors that need consideration. If data are pooled for patients with carotid artery obstructions the presence of several other pathogenic factors is frequently decisive whether the patient will suffer from a major stroke or not. Whether the middle cerebral artery remains open or is obstructed by the end of the carotid artery thrombus or by an embolus is of equal relevance for the occurrence of an infarction as the patency of the communicating arteries of the circle of Wilis or of the other large neck arteries.

It is therefore necessary that the PET units are not conducting their own research in isolation but that the results are critically evaluated in context with the information provided by other methods and of the clinical state of the patient.

The results on the examination of brain tumors gain increasingly more clinical significance. It seems to be possible to approximate the stage of the malignancy of the tumor and to measure alterations in protein synthesis after therapy. The distinction between radiation necrosis and tumor regrowth is another differential diagnostic aspect which can not be solved by any other method. The detection of hypometabolic foci in about 70 to 80 % of patients with partial complex seizures that can be measured in the interictal state has reached diagnostic significance in epilepsy.

The metabolic studies on basal ganglia disorders, although partly controversial, showed no significant alterations. This may be due to the fact that the major abnormality in the mild or moderate cases are altered states of functional activity rather than an over all reduction in neuronal activity. But there are other candidates for negative results. One of them is patient selection. Parkinsonian patients are grossly different not only with respect to the severity and duration of the disease, but also to the preponderance of the clinical signs. Symmetrical akinetic cases without tremor may have different metabolism than patients with solely unilateral tremor. Strong unilateral tremor or other focal hyperkinetic activities would be likely candidates for increased metabolism in some parts of the brain including the basal ganglia if these hyperkinesiae persist during the measurement and thus yield different results than patients without involuntary movements during the examination.

The possibility to study the binding of different ligands to dopamine receptors and to examine the effects of antagnostic agents opens new avenues for research on the role of neurotransmitters and their neuropharmacological modulation, including the monitoring of the effects of therapy on the receptors. This approach can be used for the investigation of extrapyramidal motor disorders and of animal models as the MPTP model of Parkinson's disease. This type of studies can be extended for combined subcortical and cortical pathology such as the Parkinson dementia complex or the dementia in Huntington's disease.

Cortical movement disorders have not been discussed at this meeting. PET scanning has considerably contributed to the advancement of knowledge on certain areas of cortical motor function. The role of the supplementary motor area for the initiation of movement, the involvement of parietal areas in motor control or the investigations on the frontal eye fields are some examples of this line of research. In contrast to the studies conducted so far on subcortical motor structures PET scanning has contributed to a better understanding of these aspects of brain function.

The progress in research on brain function may have valuable applications for clinical practise. Selective activation of certain brain areas with concomitant metabolic increase may become a routine method in many laboratories for testing the functional reserve capacity in patients with cerebrovascular disease. PET scanning could thus be used along the lines of classical neurology by relating functional tests with altered states of regional brain activities. For future aspects, the improvement in spatial resolution and scanning time together with the progress in radiochemistry leaves us to expect a broader application for the elucidation of brain function and neurotransmitter pathology. Selective activation of brain areas or circuitries is one of the most faszinating aspects of PET scanning for the neurosciences. It seems possible to study human brain function thereby complementing the information provided from animal studies in particular from neuro-physiological, anatomical, and audioradiographic data on the monkey. The full potential of the PET technology with respect to clinical application can only be used if the functional aspects are evaluated in context with the other data provided by other fields of the neurosciences.

Surprisingly, receptor studies of psychiatric disorders have
revealed that the only consistent abnormalities were seen in the basal
ganglia. As in Parkinson's disease it is possible to monitor the changes
in receptor occupancy and density in the striatum after neuroleptic
treatment. These observations may stimulate new insights and approaches
in the study of psychiatric and neurological disorders. The psychic and
the motor aspects of diseases of the brain are frequently associated.
The major outputs of the basal ganglia are part of a cortical-sub-
cortical motor loop but also of a limbic loop. Alterations of dopamine
receptors in subcortical movement disorders and certain psychiatric
diseases point to this dual aspect of basal ganglia function.

In summary PET scanning has reached a level of significance for
clinical diagnosis and the evaluation of prognosis and therapy particular in the field of cerebrovascular disease that it can no longer be
regarded as a pure research tool. By this reason, a wider application
for clinical neurology is desirable and seems to occur. Its enormous
potential for a better understanding of brain function, of neurotransmitters and their modulation by neuropharmacological agents and the
visualization of protein synthesis in brain tumors - in addition to
their impact for the neurosciences - may open new areas of application
in the near future.

SUMMARY of the Discussion on Brain I

C. Beckers, Université Catholique de Louvain, Faculté de Médecine,
Centre de Médecine Nucléaire, Brussels, Belgium

As pointed out by Dr. Frackowiak, London, the interest in PET
studies is not related to large series of patients, but to the exquisite
capability of physiological tracers to be used in various pathological
conditions such as cerebro-vascular diseases. All the data presented
also have stressed the non-invasive aspect of PET investigations which
allow to open many windows in the early diagnosis and the follow-up of
treatment of patients with brain diseases.

Ischemic stroke is a fairly frequent problem. The data that can be
obtained by independent methods for measuring in the brain oxygen
consumption and glucose utilization were discussed by Dr. Baron, Orsay,
particularly in the relationship of the prognostic significance of
enhanced anaerobic glycolysis in response to ischemia. While the data
related to the cerebral flow measurements and the metabolic rate of O2
and glucose display similar regional features in control subjects, many
puzzling findings are found in ischemic brain patients. As pointed out
by Dr. Frackowiak, London, the 15-0/C-15-0-2 continuous inhalation
technique has received considerable experimental validation. Largely
thanks to this methodology, the largest contribution of PET to
neurological clinical problems has probably been the elucidation in vivo
of the development of cerebrovascular ischemia to infarction. This
conclusion is supported by the data discussed by Dr. Baron, Orsay, Dr.
Pawlik, Cologne, and Dr. Samson, Orsay, as also pointed out by Dr.
Lenzi, Rome. This last author stressed the fact that the recognition of
patients with critical perfusion syndrome, altogether with their
evaluation after therapy, represents a major achievement of PET studies
in clinical medicine. The identification of patients at risk of stroke
due to critically decreased perfusion pressure remain a goal that can be
achieved by PET if not some day by SPECT.

At different stages of the discussion, the problem of the
availability of PET equipment to clinical neurology was stressed. The
opinion was quite clear from the audience: for many years the PET camera
was located in a research center far away from the hospital. In these
days, already installated clinical PET centers permit the accurate
evaluation of the clinical efficiency of PET. Many participants stressed
the importance of coupling the oxygen metabolism studies with 15-0 to
glucose uptake measurements with 18FDG or other analogs.

Conditions other than cerebral vascular diseases were also
discussed. Data presented by Dr. Schuier, Düsseldorf, indicate that FDG
studies can detect patients at risk of movement disorders as
Huntington's disease or Parkinson's disease. PET studies allow to
evaluate the efficacy of a given treatment. Another field of application
is neuropharmacology as illustrated by research on the dompaniergic
system performed in the rhesus monkey (Dr.Aquilonius, Uppsala) and in
man (Dr.Leenders, London). Much remains to be done in this field as soon
as the radiochemistry of these compounds will make them readily
available to various PET centers.

As stressed by Dr. Freund, Düsseldorf, PET methodology is an
expensive tool but we probably underestimate its clinical efficacy
because the neurologists just start to be aware of the clinical
possibilities offered by a non-invasive technique that allows a
quantitative evaluation of metabolic disturbances in various conditions

where CT-scan or magnetic nuclear resonance give normal features.

As pointed out by Dr. Beckers, Brussels, many results presented in this session stress the major role that PET can play in the future in the early detection of brain abnormalities and in the follow-up studies of patients. PET offers metabolic information which at first sight looks very expensive but on a long run may have a cost/benefit ratio that fits with the economical problems of our society. Similar difficulties have been previously met with the screening of congenital diseases of which the cost effectiveness is now very well recognized.

B R A I N

Epilepsy and Pediatric Neurology

LOCALIZING EPILEPTIC FOCI BY PET

K. Herholz, G. Pawlik, W. Staffen, P. Ziffling, I. Hebold, W.-D. Heiss

Max-Planck-Institut für neurologische Forschung
Cologne, FRG

In most experimental models of focal and generalized epileptic seizures a substantial increase of glucose metabolism has been observed in those brain structures which were involved in the pathological activity. Even in focal seizures this activity and the increase of metabolism was frequently spread intracortically, transcallosally, and to basal structures (Collins et al., 1976). The increase of metabolism appears to be mainly due to the metabolic requirements of increased electric activity, transmitter synthesis, and ion pumping. If the seizure is sustained for longer than a few minutes, it leads to a depletion of cell energy storage and to accumulation of lactate which is a major factor in the development of severe and eventually irreversible cell damage.

The advent of positron emission tomography (PET), and the adaption of the autoradiographic deoxyglucose method to this noninvasive in-vivo technique (Reivich et al., 1979) opened new possibilities for diagnosis and pathophysiological investigation of focal epilepsy. It closes a gap between the high-resolution techniques X-ray CT and magnetic resonance imaging (MRI) which yield morphological but not functional information, and the electroencephalogram (EEG) which demonstrates specific electrical alterations but is only of poor localizing value.

Focal epilepsy is often a symptom of focal brain abnormalities, e.g. tumors. In most cases, the localization of these abnormalities can be determined by clinical observations (e.g. Jacksonian focal motor seizures), or by CT or MRT scans. In complex partial seizures, however, these tools frequently fail. Surface EEG recordings, even if 24 h-monitoring is performed, also may yield ambiguous results as to the localization of the primary focus. Thus, as yet, depth electrode recordings are usually required for exact localization, but they carry all risks of an invasive technique. Therefore, this report summarizes the results of published PET studies of focal seizures with particular reference to complex partial seizures, including some observations made in our own laboratory.

128

METHODS

As in experimental studies, the deoxyglucose method is most fre-
frequently used for the investigation of epileptic foci with PET. Details of this method as it is used in our laboratory were described by
Heiss et al. (1984). Because of the relatively low positron energy of
^{18}F, and the stable distribution of the tracer 30 minutes after injection, this method gives a better spatial resolution than other
techniques involving the isotopes ^{15}O or ^{11}C. However, the accumulated tracer activity represents a weighted sum of all metabolic
activities within approx. 30 minutes, where the first minutes after
bolus injection have the highest weight. This does not cause problems
under the stable conditions of interictal studies, but compromises to
some extent the results of ictal studies.

RESULTS
Ictal studies

Engel et al. (1983) performed ictal studies in 4 patients with
spontaneous recurrent partial seizures, one with epilepsia partialis
continua, and one with a single partial seizure induced by electrical
stimulation of the hippocampus. They observed variable patterns of hypermetabolism which was a high as 6 times the interictal rate in one
study and apparently represented the extent of the structures involved
in the pathological electric activity. In the patient with epilepsia
partialis continua the metabolic activity of the entire brain was increased with accentuation in the right frontal and temporal lobes, but
the suspected focus (right central area, corresponding to continuous
clonic movements, of the left arm and leg) was not as active as other
brain regions. We did not observe any hypermetabolic areas in a patient
with continuous clonic movements of the right hand, but moderate wide
spread hypometabolism of the left cerebral hemisphere (Fig. 1). These
findings could be explained by metabolic exhaustion, or could indicate
that the pathophysiology of epilepsia partialis continua differs substantially from other partial epilepsies.

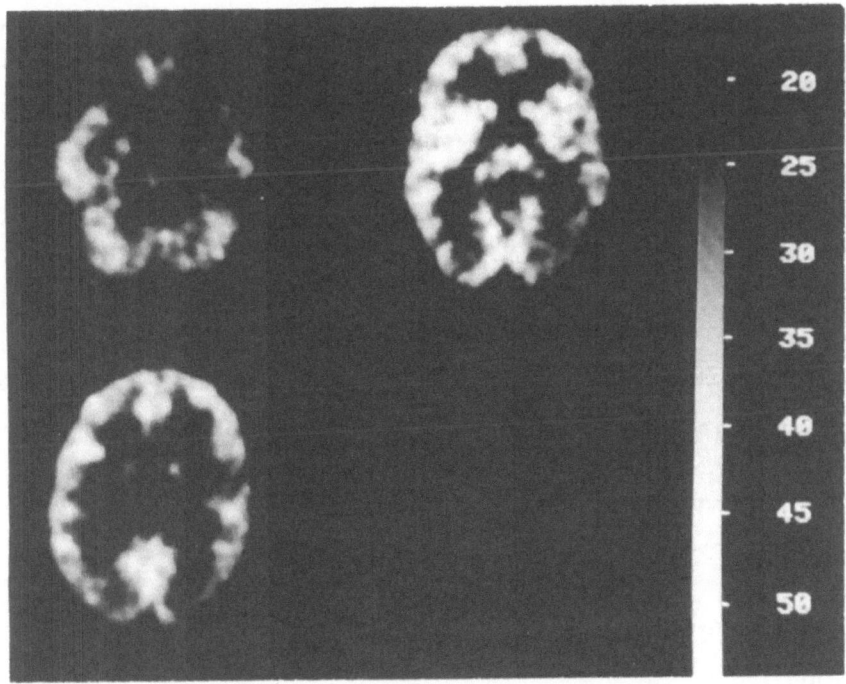

Fig. 1   Hypometabolism of left central cortex, to a lesser degree
also of left temporal and parietal cortex in a 23-year old male
with epilepsia partialis continua of the right hand.
(Viewer's right is patient's left in all figures).

Theodore et al. (1983) reported hypometabolic areas in ictal scans
obtained from 3 patients with complex partial seizures. These areas
were located in the left temporal lobe in two cases, and in the right
frontal lobe in one case. Interictal scans showed hypometabolism in the
same areas which had been hypermetabolic during the seizures.
EEG recordings during the scans showed left temporal onset in the two
cases with temporal abnormality and paroxysmal diffuse theta-activity
in the other case.

Interictal studies

As shown in table 1 hypometabolic areas were frequently found in
interictal studies of patients with focal epilepsy. Their frequency

ranges between 40 and 100%, probably depending on evaluation criteria and patients' selection. In some studies only patients with normal CT scans were included (Theodore et al., 1983; Sperling et al., 1986), and in all studies the sensitivity of PET was higher than that of X-ray CT or MRI. In order to minimize subjective influences, a regional quantitative analysis should be used for evaluation of the scans. In good correspondence with our own experience most authors report, that side to side differences of more than 15% between corresponding temporal regions of both hemispheres can be regarded as pathological.

TABLE 1   Frequency of hypometabolic areas in patients with focal
with focal epilepsy

Authors	N	Frequency (%) of scans with hypometabolic areas	Corresponding X-ray CT and MRI findings
Kuhl et al. 1980	17	82 %	29 % CT path.
Engel et al. 1982a	50	70 %	
Theodore et al. 1983	20	80 %	CT all normal
Yamamoto et al. 1983	14	100 %	
Shimizu et al. 1985	18	83 %	
Theodore et al. 1986	26	80 %	44 % CT path., 77 % MRI path.
Sperling et al. 1986	30	40 %	CT all normal, 10 % MRI path.
Böcher-Schwarz et al., 1986	10	100 %	80 % MRI path.

The most frequent histopathological finding underlying mesial
temporal lobe hypometabolism is mesial temporal sclerosis (Table 2).
The sensitivity of MRI for this frequent source of partial complex seizures is controversial: some authors claimed a good sensitivity, while in
the study of Sperling et al., (1986) this finding was missed in all 18
patients with mesial temporal sclerosis and positive PET scan.

TABLE 2   Histopathological findings in hypometabolic areas

Kuhl	hippocampal sclerosis 5, meningioma 1,
et al. 1980	tuberous sclerosis 1
Engel	mesial temporal sclerosis 15, tumors 2, angioma 1,
et al. 1982b	heterotopia 1, normal 3*
Yamamoto	temporal sclerosis 4
et al. 1983	
Sperling	mesial temporal sclerosis 18
et al. 1986	

*including 2 artifacts caused by depth electrodes

In principle, the specificity of hypometabolic areas in PET scans
is low, because they are also observed in a variety of non-epileptic
brain disorders (e.g. infarcts, hemorrhages, low-grade tumors). However,
Engel et al. (1982a) conclude, that in those patients where the localization of an hypometabolic area in interictal PET scan, interictal spikes,
begin of ictal activity and other focal surface EEG abnormalities are
corresponding, the reliability of these combined findings is as high as
with depth electrode recordings.
    The hypometabolic areas are always larger than the extent of the
underlying histopathological alterations. Since the same effect was
also observed in autoradiographic examinations of experimental focal
brain lesions, it does not appear to be due to the limited spatial resolution of PET scanners. It is unlikely that it represents active inhibition in the surrounding of the focus, because that would cause increased metabolic demand (Ackermann et al., 1984). It might therefore
reflect reduced input to structurally normal brain regions from damaged
and inhibited areas. Despite this blurring effect, we were able in most

cases to determine not only the side left/right of a focus in temporal lobe epilepsy, but also to decide whether the lateral, polar or mesial temporal cortex was most effected (Böcher-Schwarz et al., 1986). Further contrast enhancement can be achieved by active speech stimulation which leads to a widespread metabolic activation of the brain (Pawlik et al., in preparation): the hypometabolic epileptogenic focus does not participate in this activation and is therefore more clearly depicted (Fig. 2).

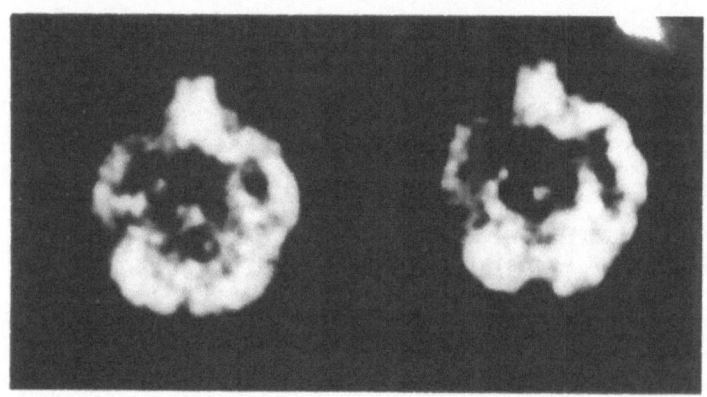

Fig. 2   26-year old female with complex partial seizures at rest (left, gray scale range 3 to 48 μmol glucose/100g tissue/min) and during speech activation (right, gray scale range 10 to 60). Right mesial temporal hypometabolic focus shown with better contrast in the activated study.

COMMENT

The referred studies indicate in accordance with our own experience that interictal PET scans with FDG are a sensitive and reliable tool for localization of the responsible focus in partial complex seizures. Besides, PET studies also yield information if other potentially epileptogenic foci are present. E.g., secondary foci can develop in long standing focal epilepsy. They have been suspected in some cases where further seizures occurred after successful removal of an epileptogenic focus by surgery (Morrell, 1985). There are further diseases with multiple potentially epileptogenic foci. Tuberous sclerosis, e.g., is characterized by multiple cortical lesions, the tubers, which are usually not detected on X-ray CT scans but show up as hypometabolic foci in

FDG-PET (Szelies et al., 1983). In this disease seizures tend to gene-
ralize, and surgical removal of one focus is of no beneficial effect.

In contrast to the interictal scans, ictal studies suffer at
present from considerable methodological problems. Because of the 30
minute tracer accumulation phase of FDG, as mentioned earlier, the
usually short periods over which epileptic discharges can be maintained
without being potentially harmful to the patient are not adequately
represented in the result. Therefore, the "ictal" images usually represent a mixture of ictal and postictal states. Corresponding to the
depression of electrical activity the cerebral metabolism is also depressed immediately after a seizure (Fig. 3).

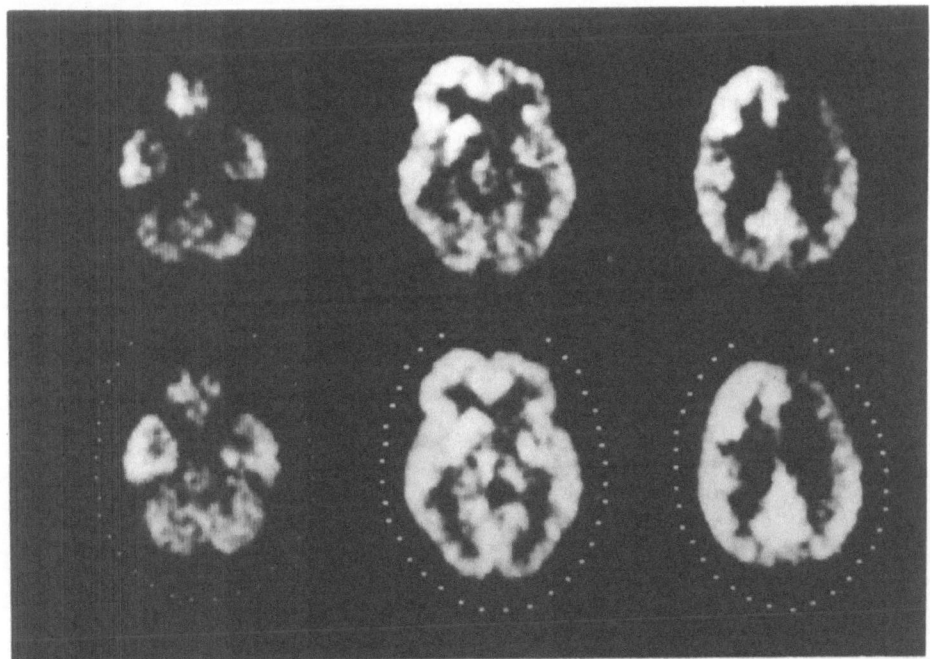

Fig. 3   47-year old male with a left frontal defect due to resection of an angiom several years ago. Immediately after a focal
seizure with generalization depression of glucose metabolism (top
row, gray scale range 3 to 55 µmol/100g/min) and postictal aphasia.
Normalization of metabolic level (bottom row, same scale) after recovery.

134

Therefore, ictal scans which are much more difficult to perform for
practical reasons are apparently also less reliable and reproducible.
Nevertheless, the ictal phase would be more interesting for pathophysiological investigations and shows apparently more specific
alterations than the interictal one. It remains to be determined if
measurements of cerebral blood flow with PET which can be performed in a
much shorter time (e.g. within 40 sec. after intravenous bolus injection
of ^{15}O-water, (Raichle et al., 1983) than FDG-scans will overcome these
problems.

Besides the localization of epileptic foci PET-studies with FDG
yield some information about the functional status of the rest of the
brain. This might be important in children with severe hemiparesis and
intractable seizures due to perinatal brain damage if aggressive surgery
like hemispherictomy or callosotomy is considered to control seizures.
In these cases the residual metabolism of the affected hemisphere might
serve as an estimate of its functional capabilities. Another finding of
clinical importance is the observation of severe cerebellar hypometabolism in patients treated with phenytoin over a long time (Fig. 4). It
It can be observed before the clinical manifestation of cerebellar
symptoms.

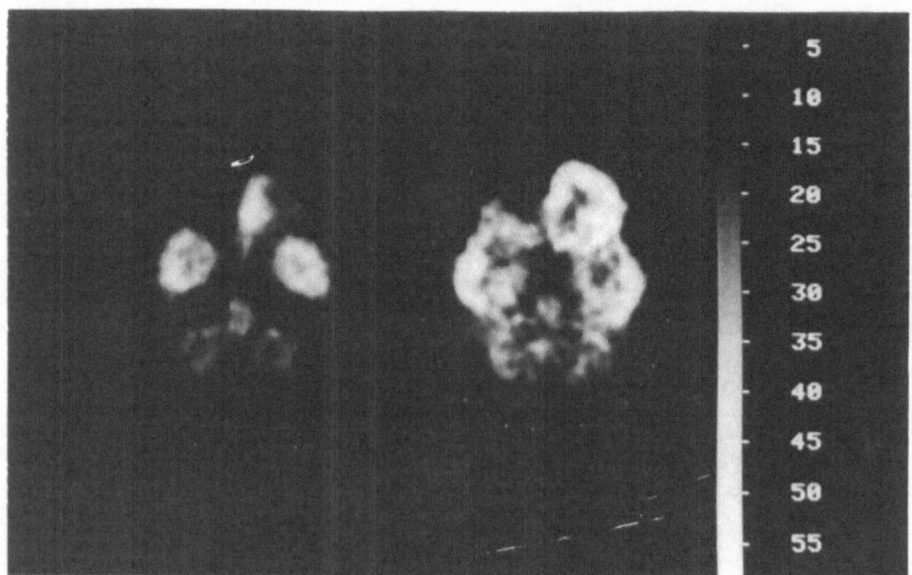

Fig. 4   Severe cerebellar hypometabolism due to long-term phenytoin
treatment in a 15-year-old male. Right frontal defect due to unsuccessful surgery for intractable focal epilepsy.

The rapid development of new radio-labelled receptor ligands may also open new perspectives for diagnosis and pathophysiological investigation of focal epilepsy. Preliminary studies with ^{11}C-carfentanil indicate an increased binding capacity of μ-opiate receptors in amygdala, temporal cortex, and thalamus in patients with temporal lobe epilepsy (Frost et al., 1985 and 1986). Other potentially useful agents are ^{18}F-3-acetylcyclofoxy (Larson and DiChiro, 1985) also for opiate receptor imaging, and ligands for imaging of benzodiazepine receptors, e.g. ^{11}C-RO-15-1788 (Persson et al., 1985).

REFERENCES

Ackermann, R.F., Finch, D.M., Babb, T.L., et al. 1984. Increased glucose metabolism during long-duration recurrent inhibition of hippocampal pyramidal cells. J. Neuroscience, 4, 251-264.

Böcher-Schwarz, H.G., Stefan, H., Pawlik, G., et al. 1986. Das Bild der "Temporallappenepilepsie" in der Positronen-Emissions-Tomographie. Neue diagnostische Möglichkeiten zur Lokalisation des epileptogenen Focus. 37. Jahrestagung der Deutschen Gesellschaft für Neurochirurgie. Bonn, 5. - 7. Mai.

Collins, R.C., Kennedy, C., Sokoloff, L., et al. 1976. Metabolic anatomy of focal motor seizures. Arch. Neurol., 33, 536-542.

Engel, J.Jr, Kuhl, D.E., Phelps, M.E., et al. 1982a. Comparative localization of epileptic foci in partial epilepsy by PCT and EEG. Ann. Neurol., 12, 529-537.

Engel, J.Jr, Brown, W.J., Kuhl, D.E., et al. 1982b. Pathological findings underlying focal temporal lobe hypometabolism in partial epilepsy. Ann. Neurol., 12, 518-528.

Engel, J.Jr, Kuhl, D.E., Phelps, et al. 1983. Local cerebral metabolism during partial seizures. Neurology (Cleveland), 33, 400-413.

Frost, J.J., Wagner, H.N.Jr, Dannals R.F., et al. 1985. Imaging opiate receptors in the human brain by positron tomography. J. Cereb. Blood Flow Metab., 9, 231-236.

Frost, J.J., Mayberg, H.S., Fisher, J., et al. 1986. Relationship of opiate receptor binding and temporal lobe epilepsy using C-11 carfentanil. J. Nucl. Med., 27, 1027.

Heiss, W.-D., Pawlik, G., Herholz, K., et al. 1984. Regional kinetic constants and cerebral metabolic rate for glucose in normal human volunteers determined by dynamic positron emission tomography of (18F)-2-fluoro-2-deoxy-D-glucose. J. Cereb. Blood Flow Metab., 4, 212-223.

Kuhl, D.E., Engel, J.Jr, Phelps, M.E. et al. 1980. Epileptic patterns of local cerebral metabolism and perfusion in humans determined by emission tomography of 18-FDG and 13-NH-3. Ann. Neurol., 8, 348-360.

Larson, S.M. and Di Chiro, G. 1985. Comparative anatomo-functional imaging of two neuroreceptors and glucose metabolism: A PET study performed in the living baboon. J. Comput. Assist. Tomogr., 9, 676-681.

Morell, F. 1985. Secondary epileptogenesis in man. Arch. Neurol., 42, 318-335.

Persson, A., Ehrin, E., Eriksson, L., et al. 1985. Imaging of 11-C-labelled Ro-15-1788 binding to benzodiazepine receptors in the human brain by positron emission tomography. J. psychiat. Res., 19, 609-622.

Raichle, M.E., Martin, W.R.W., Herscovitch, P., et al. 1983. Brain blood flow measured with intravenous H-2-15-O. II. Implementation and validation. J. Nucl. Med., 24, 790-798.

Reivich, M., Kuhl, D., Wolf, A., et al. 1979. The (18-F)fluorodeoxy-glucose method for the measurement of local cerebral glucose utilization in man. Circ. Res., 44, 127-137.

Shimizu, H. and Ishijima, B. 1985. Diagnosis of temporal lobe epilepsy by positron emission tomography. Folia Psychiat. Neurol. Jpn., 39, 251-256.

Sperling, M.R., Wilson, G., Engel, J.Jr, et al. 1986. Magnetic resonance imaging in intractable partial epilepsy: Correlative studies. Ann. Neurol., 20, 57-62.

Szelies, B., Herholz, K., Heiss, W.-D., et al. 1983. Hypometabolic cortical lesions in tuberous sclerosis with epilepsy: Demonstration by positron emission tomography. J. Comput. Assist. Tomogr., 7, 946-953.

Theodore, W.H., Newmark, M.E., Sato, S., et al. 1983. (18-F)fluoro-deoxyglucose positron emission tomography in refractory complex partial seizures. Ann. Neurol., 14, 429-437.

Theodore, W.H., Dorwart, R., Holmes, M., et al. 1986. Neuroimaging in refractory partial seizures: Comparison of PET, CT, and MRI. Neurology, 36, 750-759.

Yamamoto, Y.L., Ochs, R., Gloor, P., et al. 1983. Pattern of rCBF and focal energy metabolic changes in relation to electroencephalo-graphic abnormality in the inter-ictal phase of partial epilepsy. In: "Cerebral Blood Flow, Metabolism and Epilepsy" (Eds. M. Baldy-Moulinier, D.H. Ingvar and B.S. Meldrum). (John Libbey, London-Paris). pp 51-62.

CLINICAL APPLICATIONS OF PET: STUDIES OF BRAIN GLUCOSE METABOLISM IN PEDIATRIC NEUROLOGY

A.M. Goffinet, A.G. Devolder, A. Bol, C. Michel, M. Cogneau

Positron Tomography Laboratory
University of Louvain
2, Chemin du Cyclotron
Louvain-la-Neuve, Belgium

So far, positron emission tomography (PET) has not been applied extensively in pediatric neurology, possibly due to difficulties inherent in radioisotope analyses in children. This situation is subject to change, however, with the continuous improvement in the sensitivity of PET cameras. In this chapter, data from the literature and our recent experiences with the use of FDG in children are summarized. Studies with other tracers are reviewed elsewhere (Phelps and Mazziotta, 1985; Perlman et al., 1985) and will not be considered.

PROBLEMS SPECIFIC TO STUDIES IN CHILDREN

Various difficulties arise when working with children, both at the technical level and regarding data interpretation. First, what can be considered as a "safe" radioisotope dose? The most widely used dose is between 100 and 150 µCi/kg body weight. However, even that small amount cannot be administered to normal children, so that appropriate controls cannot be obtained. Chugani and Phelps (1986) introduced the use as controls of subjects with minimal abnormalities. We take an analogous approach, employing those studies as reference, where changes are either absent or limited to a clearly defined region.

Rate constants and the lumped constant for FDG have never been measured in child brain. Adult values (Phelps et al., 1979) are used, and there is reason to believe that they are satisfactory, at least after the second year of age. This problem should, however, always be kept in mind.

Children are often agitated during PET studies, so that some medication usually must be given. In our experience, intramuscular dehydrobenzperiodol (DHB) is quite effective and has minimal effects on brain metabolism. The drug does, however, increase striatal glucose utilization to a varying extent. Interestingly, this effect is prevented by a small oral dose of etybenzatropine (Fig. 1).

138

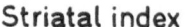

Striatal index

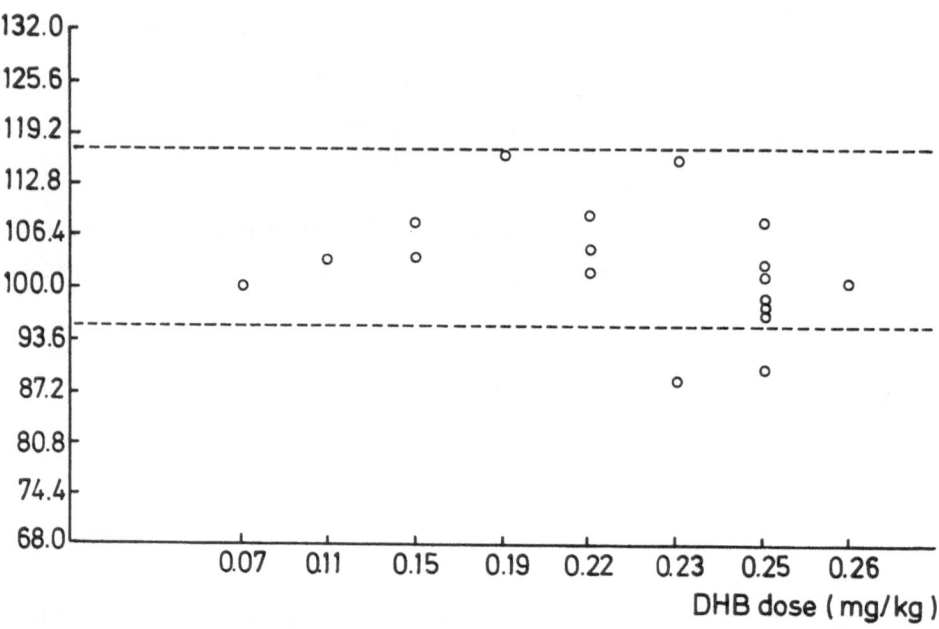

Fig. 1 Effect of dehydrobenzperidol on brain metabolism. The ratio
of glucose metabolism in the striatum versus neocortex (striatal
index) is plotted against drug dose. An activation of the striatum
is present at low drug doses, which is not found at higher dosages
when oral etybenzatropine is given concomitantly.

The developmental physiology of brain glucose metabolism is largely
unknown. Established curves start in early adulthood (Kuhl et al.,
1982; Duara et al., 1984). Recent data show that glucose metabolism is
consistently higher in children than in adult subjects (Phelps et al.,
1986), a feature which is confirmed in our control group (Fig. 2). This
increased metabolic rate has been attributed to the increased synaptic
density in the cerebral cortex of children (Huttenlocher, 1979). In our
experience, the state of agitation or of alertness of the subject has a
large influence on brain metabolism. It is our impression that age-
related metabolic activations may be accounted for by the increased
agitation or alertness of the child during a procedure, which is not so
benign after all. The evolution with age of the regional metabolic

pattern is also hardly known, and observations are to some extent
contradictory (Doyle et al., 1983; Chugani and Phelps, 1986). An
accepted finding is that the adult pattern becomes normally established
before one year.

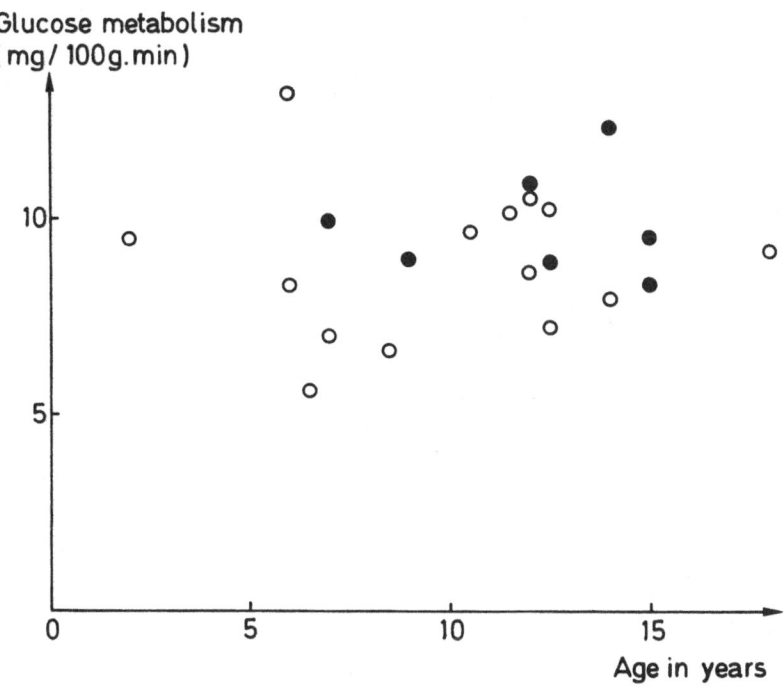

Fig. 2   Brain glucose metabolism as a function of age in control
(full circles) and autistic (open circles) children. Metabolic
rates are high compared to those in adult subjects, but there are
no differences between the two groups of children.

AUTISTIC SYNDROME AND RETT SYNDROME
      The first clinical problem that we chose to investigate was that of
childhood autism defined according to the criteria of DSM III (1980).
So far, we found that global brain glucose utilization is apparently
not different from that in control children (Fig. 2). The regional
pattern of glucose metabolism is also normal in the majority of these
patients (Fig. 3).

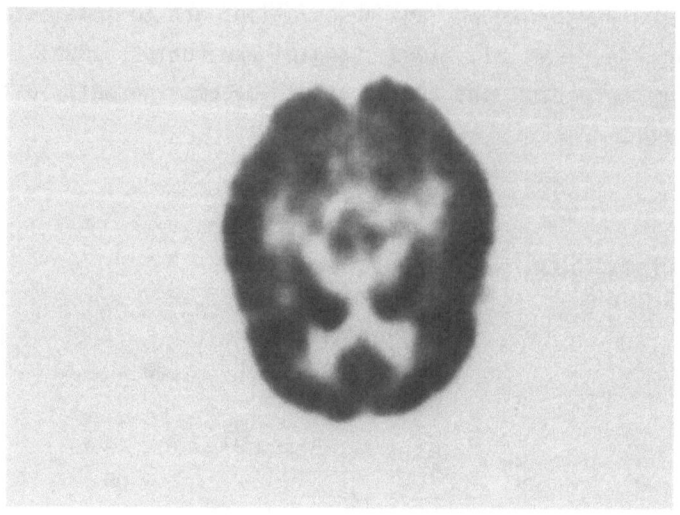

Fig. 3   Example of autism with normal metabolic map.

In about one third of the studies, there was a relative activation in prefrontal versus parieto-occipital cortical areas (Fig. 4), whereas the reverse pattern (i.e., hypofrontality) was rarely observed. No correlations were found between metabolic pattern, clinical data, blood serotonin levels, or any other parameter. We conclude from this limited sample that brain glucose metabolism is largely unaffected in patients with autism and mental retardation, at least when no anatomic lesions are seen with CT or MRI. These data do not confirm the global hypermetabolism reported in adult autistic subjects by Rumsey et al., (1985), but they are in agreement with the study of Herold et al., (1985).

We also had the opportunity to study one girl aged 2 years with Rett syndrome. In this case, global glucose metabolism was low, and the regional pattern showed a decreased FDG uptake in posterior cortical territories. Further studies are obviously needed before any conclusions can be drawn.

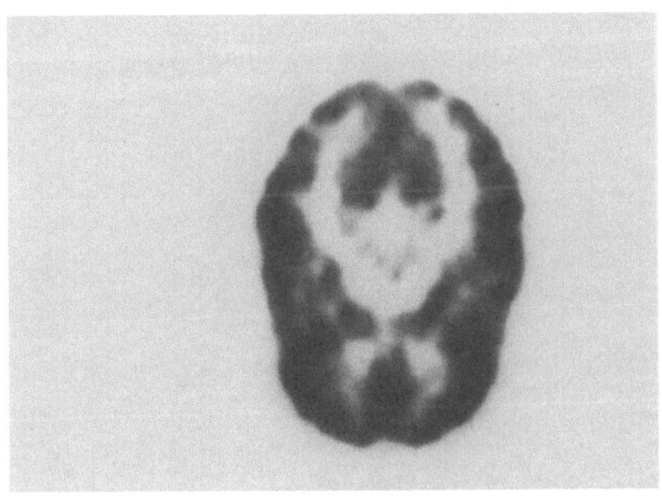

Fig. 4   Autistic child with relative hyperfrontality.

EPILEPSY

Several studies have focused on epilepsy in adult patients (see Phelps and Mazziotta, 1985, for review). Therefore, only a few selected aspects specific to children are considered here. Despite its poor spatial resolution, PET appears extremely sensitive for the detection of epileptic foci. Data interpretation obviously necessitates the availability of EEG recordings during the PET study. In a "non-hospital" environment, we find the use of cassette recordings quite satisfactory.

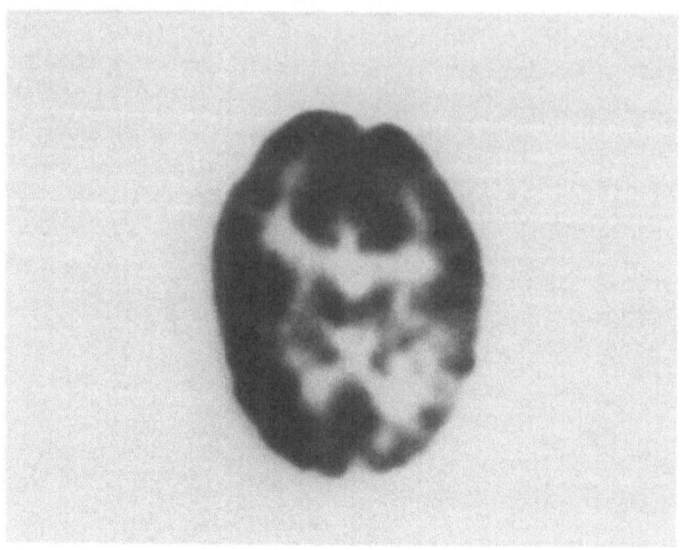

Fig. 5   Focal epilepsy in a 13-year-old girl. Clinical signs were minimal (apart from epilepsy); CT scan was normal. PET reveals a large hypometabolic area in the anterior right hemisphere.

In focal epilepsy, large lesions, most often hypometabolic, are often found in "anatomically" normal or minimally affected brains as defined by CT or MR structural imaging. The extent of the metabolic defects is also in contrast with the clinical deficits, which are sometimes very mild (Fig. 5). In "petit mal" epilepsy, a large increase in brain glucose utilization can be elicited by the induction of spike-wave discharges (hyperpnea) as initially described by Engel et al., (1984).

An interesting, albeit isolated, observation is that diphenyl-hydantoin toxicity can be demonstrated with PET (cerebellar hypometab-olism) before obvious clinical signs appear (Fig. 6).

143

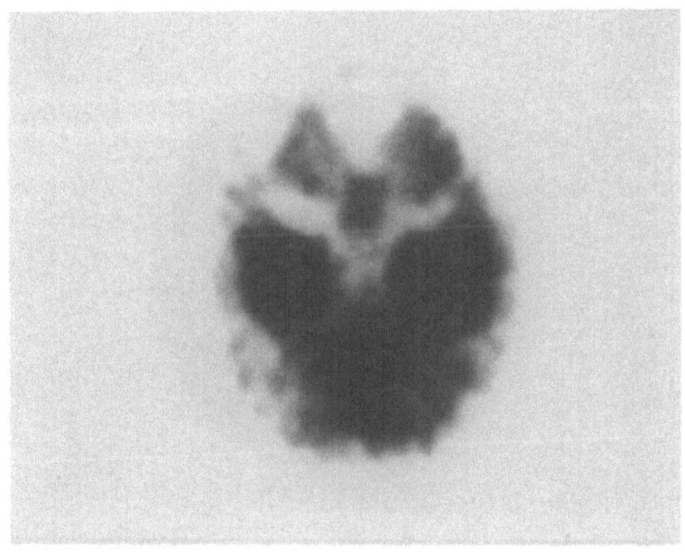

Fig. 6   Subclinical diphenylhydantoin intoxication. Note the
striking hypometabolism of cerebellum.

TUMORS

According to studies performed mainly at the NIH (DiChiro et al.,
1984), brain tumors are characterized by an increased uptake of FDG,
apparently related to malignancy, an observation which is thought to
reflect the well-known "Warburg effect". To our knowledge, no studies
have been performed in children. In the two cases that we examined, no
increased FDG utilization was found.

MOYA-MOYA DISEASE

Moya-Moya syndrome is a frequent cause of cerebrovascular disease
in children. In two patients, analysis of glucose utilization at a
distance from the site of a cerebrovascular accident provided some
estimate of the extent of parenchymal involvement (Fig. 7). In this
limited experience, PET did not provide any obvious advantage over CT.
Measurements of CBF and oxygen extraction would probably be more
interesting in this pathology.

144

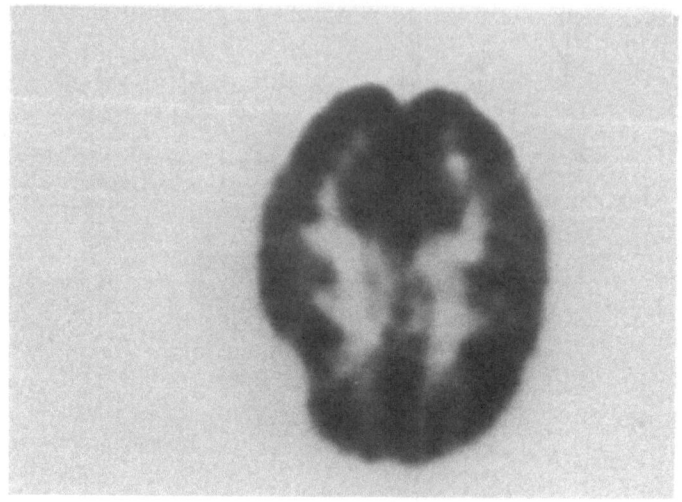

Fig. 7   Moya-Moya disease. The focus corresponding to the previous ischemic accident is visible.

HUNTINGTON'S DISEASE

We had the opportunity to study one boy with Huntington's disease at the age of 14. In this case, glucose metabolism was normal in all brain areas except in the striatum, which showed a drastic (45%) metabolic reduction. Huntington's disease apparently yields the same pattern of alterations in young subjects as it does in adults (Fig. 8).

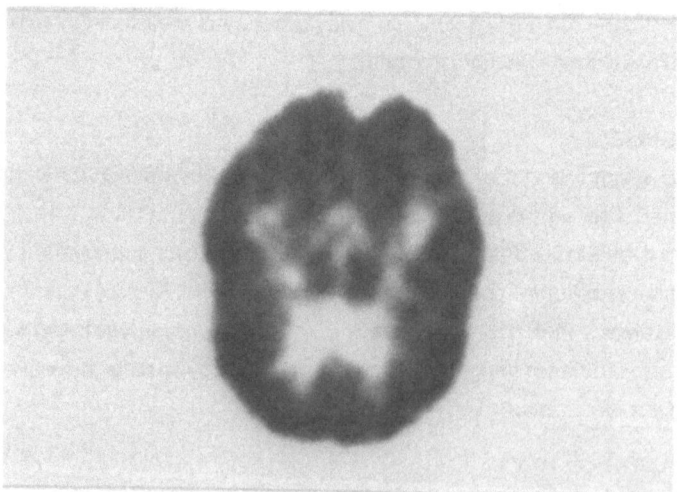

Fig. 8   Huntington's disease in a 14-year-old boy. Note the profuse metabolic defect in the striatum.

SPECIFIC METABOLIC DISEASES

Provided patients are well-selected, PET seems to offer significant prospects for the diagnosis of brain dysfunction in metabolic diseases. In one patient with adenylosuccinase deficiency, a recently described anomaly of purine metabolism (Jaeken and Van den Berghe, 1984), widespread hypometabolism was found in all cortical areas, whereas the thalamus, striatum and cerebellum were normal (Fig. 9).

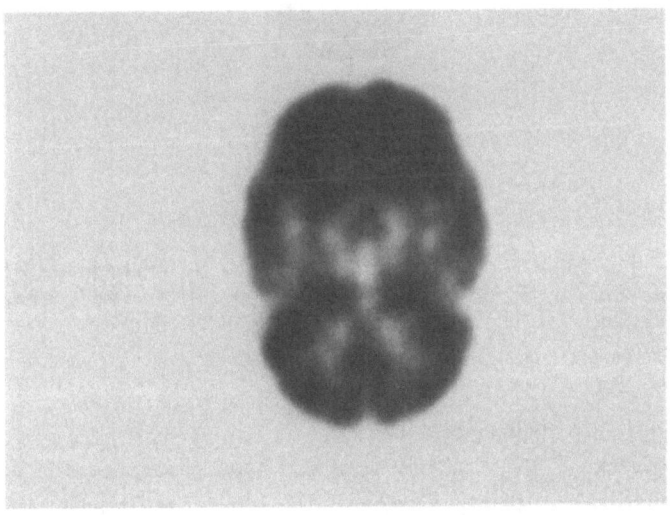

Fig. 9 Adenylosuccinase deficiency in a 5-year-old girl. There is marked hypometabolism in all cortical areas, with preservation of cerebellum. CT scan normal.

Another subject, by contrast, who had very low CSF levels of GABA, exhibited selective hypometabolism of the cerebellar cortex. Cerebellar nuclei and other CNS structures had apparently normal FDG uptake (Fig. 10).

These observations demonstrate that metabolic disorders, which often cause rather similar clinical pictures, can lead to very different metabolic patterns. Possibly, the distribution of parenchymal involvement reflects local sensitivity to abnormal metabolic products. It will be interesting to correlate the PET metabolic maps with biochemical findings, such as the topography of enzyme deficiencies.

146

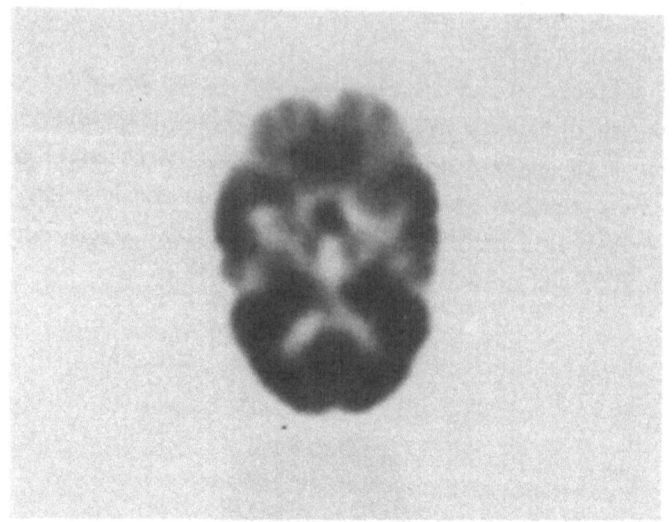

Fig. 10   Boy aged 4, with GABA deficiency of unknown origin: the cerebellar cortex is selectively affected, while other areas and central cerebellar nuclei are normal. CT scan normal.

NEUROPSYCHOLOGIC DISTURBANCES

To our knowledge, PET studies have not been published in cases of learning disabilities, subtle language disorders, and borderline behavioral abnormalities, e.g., minimal brain dysfunction. In three patients, we were unable to find any focal anomalies with the FDG method. Despite great hope that PET might help clinicians to get important information on these problems, the first impression is not optimistic. Obviously, more studies are needed. Possibly, the use of other tracers, or of specific stimuli, may reveal dysfunctions that are not seen with the rather crude method used so far. However, the great variability among subjects will always impose stringent limitations on the interpretation of subtle abnormalities.

REFERENCES

Chugani, H.T. and Phelps, M.E. 1986. Maturational changes in cerebral function in infants determined by (18F)-FDG positron emission tomography. Science, 231, 840-843.
Diagnostic and Statistical Manual of Mental Disorders, 3rd Edition. 1980. Washington, D.C., American Psychiatric Association.

DiChiro, G., Brooks, R.A., Patronas, N.J., et al. 1984. Issues in the
    in vivo measurement of glucose metabolism of human central nervous
    system tumors. Ann. Neurol., 15, (Suppl.), S138-S146.
Doyle, L.W., Nahmias. C., Firnau, G., et al., 1983. Regional cerebral
    glucose metabolism of newborn infants measured by positron
    emission tomography. Develop. Med. Child Neurol., 25, 143-151.
Duara, R., Grady, C.L., Haxby, J., et al. 1984. Human brain glucose
    utilization and cognitive function in relation to age. Ann.
    Neurol., 16, 702-713.
Engel, J.Jr., Lubens, P., Kuhl, D.E., et al. 1985. Local cerebral
    metabolic rate for glucose during petit mal absences. Ann. Neurol.,
    17, 121-128.
Herold, S., Frackowiak, R.S.M., Rutter, M., et al. 1985. Regional
    cerebral blood flow, oxygen and glucose metabolism in young
    autistic adults. J. Cereb. Blood Flow Metab., 5, (Suppl. 1),
    S189-S190.
Huttenlocher, P.R. 1979. Synaptic density in human frontal cortex:
    developmental changes and effects of aging. Brain Res., 163,
    195-205.
Jaeken, J. and Van den Berghe, G. 1984. An infantile autistic syndrome
    characterized by the presence of succinylpurines in body fluids.
    Lancet, 1, 1058-1061.
Kuhl, D.E., Metter, E.J., Riege, W.H., et al. 1982. Effects of human
    aging on patterns of local cerebral glucose utilization determined
    by the 18-F-fluorodeoxyglucose method. J. Cereb. Blood Flow
    Metab., 2, 163-171.
Perlman, J.M., Herscovitch, P., Kreusser, K.L., et al. 1985. Positron
    emission tomography in the newborn: Effect of seizure on regional
    cerebral blood flow in an asphyxiated infant. Neurology, 35, 244-
    247.
Phelps, M.E., Chugani, H.T. and Mazziotta, J.C. 1986. Functional
    development of human brain from 5 days to 20 years of age. J.
    Nucl. Med., 27, 901.
Phelps, M.E., Huang, S.C., Hoffman, E.J., et al. 1979. Tomographic
    measurement of local cerebral glucose metabolic rate in humans
    with (18-F)2-fluoro-2-deoxy-D-glucose: Validation of method.
    Ann. Neurol., 6, 371-388.
Phelps, M.E. and Mazziotta, J.C. 1985. Positron emission tomography:
    Human brain function and biochemistry. Science, 228, 799-809.
Rumsey, J.M., Duara, R., Grady, C., et al. 1985. Brain metabolism in
    autism. Arch. Gen. Psychiat., 42, 448-455.

THE VALUE OF PET IN THE CLINICAL EVALUATION OF EPILEPTIC PATIENTS

H.-G. Wieser, Universitätsspital, Neurologie/EEG, Zürich, Switzerland

Whereas defining the epileptic nature, classifying the seizure
type, and exclusion of a tumor might suffice in many instances to direct
therapeutic action, identification of seizure-mediating brain structures
is the crucial step if surgical treatment has to be contemplated because
of drug-resistance. The diagnostic tests most commonly included in presurgical evaluation protocols designed to localize a resectable epileptogenic lesion, might be divided into those which test for structural
lesions, and those which test for cerebral function. The latter
encompass tests of epileptic excitability, confirmatory tests of focal
functional deficits, and functional mapping (Engel, 1987a).

Radiographic studies, particularly X-ray computed tomography (CT)
and, more recently, magnetic resonance imaging (MRI), have become
important tools for localizing structural abnormalities. Although MRI
has a greater spatial resolution than CT and thus helps considerably to
point the way to an epileptogenic zone, EEG evidence of epileptic
excitability is still essential because CT- and MRI-demonstrated lesions
are not necessarily the site of epileptic seizure generation. In
addition, in many patients with recurrent seizures these examinations
are normal or show only "non-specific" abnormalities such as temporal
lobe atrophy, suggested by asymmetries in ventricular or middle fossa
size, or some calcifications.

Therefore, most centres view the careful analysis of the ictal
behaviour together with a reliable EEG recording of the ictal event, as
the most important constituent of the presurgical evaluation. Of course,
interictal EEG data are also taken into account and indeed play the
determining role in the protocols of those few centres which emphasize
intra-operative electrocorticography. Since surface EEG recordings have
severe limitations, direct intracranial recording techniques (stereotactic depth and foramen ovale electrode recordings, subdural strips and
grids) have very often to be employed (Wieser, 1987). Such procedures
are invasive and are therefore not without risks.

For this reason, new non-invasive "tests of focal functional deficit" have been developed with the aim of substituting for invasive procedures. Along with modern functional imaging techniques, the more traditional tests of functional deficits are included such as epilepto-logical-neurological data (history, local neurological signs, interictal performance, behavioral traits), refined psychometric testing (including intracarotid or selective amytal test), non-epileptiform EEG background abnormalities (including pharmacological tests), and tests of functional hypo-excitability (afterdischarge thresholds, evoked potentials).

Of the functional imaging techniques now available, PET without any doubt has the greater potential but, because of the requirement of a cyclotron, single photon emission tomography (SPECT) currently enjoys a more widespread application (Sperling et al., 1987). This is true also for our hospital which has at its disposal SPECT but not yet PET. The following discussion, therefore, is limited to reviewing the experience with PET at other surgical epilepsy centres, in particular UCLA and Montreal Neurological Institute. However, some patients evaluated and operated at our institution had undergone PET studies elsewhere.

Has PET changed the presurgical protocol?

To date, the leading centres concerned with surgical therapy of epilepsy use PET as an important confirmatory functional test procedure. This means that, in general, PET could not substitute for the invasive tests. However, in a certain percentage of the "simpler" cases, in which all non-invasive information points to an unequivocally concordant epi-leptogenic brain region, and no contradictions emerge between different categories of tests, the application of PET allowed bypassing of an invasive EEG study. For example, a patient with complex partial seizures and a typical aura, pointing to limbic structures, and a MRI finding showing some lesion in one anterior mesial temporal lobe, interictal anterior temporal lobe spikes either restricted homolaterally or at least with ipsilateral predominance, an ictal surface EEG at least compatible with ipsilateral mesiobasal limbic seizure onset, and an ipsilateral hypometabolic temporal lobe in the PET, might be considered for anterior temporal lobectomy without resorting to invasive procedures. However, it has not yet been settled whether a very selective operation like the amygdalohippocampectomy (Yasargil et al., 1985; Wieser, 1986) can be attempted with reasonable degree of success on the basis of such a constellation of findings.

According to recent published studies of the UCLA group 28 % of
their patients in this new protocol no longer undergo invasive depth
recordings (Engel et al., 1987).

Interictal PET findings using the doexyglucose method
    Engel et al. (1987), Theodore et al. (1983), and Yamamoto et al.
(1983) using 18-FDG PET in patients suffering from partial epilepsies,
reported a good correlation in most cases between the site of focal
hypometabolism during the interictal state and the epileptic focus
determined by the combined results of all electrophysiological studies.
Seventy percent of 50 patients (Engel et al., 1987) and 79 % of 28
patients (Theodore et al., 1983) had a hypometabolic zone. The FDG study
of Yamamoto et al. (1983) indicated that there were at least five
different patterns of abnormal rCMRGl findings: I. Unilateral focal
hypometabolism; II. Focal with ipsilateral local extension of hypometabolism; III. Bilateral focal hypometabolism; IV. Unilateral focal
hypometabolism and contralateral focal hypermetabolism; V. Bilateral
diffuse hypometabolisms with unilateral maximum focal hypometabolism.
These authors, however, stated that when they calculated relative
hypometabolism between the region of interest and the contralateral
homotopic, they did not find any significant relative hypometabolism in
the region of interest in types III and V where symmetrical reduction of
rCMRGL was observed in both cerebral hemispheres. Yamamoto et al. (1983)
found a similar tendency towards reduced rCBF and rCMRO in the zone of
glucose hypometabolism in most cases, especially in types I, II, and V.
No clear distinct patterns, however, were found in oxygen-15 studies in
the interictal phase of partial epilepsy in types III and IV. The
Montreal group confirmed the earlier findings of Engel et al. (1982a)
insofar as a good correlation was found between the degree of astroglial
proliferation and severity of glucose hypometabolism. However, no
correlation was found between glucose hypometabolism and neuronal loss
or vascular changes observed in the epileptogenic tissue removed during
surgery.
    In their recent survey of a total of 61 patients, Engel et al.
(1987) report that 36 out of 47 with pathological histological findings
had corresponding PET findings, and 11 of these had not. On the other
hand, of the remaining 14 patients without pathological histological

findings, 9 had normal PET but 5 had focal hypometabolic PET scans. Hippocampal sclerosis (HS), present in 39 out of these 61 patients, was correctly indicated by corresponding hypometabolic PET in 29 patients (74 %). HS plus small lesions were correctly indicated by PET scans in 3 out of 4 patients, and small lesions only, in 4 out of 4; no pathology in 5 out of 14 (36 %) patients. Thus, PET indicated various pathological findings correctly in 67 % in this series.

The 4 patients with focal tuberous sclerosis reported by Szelies et al. (1983) all had a corresponding hypometabolic zone. In patients with more widespread epileptogenic lesions suffering from the Lennox-Gastaut syndrome, Gur et al. (1982), Theodore et al. (1984), and Chugani et al. (1984) found various hypometabolic areas either unilateral focal or unilateral diffuse or even bilateral diffuse.

Summarizing these not specifically referenced data, and especially the correlation studies performed at UCLA, the following points should be emphasized: first, in general, good correlations between local hypometabolic PET zone and seizure originating area (as defined by depth EEG recordings) and between local hypometabolic PET zone and structural lesion in the sense of sclerosis were found. Second, the hypometabolic PET zone as a rule considerably exceeded the histologically determined structural lesion (in the resected specimen). Third, no correlation was found between the degree of hypometabolism and the EEG background activity or spike rate.

Ictal PET findings

Spontaneous ictal FDG scans of patients with partial epilepsy have been occasionally obtained by several groups (Engel et al., 1982b; Theodore et al., 1983; Ackerman et al., 1986; Franck et al., 1986). As a rule, interictally hypometabolic zones became hypermetabolic ictally. In addition, other brain areas could become hypermetabolic or instead hypometabolic. In the former instance, preferred ictal spread might be the most likely explanation. It has to be emphasized, however, that because of the long sampling time the socalled ictal scan in reality presents a mixture of interictal (hypometabolic), early ictal (hyper-metabolic focal), late ictal (hypermetabolic - propagated), and postictal (hypometabolic - "exhausted" = depressed) stages. Therefore, it is not surprising that a large variety of ictal patterns were observed. In fact, there are observations where the presumed seizure focus had normal metabolisms ictally, while the remainder of the brain was hypometabolic (Ackerman et al., 1986). Franck et al. (1986) have reported 5 patients during status epilepticus. Their data confirm previous experimental findings that focal ictal status epilepticus is characterized by large increase in cerebral blood flow and metabolism, and that the increase in perfusion always exceeded that in oxygen consumption, resulting in a significant decrease in the oxygen extraction ratio.

Concerning generalized seizures, Engel et al. (1985) have reported 4 petit mal patients with a global increase in glucose utilization when petit mal seizures occurred during a scan. This increase exceeds that found with generalized convulsive seizures following electroconvulsive therapy (ECT). The most likely explanation for this is that petit mal seizures are not followed by electroencephalographic or behavioural postictal depression, whereas the convulsive seizures are followed by one that is profound, so that ictal increase is counter-balanced by postictal metabolic decrease.

It is obvious that, because of the usually unpredictive nature of the seizures, ictal information except in status epilepticus patients or in those patients with a reliable trigger mechanism, is not usually available. This limits the practical application of metabolic PET studies for defining seizure-originating structures, even if sampling times could be shortened to the period of a seizure.

Future perspectives

At least 6 points might be of great promise for the future of PET in epilepsies and especially in their presurgical evaluation:
1. Better spatial resolution (although in the interictal scans the size of the hypometabolic areas seems not to be so much a question of spatial resolution but of the decreased metabolism in the projection areas of the inhibited principle neurons).
2. Identification of distinct abnormal metabolic patterns, and correlating them with all other hitherto used non-invasive and invasive presurgical evaluation techniques, might allow the finding of specific patterns which suggest certain epileptic syndromes suitable for specific surgical approaches (for example, identification of candidates for

154

anterior corpus collosum section).

3. Behavioural activation methods able to activate specific brain regions in a distinct way could probably augment considerably the sensitivity and thereby the diagnostic value of PET.

4. Better time resolution would allow the study of the dynamics of seizures.

5. Great expectations are based on the possibility of studying protein synthesis, blood-brain barrier, diffusion pH and water content (Syrota, 1985) which, according to animal experiments, may be disturbed in the epileptic focus.

6. Moreover, PET techniques have been developed which measure receptor binding sites: The study of dopamin (Garnett et al., 1983), benzo-diazepin (Comar et al., 1979), and opiate receptor binding (Maziere et al., 1981), as well as that of brain metabolism of antiepileptic drugs (Baron et al., 1983; Mintun et al., 1983; Phelps et al., 1982, 1983) offer a new avenue to the better understanding of the basic mechanisms of epilepsy in humans (Delgado-Escueta et al., 1986; Engel, 1987b).

One of the further advantages offered by PET is the fact that this method allows the use of the same radio-isotope techniques in humans which have been applied in animal experiments using contact auto-radiography. Consequently, this should improve direct comparison between animal experimental data and the clinical situation and its direct transference.

REFERENCES

Ackerman, R.F., Engel, J.Jr., Phelps, M.E. 1986. Identification of seizure-mediating brain structures with the deoxyglucose method: studies of human epilepsy with positron emission tomography and animal seizure models with contact autoradiography. In "Advances in Neurology". (Eds. A.V. Delgado-Escueta, A.A. Jr., Ward, D.M. Woodbury, R.J. Porter). (Raven Press, New York). pp 921-934.
Baron, J.C., Comar, D., Crouzel, C. et al. 1983. Brain regional pharmacokinetics of 11-C-labeled diphenylhydantoin and pimozide in man. In "Positron Emission Tomography of the Brain". (Eds. W.-D. Heiss, M.E. Phelps). (Springer, Berlin, Heidelberg, New York). pp. 212-224.
Chugani, H.T., Engel, J.Jr., Mazziotta J.C. et al. 1984. 18-F-2-fluoro-deoxyglucose positron emission tomography in medically refractory childhood epilepsy. Neurology, 34, (Suppl. 1), 107.
Comar, D., Maziere, M., Gadot, J.M. et al. 1979. Visualization of 11-C-flunitrazepam displacement in the brain of the live baboon. Nature, 280, 329-331.
Delgado-Escueta, A.V., Ward, A.A.Jr., Woodbury, D.M. et al. 1986. New wave of research in the epilepsies. In "Advances in Neurology".

(Eds. A.V. Delgado-Escueta, A.A.Jr. Ward, D.M. Woodbury, R.J.
    Porter). (Raven Press, New York). pp. 3-55.
Engel, J.Jr. 1987a. Approaches to localization of the epileptogenic
    lesion. In "Surgical Treatment of the Epilepsies". (Ed. J.Jr.
    Engel). (Raven Press, New York). pp. 75-96.
Engel, J.Jr. 1987b. New concepts of the epileptic focus. In "The
    Epileptic Focus". (Eds. H.-G. Wieser, E.-J. Speckmann, J.Jr.
    Engel). (John Libbey, London, Paris). pp. 83-94.
Engel, J.Jr., Brown, W.J., Kuhl, D.E. et al. 1982a. Pathological
    findings underlying focal temporal lobe hypometabolism in partial
    epilepsy. Ann. Neurol., 12, 518-528.
Engel, J.Jr., Kuhl, D.E., Phelps, M.E. 1982b. Patterns of human local
    cerebral glucose metabolism during seizures. Science, 218, 64-66.
Engel, J.Jr., Lubens, P., Kuhl, D.E. et al. 1985. Local cerebral
    metabolic rate for glucose during petit mal absences. Ann.
    Neurol., 17, 121-128.
Engel, J.Jr., Cahan, L.D., Sutherling, W.W. et al. 1987. The use of
    positron emission tomography in the surgical treatment of
    epilepsy. In "Presurgical Evaluation of Epileptics". (Eds. H.-G.
    Wieser, C.E. Elger). (Springer, Berlin, Heidelberg, New York). in
    press.
Franck, G., Sadzot, B., Salmon, E. et al. 1986. Regional cerebral blood
    flow and metabolic rates in human focal epilepsy and status
    epilepticus. In "Advances in Neurology". (Eds. A.V. Delgado-
    Escueta, A.A.Jr. Ward, D.M. Woodbury, R.J. Porter). (Raven Press,
    New York). pp. 935-948.
Garnett, E.S., Firnau, G., Nahmias, C. 1983. Dopamine visualized in the
    basal ganglia of living man. Nature, 305, 137-138.
Gur, R.C., Sussman, N.M., Alavi, A. et al. 1982. Positron emission
    tomography in two cases of childhood epileptic encephalopathy
    (Lennox-Gastaut syndrome). Neurology, 32, 1191-1195.
Maziere, M., Berger, G., Godot, J.M. et al. 1981. Etorphine 11-C: A new
    tool of the "in vivo" study of brain opiate receptors. J. Label.
    Compounds Radiopharm., 18, 15-16.
Mintun, M.A., Wooten, F., Raichle, M.E. 1983. A quantitative model for
    the in vivo assessment of drug-binding sites with PET. J. Cereb.
    Blood Flow Metabol., 3, (Suppl. 1), 566-567.
Phelps, M.E., Mazziotta, J.C., Huang, S.C. 1982. Study of cerebral
    function with positron computed tomography. J. Cereb. Blood Flow
    Metabol., 2, 113-162.
Phelps, M.E., Schelbert, H., Mazziotta, J.C. 1983. Positron emission
    computed tomography in the study of myocardial and cerebral
    function. Ann. Intern. Med., 98, 339-359.
Sperling, M.R., Sutherling, W.W., Nuwer, M.R. 1987. New techniques for
    evaluating patients for epilepsy surgery. In "Surgical Treatment
    of the Epilepsies". (Ed. J.Jr. Engel). (Raven Press, New York).
    pp. 235-258.
Syrota, A. 1985. Measurement of cerebral protein synthesis and intra-
    cellular pH in man by positron emission tomography. In "Functional
    Mapping of the Brain in Vascular Disorders". (Ed. W.-D. Heiss).
    (Springer, Berlin, Heidelberg, New York, Tokyo). pp 107-121.
Szelies, B., Herholz, K., Heiss, W.-D. et al. 1983. Hypometabolic
    cortical lesions in tuberous sclerosis with epilepsy:
    demonstration by positron emission tomography. J. Comput. Assist.
    Tomogr., 7, 946-953.
Theodore, W.H., Newmark, M.E., Sato, S. et al. 1983. 18-F-fluorodeoxy-

glucose positron emission computed tomography in refractory complex partial seizures. Ann. Neurol., 14, 429-437.

Theodore, W.H., Brooks, R.D., Patrones, N. et al. 1984. Positron emission tomography in the Lennox-Gastaut syndrome. Neurology, 34, (Suppl. 1), 106-107.

Wieser, H.G. 1986. Selective amygdalohippocampectomy: indications, investigative technique and results. In "Advances and Technical Standards in Neurosurgery". (Ed. L. Symon). (Springer, Vienna, New York). pp. 39-133.

Wieser, H.G. 1987. Data analysis. In "Surgical Treatment of the Epilepsies". (Ed. J.Jr. Engel). (Raven Press, New York). pp. 335-360.

Yamamoto, Y.L., Ochs, R., Gloor, P. et al. 1983. Patterns of rCBF and focal energy metabolic changes in relation to electroencephalo-graphic abnormality in the inter-ictal phase of partial epilepsy. In "Current Problems in Epilepsy 1: Cerebral Blood Flow, Metabolism and Epilepsy". (Eds. M. Baldy-Moulinier, D.H. Ingvar, B.S. Meldrum). (John Libbey, London, Paris). pp. 51-62.

Yasargil, M.G., Teddy, P.H., Roth, P. 1985. Selective amygdalo-hippocampectomy. 1: Operative anatomy and surgical technique. In "Advances and Technical Standards in Neurosurgery". (Ed. L. Symon). (Springer, Vienna, New York). pp. 93-123.

B R A I N

Dementias

ENERGY METABOLISM AND NEUROTRANSMITTER FUNCTION IN AGEING AND THE DEMENTIAS

R.S.J. Frackowiak

MRC Cyclotron Unit, Hammersmith Hospital and
National Hospital for Nervous Diseases, Queen Square
London, U.K.

The study of the dementias must be viewed in the context of the physiology of normal ageing. One of the questions that dominated dementia research for a time was whether dementia of the degenerative type constituted an acceleration of the normal ageing process. Other questions in the pathophysiological study of the dementias relate to the relationship between cerebral ischemia and the pathogenesis of multi-infarct disease and the possibility of in vivo aetiological diagnosis using an objective biological test. PET has addressed these questions in a number of ways. Studies of energy metabolism have appeared since 1981, firstly in terms of oxygen metabolism and haemodynamics and then glucose metabolism. Correlations of energy metabolism with type and severity of dementia have been attempted. The distribution of abnormalities of energy metabolism has been correlated with the functional disturbances measured clinically. Specific patterns of disturbed metabolism have been sought in relation to cortical and subcortical dementias and dementias of vascular aetiology. Finally, studies of neurotransmitter function have been undertaken with the dual aim of elucidating pathogenic factors and also developing more specific diagnostic markers.

The diagnosis of dementia is a clinical one. However, its aetiological precision in the earliest stages of disease has always been difficult if only because of the frequent coexistence of Alzheimer's disease and multi-infarct dementia. Dementia may be considered as an end organ failure syndrome with multiple subtending pathogenic mechanisms and aetiologies. PET has been used in an attempt to obtain new insights into these mechanisms in vivo in man. These studies will be briefly reviewed in this report.

PHYSIOLOGY OF AGEING - ENERGY METABOLISM

PET studies in normal ageing have concentrated on defining the normal regional changes in cerebral metabolism and haemodynamics and describing the regional metabolic responses of the brain to physiological stimuli. In relation to energy metabolism the picture remains surprisingly confused, given the quantitative and spatial accuracy afforded by PET technology. A considerable part of the confusion may be ascribed to technical factors as measurements have been made and reported concurrently with rapid advances in their technical precision.

Flow/metabolism relationships

The OER is an expression of the relationship between CBF (i.e. oxygen supply) and $CMRO_2$ (i.e. its utilization). The product of OER and the stable arterial oxygen content is the arterio-venous oxygen difference. The OER expresses the fractional extraction of oxygen, whereas the AVO_2 expresses the absolute oxygen extraction in mlO_2 per ml of blood. It has been clearly demonstrated that the coupling of flow to metabolism is a general phenomenon in the normal brain (Frackowiak et al., 1980; Lebrun-Grandie et al., 1983). The fractional oxygen extraction (OER) is uniformly about 40% (Lammertsma et al., 1983; Lenzi et al., 1983). Changes in OER consequent on variations of oxygen content or p_aCO_2 of arterial blood are likewise generalised phenomena, with no regional emphasis. There have been independent publications from two laboratories which indicate a significant decline of CBF with age in grey matter (Pantano et al., 1984). There is no change in white matter CBF however (Frackowiak, 1982). The variability of the CBF measured in young subjects is considerably greater than in the elderly. On the other hand, measurement of $CMRO_2$ in grey matter has shown an insignificant trend to decline with age in the two largest series reported, despite a coefficient of variation in the measurements of under 10%. The slope of the linear regression of $CMRO_2$ with the age reported from Hammersmith (Frackowiak, 1982) and Orsay (Pantano et al., 1984) was 0.02 ml/100ml/min. This finding is of interest because it constitutes evidence of a small resetting of the CBF: metabolism couple with advancing age.

An increase in the fractional extraction of oxygen from early infancy to adulthood has been recognised in grey matter. This ranges from about 25% in young infants (determined by Kety-Schmidt techniques; Kennedy and Sokoloff, 1957) to 35 - 40% in adults to 45 - 50% in old age (Frackowiak et al., 1984). The significance, in physiological terms, of this slight rise in OER from infancy to old age is difficult to be certain of. It does not represent ischemia as a more than twofold excess of oxygen for metabolic requirements is supplied to the tissue, which constitutes a considerable reserve. The increase is unaccompanied by any alteration of the CBF/CBV ratio (unpublished results from our laboratory), a measure of haemodynamic reserve (Gibbs et al., 1984) which indicates the capacity of the cerebral vessels to dilate in response to a fall in perfusion pressure. There is therefore a normal capacity to autoregulate which regional CBF studies have also demonstrated (Simard et al., 1971) in normal ageing. The basis for the resetting is not precisely known but is probably anatomical. Normal white matter has a metabolic activity and blood flow about quarter that of the grey matter. The difference in capillary density in the two tissues differs by approximately the same amount. It is therefore reasonable to postulate that the slight rise in OER in the face of normal vascular reactivity and autoregulation, represents a gradual decrease in the capillary density with age. The mechanism of such a postulated change can only be conjectural at this stage of our knowledge, but may represent the result of random local occlusions of capillaries for diverse reasons. This would result in an increase in the mean tissue intercapillary distance which governs the shape of the oxygen diffusion gradient and consequently the OER.

Glucose metabolism

Glucose metabolism has been measured in ageing using variations of Sokoloff's deoxyglucose technique (Reivich et al., 1979; Sokoloff, 1981; Sokoloff et al., 1977). This is an analog method which depends on an adequate description of the relationship between the handling of the analog and natural substrate (glucose) by the tissue. If this description is readily quantified the use of the analog (e.g. ^{18}FDG) will result in an accurate measure of the consumption of glucose. The measurement of glucose consumption (CMRGlu) in ageing has not provided consistent results. Thus Kuhl and his colleagues reported a decline in CMRGlu (Kuhl et al., 1982). On the other hand, Rapoport and his colleagues in NIA have reported no significant decline in glucose consumption with age (Duara et al., 1983, 1984). Their study seems to be consistent with the 1960's NIH study with A-V difference techniques (Dastur et al., 1963). The latter study was at variance with most other workers at the time and the discrepancy was attributed to the highly rigorous selection criteria for normality. Similar criteria have been used in the subsequent PET study. Whether the "super-normal" and "normal" aged have different cerebral physiology is one question, the significance of this is another. Studies from Brookhaven also suggest no decline in CMRGlu with normal ageing (DeLeon et al., 1984). It is important to realise that the coefficient of variation of the measurements in the studies from these two centres is of the order 20 - 25%, compared with an 8 - 10% COV in $CMRO_2$ in normal populations. This makes the demonstration of a small, though significant negative correlation between CMRGlu and age difficult. There are still technical factors which require solution before definitive data concerning CMRGlu and normal ageing are produced.

Stoichiometry of energy metabolism

A further problem relating to energy metabolism in normal ageing is whether glucose and oxygen are handled differently by the ageing brain. Kuhl, comparing his results on glucose consumption to the Hammersmith data on oxygen metabolism, showed that the age related decline in CMRGlu was more pronounced than that of $CMRO_2$ (Kuhl et al., 1984). This suggests that the brains of elderly subjects use energy substrates other than glucose (e.g. ketones). Some evidence for such a hypothesis had already been suggested by Gottstein using arterio-venous techniques (Gott-stein et al., 1971). Unfortunately a study of the metabolism of both energy substrates in the same subjects has not been published, though the technical feasibility of making such combined measurements has been demonstrated (Baron et al., 1982)

Atrophy and metabolic measurements

The interpretation of changes in cerebral metabolism in ageing (and dementia) is made difficult because of the possible influence of atrophy on metabolic measurements. Metabolic measurements are made from regions (volumes) of interest defined by the axial resolution of the scanned

tomographic plane and the transaxial area defined in analysis. Such
volumes contain varying proportions of CSF, grey matter, white matter
and other intracranial contents. The choice of regions in making measurements must take cognisance of this fact. Atrophy of cortex which
significantly alters its volumetric dimensions may result in regions of
interest containing smaller or larger proportions of grey and white matter with a resultant apparent decline in cortical metabolism. Herscovitch and his colleagues have described a method of attempted correction
for atrophy based on CT scanning and reported an expected 11% decrease
in metabolism due to atrophic changes associated with normal ageing
(Herscovitch et al., 1984). That this is not the whole story is demonstrated by the fact that CBF and $CMRO_2$ appear to decline at different
rates with age. In any event the site of pathology, whether due to
intrinsically decreased cellular metabolism or cell death, is clearly
demonstrated. The resolution of the problem will come if a general tracer of living neurones can be developed and metabolic rates quoted regionally in terms of neuronal density rather than volume. Correlations
of structural and metabolic abnormalities have been attempted and reported in preliminary form. The different resolution of the two imaging
modalities makes interpretation difficult and too few patients have been
reported to draw firm conclusions (DeLeon et al., 1983a).

Regional function

In terms of regional information, PET has provided accurate regional
distribution of CBF and energy metabolism in different cerebral structures. The hyperfrontal pattern described by Ingvar (1979) in the awake,
alert, normal individual is much less frequently seen than with the
intracarotid ^{133}Xe technique. The reason is probably methodological
and relates to siting of detectors and distribution of the ^{133}Xe after
intracarotid injection. It appears that most cortical regions have similar perfusion and the major difference lies between grey and white matter. The small differences registered by PET between different cortical
areas may be partly explicable in terms of the resolution of the PET
cameras. The cortical strip with a width averaging 3 - 4 mm has been examined to date by instruments with transaxial resolutions averaging 1 -
3 cm². Recently Horwitz has reported that changes in the metabolic
inter-relationships between different brain regions occur with ageing

(Horwitz et al., 1986). The physiological significance of these statistical correlations remains to be elucidated (Ford, 1986)

Physiological stimulation

PET studies of energy metabolism have described perturbations of the normal pattern of distribution of energy metabolism by specific physiological stimuli. Mazziotta, Phelps and colleagues have demonstrated focal increases in cortical metabolism in response to visual, auditory and alerting stimuli during the performance of memory and auditory discrimination tasks (Mazziotta et al., 1981, 1982a, 1982b, 1984; Phelps et al., 1981). This disturbance of the resting state pattern in the normal individual, provides the opportunity for working out intracerebral connections subserving complex functions in the brain. This is an exciting prospect both for the field of normal and diseased neuropsychology. Of particular importance to the study of ageing will be the comparison between the young and elderly of focal patterns and the capacity to augment cerebral metabolism locally in response to standard physiologial stimuli. A disappointment till now has been the apparent inability to describe the effects of stimulation by absolute measures of energy metabolism in the majority of cases. Many of the reports present results in terms of ratios of metabolism - either right/left, anterior/posterior, lobe/lobe or local/global ratios. There are however studies which show a correlation between a graded physiological stimulus and increases in metabolism. Interestingly the physiological response is not always linear (Mazziotta et al., 1982b; Fox and Raichle, 1984, 1985).

VASCULAR DEMENTIA

Multi-infarct dementia constitutes a relatively small cause of mental deterioration in the elderly, though it may coexist with other degenerative diseases and particularly Alzheimer's dementia (Tomlinson et al., 1970). It assumes importance because therapeutic efforts can be made to attempt to halt its course. The study of vascular dementias cannot be considered in isolation from the pathophysiology of acute ischemic brain disease nor an appreciation of the homeostatic mechanisms which normally prevent ischemia in the face of acute or chronic falls in cerebral perfusion. Reviews of insights into these normal and pathological mechanisms obtained with PET have appeared recently (Frackowiak, 1985a, 1985b, 1986) and in this volume.

Chronic ischaemia

Studies of the ischemic pathogenesis of multi-infarct dementia have concentrated on establishing the relationship between CBF and $CMRO_2$ in terms of oxygen extraction (Frackowiak et al., 1981; Gibbs et al., 1986). In a comparison of patients with multi-infarct and degenerative dementia no evidence has been found for a disturbance of the normal balance between CBF and $CMRO_2$ in either group of patients. All the patients with multi-infarct disease were examined in a stable phase of their disease, between acute ischemic events. The observation of a normal OER was true both regionally and globally. This was clear evidence for the absence of any pathogenic mechanism which might be termed "chronic ischaemia". Ischaemia is the pathological state in which energy metabolism and hence function is perfusion limited. The blood supply to the brain is normally considerably in excess to metabolic requirements, hence the extraction of oxygen is normally only 40% or so. The remainder constitutes a reserve which acts to buffer metabolism from normal moment to moment physiological fluctuations of blood flow. Before ischaemia can occur, this reserve must be totally exhausted and oxygen extraction maximal, at which point delivery becomes limiting to metabolism.

We know from pathological studies that the substrate for vascular dementia is the accumulation of ischaemic infarctions, usually beyond a threshold volume and sometimes with strategic placement (Tomlinson et al., 1970). The pathophysiological sequence in these acute events is a fall in perfusion pressure and flow to levels below half of normal. At this stage OER is maximal and ischemia is established. Depending on the depth and duration of ischemia, cell death and/or frank infarction occur. This phase is characterised by low $CMRO_2$ with high OER which rapidly changes to low $CMRO_2$ and low OER with neuronal destruction. Eventually with time, tisssue reparative processes lead to a recoupling of CBF and $CMRO_2$ and hence normalization of OER. If large infarctions occur, OER may remain subnormal. It is of interest in this context that of the 23 patients with multi-infarct dementia studied in our laboratory in the stable inter-ischemic phase of disease, none exhibited global abnormalities of OER.

In certain rare and specific cases patients presenting primarily with dementia have been observed who have demonstrated a chronic focal elevation of OER in the territories of occluded cervical arteries (Gibbs et al., 1986). Such patients invariably have very extensive neck vessel occlusions. The OER lies at submaximal levels of 50 - 70%. This is therefore a precarious situation in which CBF is low and close to ischemic levels. The maintenance of cerebral oxygen delivery is entirely dependent on the small residual arterial oxygen reserve. The capacity for further ischemic episodes to occur would seem a priori to be great in such patients. This pathophysiological situation is rare, dangerous but also potentially amenable to treatment by revascularisation.

DEGENERATIVE DEMENTIA

From the earliest studies of Alzheimer's dementia with PET, changes have been described in energy metabolism (Frackowiak et al., 1981) which have subsequently been confirmed by all laboratories studying both oxygen and glucose consumption (DeLeon et al., 1983b; Duara et al., 1986; Foster et al., 1983, 1984, 1986; Friedland et al., 1983). The principle findings have been a progressive decline of grey matter $CMRO_2$, CMRGlu and CBF with increasing severity of dementia. White matter $CMRO_2$ correlates with the severity of dementia but not the degree of atrophy seen on CT scanning. Patients with mild to moderate dementia exhibit an average 20% decrease in metabolic activity and those with severe disease a 40% decline compared to normal, age-matched subjects (Frackowiak et al., 1981). No correlation has been demonstrated between grey matter CBF and $CMRO_2$ and clinico-pathological type of dementia. This is a finding at variance with the earlier (non-PET) CBF literature which suggested that changes in CBF in early cases of dementia distinguished degenerative from multi-infarct disease (Harrison et al., 1979).

Temporo-parietal metabolism

Focal CBF and $CMRO_2$ abnormalities are seen in degenerative dementia of Alzheimer type. The most characteristic, seen in early to moderate disease, is a depression of metabolism in the posterior temporal-parietal regions bilaterally (Frackowiak et al., 1981). This region shows the smallest age related decline in $CMRO_2$ (9% decline in normal ageing with a further 29% fall in dementia). With increasing severity of disease, the frontal regions also show striking depression of metabolism. There is relative sparing of occipital and primary motor-sensory cortices within the context of a generalised global decline in cortical energy metabolism. The basis for this focal emphasis of pathology is not entirely clear.

Studies of glucose consumption show similar changes (Duara et al., 1986). The most commonly reported is the focalized posterior temporal-parietal depression. Some reports suggest that the expression of cortical metabolic activity as a frontal to parietal ratio provides an index with high sensitivity to the presence of dementia (Friedland et al., 1983). In the patients with mild to moderate disease it is claimed that the ratio will distinguish disease from normal ageing with no overlap between the groups. The frontal decline in energy metabolism seen in advanced disease has been confirmed recently in terms of CMRGlu (Duara et al., 1986).

Studies of glucose consumption have also addressed the question of the sensitivity of metabolic changes to dementia (Cutler et al., 1985a; Haxby et al., 1985). There are reports that patients with mild, but clinically evident dementia do not show a fall in cortical metabolism in comparison to normal volunteers. This is at variance with the reports measuring $CMRO_2$ in which a negative linear correlation has been demonstrated with disease severity. It is possible that small depressions in CMRGlu have not been recognised because of the large coefficient of variation in the normal CMRGlu data.

Metabolism/functional correlation

Focal abnormalities have been correlated with functional changes determined clinically (Chase et al., 1984; Foster et al., 1984, 1986). In particular, aphasia, apraxia and visuo-spatial function have been correlated with changes in CMRGlu in the appropriate hemisphere. Such lobar changes have also been reported in terms of $CMRO_2$, but were demonstrated to be bilateral with some increased emphasis on the appropriate side (Frackowiak et al., 1981). The resolution of earlier generation tomographs with which many of these studies were performed was poor and it is likely that with newer cameras such focal structure-function relationships may become more precisely defined.

Rare patients with apparent degenerative dementia of Alzheimer type have been described with remarkably asymmetrical abnormalities of parietal metabolism (CMRGlu) (Chase et al., 1984) and different hemispheric asymmetries have been reported in early and late onset Alzheimer's disease (Koss et al., 1985). No specific reports of cases with atypical presentation of Alzheimer's disease with focal disability (such as slowly progressive aphasia) have been reported. Members of a family with Alzheimer disease have been studied and posterior temporal-parietal changes, indistinguishable from those seen in sporadic cases of the disease have been described in affected individuals (Cutler et al., 1985b). There has been insufficient length of follow-up to determine whether at-risk individuals who develop disease show progressive metabolic changes and whether they differ from at-risk subjects who do not develop dementia.

Diagnosis

The question of the specificity of changes in energy metabolism in Alzheimer's disease has been the subject of a number of studies. Kuhl has shown posterior temporal-parietal hypometabolism in patients with Parkinsonism and dementia (Kuhl et al., 1985a). A striking case study in this report demonstrates a normal pattern of CMRGlu in a patient with normal mentation and Parkinsonism, which becomes abnormal four years later, coincidentally with the development of dementia.

Patients with dementia associated with progressive supranuclear palsy show a marked decline in frontal CMRGlu without posterior changes (D'Antona et al., 1985). This pattern has also been demonstrated in terms of oxygen metabolism (Leenders et al., 1986a). A similar pattern has been described in patients with Pick's disease (Chase - communicated at a meeting on dementia - Heidelberg 1986). Patients with Huntington's disease demonstrate global cortical hypometabolism without focal cortical emphasis but with marked metabolic depression in the caudate even when it appears structurally normal in CT (Hayden et al., 1986; Kuhl et al., 1985b). There are suggestions that the caudate metabolic changes may antedate the development of symptoms of the disease and therefore act as a marker of Huntington gene carrier status. More studies are needed to confirm whether this impression is true. Jacob-Creutzfeldt dementia has been reported to show changes similar to Alzheimer's disease (Friedland et al., 1984). Systematic studies of patients with pseudodementia (dementia of depression) are however lacking. Normal pressure hydrocephalus has been differentiated from Alzheimer's disease in metabolic terms also (Jagust et al., 1985).

Clearly, abnormalities of posterior temporal-parietal energy metabolism are not very specific for Alzheimer's disease on their own, though in clinical context the changes assume greater significance.

NEUROCHEMISTRY IN VIVO

Other functional aspects of cerebral metabolism have been examined with PET techniques in man. Studies of protein metabolism in Alzheimer's dementia, though preliminary, show a very similar distribution of defects of amino acid (methionine) incorporation into protein as the studies of energy metabolism (Bustany et al., 1983a, 1983b, 1985). There is no change in the permeability of the blood-brain-barrier to methionine, but the turnover of the free amino acid pool is greatly decreased, especially in frontal and temporo-parietal areas.

The elaboration of methods to measure neurotransmitter function are in early stages of development, but constitute an important growth area in PET of potential significance to the study of ageing and the pathogenesis of the degenerative dementias (for example, changes in dopamine and serotonin) receptors have been demonstrated to occur with normal ageing (Wong et al., 1984). There are also significant diagnostic implications. It has been shown that [76]Br-bromospiperone binding is decreased in the basal ganglia and in the frontal cortex of patients with progressive supranuclear palsy (Baron et al., 1986). This ligand is a potent dopamine D_2 receptor antagonist (with some anti-serotonin S_2 activity probably explaining the cortical changes). Studies of dopaminergic function with ^{18}F-DOPA show there is also depressed uptake and retention of this ligand at presynaptic sites in the striatum (Leenders et al., 1986a). In Parkinsonism, a number of groups have demonstrated decreased ^{18}F-DOPA associated uptake and retention in the striatum (Leenders et al., 1986b). Normal ^{11}C-methylspiperone binding has been demonstrated in this disease (Leenders et al., 1986c). In Huntington's disease ^{18}F-DOPA uptake is normal, but ^{11}C-methyl-spiperone binding is depressed (Leenders et al., 1986d).

It is clear from these preliminary observations that there are different and characteristic patterns of pre and post-synaptic dysfunction in these subcortical diseases associated with dementia. The combination of measures of energy metabolism and specific markers of neurotransmitter function seem to be a more sensitive approach to the diagnosis of specific dementing diseases and may provide important information regarding pathogenesis in the future.

REFERENCES

Baron, J.C., Lebrun-Grandie, P., Collard, P., et al. 1982. Non invasive measurement of blood flow, oxygen consumption and glucose utilisation in the same brain regions in man by positron emission tomography: concise communication. J. Nucl. Med., 23, 391-399.

Baron, J.C., Maziere, B., Loc'h, C., et al. 1986. Loss of striatal (76Br)bromospiperone binding sites demonstrated by positron tomography in progressive supranuclear palsy. J. Cereb. Blood Flow Metab., 6, 131-136.

Bustany, P., Henry, J.F., DeRotrou, J., et al. 1985. Correlations between clinical state and positron emission tomography measurement of local brain protein synthesis in Alzheimers disease, Parkinsons disease, schizophrenia and gliomas: In "The Metabolism of the Human Brain studied with Positron Emission Tomography" (Eds. T. Greitz, D. Ingvar and L. Widen). (Raven Press, New York). pp. 241-249.

Bustany, P., Henry, J.F., Sargent, T., et al. 1983. Local brain protein metabolism in dementia and schizophrenia: in vivo studies with 11-C-L-methionine and positron emission tomography. In "Positron Emission Tomography of the Brain" (Eds. W.-D. Heiss and M.E. Phelps). (Springer-Verlag, New York). pp. 208-211.

Bustany, P., Henry, J.F., Soussaline, F., et al. 1983. Brain protein synthesis in normal and demented patients - a study by positron emission tomography with 11-C-L-methionine. In "Functional radionuclide Imaging of the Brain" (Ed. P.L. Magistretti). (Raven Press, New York). pp. 319-326.

Chase, T.N., Foster, L.N., Fedio, P., et al. 1984. Regional cortical dysfunction in Alzheimers disease as determined by positron emission tomography. Ann. Neurol., 15, (Suppl. 3), S170-S174.

Cutler, N.R., Haxby, J.V., Duara, R., et al. 1985a. Clinical history brain metabolism and neuropsychological function in Alzheimer's disease. Ann. Neurol., 18, 298-309.

Cutler, N.R., Haxby, J.V., Duara, R., et al. 1985b. Brain metabolism as measured with positron emission tomography: serial assessment in a patient with familial Alzheimer's disease. Neurology, 35, 1556-1561.

D'Antona, R., Baron, J.C., Samson, Y., et al. 1985. Subcortical dementia: frontal cortex hypometabolism detected by positron tomography in patients with progressive supranuclear palsy. Brain, 108, 785-800.

Dastur, D.K., Lane, M.H., Hansen, D.B., et al. 1963. Effects of aging on cerebral circulation and metabolism in man. In "Human aging. US Public Health Service Publ. no 986" (Eds. J.E. Barren, R.N. Butler, S.W. Greenhouse et al.). (US Public Health Service Publ., Washington). pp. 59-76.

DeLeon, M., George, A.E., Ferris, S.H., et al. 1984. Positron emission tomography and computed tomographic assessment of the human brain. J. Comput. Assist. Tomogr., 8, 88-94.

DeLeon, M.J., Ferris, S.H., George, A.E., et al. 1983a. Computed tomography and positron emission transaxial tomography evaluations of normal aging and Alzheimer's disease. J. Cereb. Blood Flow Metab., 3, 391-394.

DeLeon, M.J., Ferris, S.H., George, A.E., et al. 1983b. Positron emission tomographic studies of aging and Alzheimer's disease. AJNR, 4, 568-571.

Duara, R., Margolin, R.A., Robertson-Tschabo, E.A., et al. 1983. Resting cerebral glucose utilisation as measured with positron emission tomography in 21 healthy men between the ages of 21 and 83 years. Brain, 106, 761-775.

Duara, R., Grady, C., Haxby, J., et al. 1984. Human brain glucose utilisation and cognitive function in relation to age. Ann. Neurol., 16, 702-713.

Duara, R., Grady, C., Haxby, J., et al. 1986. Positron emission tomography in Alzheimer's disease. Neurology, 36, 879-887.

Ford, I. 1986. Confounded correlations: statistical limitations in the analysis of inter-regional relationships of cerebral metabolic activity. J. Cereb. Blood Flow Metab., 6, 385-388.

Foster, N.L., Chase, T.N., Fedio, P., et al. 1983. Alzheimer's disease: focal cortical changes shown by positron emission tomography. Neurology, 33, 961-965.

Foster, N.L., Chase, T.N., Mansi, L., et al. 1984. Cortical abnormalities in Alzheimer's disease. Ann. Neurol., 16, 649-654.

Foster, N.L., Chase, T.N., Patronas, N.J., et al. 1986. Cerebral mapping of apraxia in Alzheimer's disease by positron emission tomography. Ann. Neurol., 19, 139-143.

Fox, P.T. and Raichle, M.E. 1984. Stimulus rate dependence of regional cerebral blood flow in human striate cortex demonstrated by positron emission tomography. J. Neurophysiol., 51, 1109-1120.

Fox, P.T. and Raichle, M.E. 1985. Stimulus rate determines regional brain blood flow in striate cortex. Ann. Neurol., 17, 303-305.

Frackowiak, R.S.J. 1982. Human regional cerebral blood flow and oxygen metabolism studied with oxygen-15 and positron emission tomography. MD Thesis Cambridge, 1-209.

Frackowiak, R.S.J. 1985a. The pathophysiology of human cerebral ischaemia: a new perspective obtained with positron tomography. Quat. J. Med., 57, 713-727.

Frackowiak, R.S.J. 1985b. Pathophysiology of human cerebral ischaemia: studies with positron tomography and oxygen-15. In "Brain Imaging and Brain Function" (Ed. L. Sokoloff). (Raven Press, New York). pp. 139-162.

Frackowiak, R.S.J. 1986. PET scanning: can it help resolve management issues in cerebral ischemic disease. (Editorial). Stroke, 17, 803-807.

Frackowiak, R.S.J, Lenzi, G.L., Jones, T., et al. 1980. Quantitative measurement of regional cerebral blood flow and oxygen metabolism in man using 15-0 and positron emission tomography: theory, procedure and normal values. J. Comput. Assist. Tomogr., 4, 727-736.

Frackowiak, R.S.J., Pozzilli, C., Legg, N.J., et al. 1981. Regional cerebral oxygen supply and utilisation in dementia: a clinical and physiological study with oxygen-15 and positron tomography. Brain, 104, 753-778.

Frackowiak, R.S.J., Wise, R.J.S., Gibbs, J.M., et al. 1984. Oxygen extraction in the ageing brain. Monogr. Neurol. Sci., 11, 118-122.

Friedland, R.P., Budinger, T.F., Ganz, E., et al. 1983. Regional cerebral metabolic alterations in dementia of the Alzheimer type: positron emission tomography with (18-F)-fluorodeoxyglucose. J. Comput. Assist. Tomogr., 7, 590-598.

Friedland, R.P., Prusiner, S.B., Jagust, W.J., et al. 1984. Bitemporal hypometabolism in Creutzfeldt-Jacob disease measured by positron emission tomography with (18-F)-2-fluorodeoxyglucose. J. Comput. Assist. Tomogr., 8, 978-981.

Gibbs, J.M., Wise, R.J.S., Leenders, K.L., et al. 1984. Evaluation of cerebral perfusion reserve in patients with carotid artery occlusion. Lancet, 1, 310-314.

Gibbs, J.M., Frackowiak, R.S.J. and Legg, N.J. 1986. Regional cerebral blood flow and oxygen metabolism in dementia due to vascular disease. Gerontology, 32, (Suppl. 1), 84-88.

Gottstein, U., Müller, W., Berghoff, W., et al. 1971. Zur Utilisation von nicht-veresterten Fettsäuren und Ketonkörpern im Gehirn des Menschen. Klin. Wschr., 49, 406-411.

Harrison, M.J.G., Thomas, D.J., DuBoulay, G.H., et al. 1979. Multi-infarct dementia. J. Neurol. Sci., 40, 97-103.

Haxby, J.V., Duara, R., Grady, C.L., et al. 1985. Relations between neurophysiological and cerebral metabolic asymmetries in early Alzheimer's disease. J. Cereb. Blood Flow Metab., 5, 193-200.

Hayden, M.R., Martin, W.R.W., Stoessl, A.J., et al. 1986. Positron emission tomography in the early diagnosis of Huntington's disease. Neurology, 36, 888-894.

Herscovitch, P., Gado, M., Mintun, M.A. 1984. The necessity for correcting for cerebral atrophy in global positron emission tomography measurements. Monogr. Neural. Sci., 11, 93-97.

Horwitz, B., Duara, R. and Rapoport, S.I. 1986. Age differences in intercorrelations between regional cerebral metabolic rates for glucose. Ann. Neurol., 19, 60-67.

Ingvar, D.H. 1979. Hyperfrontal distribution of the cerebral grey matter flow in resting wakefulness: on the functional anatomy of the concious state. Acta Neurol. Scand., 60, 12-25.

Jagust, W.J., Friedland, R.P., Budinger, T.F. 1985. Positron emission tomography with (18-F)fluorodeoxyglucose differentiates normal pressure hydrocephalus from Alzheimer type dementia. J. Neurol. Neurosurg. Psychiat., 48, 1091-1096.

Kennedy, C. and Sokoloff, L. 1957. An adaptation of the nitrous oxide method to the study of the cerebral circulation in children: normal values for cerebral blood flow and cerebral metabolic rate in childhood. J. Clin. Invest., 36, 1130-1137.

Koss, E., Friedland, R.P., Ober, B.A., et al. 1985. Differences in lateral hemispheric asymmetries of glucose utilisation between early and late onset Alzheimer-type dementia. Amer. J. Psychiat., 142, 638-640.

Kuhl, D.E., Metter, E.J., Riege, W.H., et al. 1982. Effects of human ageing on patterns of local cerebral glucose utilisation determined by the 18-F-fluorodeoxyglucose method. J. Cereb. Blood Flow Metab., 2, 163-171.

Kuhl, D.E., Metter, E.J., Riege, W.H., et al. 1984. The effect of normal ageing on patterns of local cerebral glucose utilisation. Ann. Neurol., 15, (Suppl.), S133-S137.

Kuhl, D.E., Metter, E.J., Benson, D.F., et al. 1985a. Similarities of cerebral glucose metabolism in Alzheimer's and Parkinsonian dementia. J. Cereb. Blood Flow Metab., 5, (Suppl. 1), S169-S170.

Kuhl, D.E., Markham, C.H., Metter, E.J., et al. 1985b. Local cerebral glucose utilisation in symptomatic and pre-symptomatic Huntington's disease. In " Brain Imaging and Brain Function" (Ed. L. Sokoloff). (Raven Press, New York). pp. 199-209.

Lammertsma, A.A., Wise, R.J.S., Heather, J.D., et al. 1983. The correction for the presence of intravascular oxygen-15 in the steady state technique for measuring regional oxygen extraction ratio in the brain. II. Results in normal subjects, brain tumour and stroke patients. J. Cereb. Blood Flow Metab., 3, 425-431.

Lebrun-Grandie, P., Baron, J.C., Soussaline, F., et al. 1983. Coupling between regional blood flow and oxygen utilisation in the normal human brain. Arch. Neurol., 40, 230-236.

Leenders, K.L., Frackowiak, R.S.J. and Lees, A.J. 1986a. Steele-Richardson-Olszweski syndrome: brain energy metabolism, blood flow and fluorodopa uptake measured by positron emission tomography. Brain, submitted.

Leenders, K.L., Palmer, A.J., Quinn, N., et al. 1986b. Brain dopamine metabolism in patients with Parkinson's disease measured with positron emission tomography. J. Neurol. Neurosurg. Psychiat., 49, 853-860

Leenders, K.L., Palmer, A., Turton, D., et al. 1986c. DOPA uptake and dopamine receptor binding visualised in the human brain in vivo. In "Recent Developments in Parkinsons disease" (Eds. S. Fahn, C.D. Marsden, J. Jenner, et al.) (Raven Press, New York). pp. 103-113.

Leenders, K.L., Frackowiak, R.S.J., Quinn, N., et al. 1986d. Brain energy metabolism and dopaminergic function in Huntington's disease measured in vivo using positron emission tomography. Movement Disorders, 1, 69-77.

Lenzi, G.L., Gibbs, J.M., Frackowiak, R.S.J., et al. 1983. Measurement of cerebral blood flow and oxygen metabolism by positron emission tomography und the 15-O steady state technique aspects of methodology, reproducibility and clinical application. In "Functional Radionuclide Imaging of the Brain" (Ed. P.L. Magistretti). (Raven Press, New York). pp. 291-304.

Mazziotta, J.C., Phelps, M.E., Miller, J., et al. 1981. Tomographic mapping of human cerebral metabolism: normal unstimulated state. Neurology, 31, 503-516.

Mazziotta, J.C., Phelps, M.E., Carson, R.E., et al. 1982a. Tomographic mapping of human cerebral metabolism: auditory stimulation. Neurology, 32, 921-937.

Mazziotta, J.C., Phelps, M.E., Carson, R.E., et al. 1982b. Tomographic
    mapping of human cerebral metabolism: sensory deprivation. Ann.
    Neurol., 12, 435-444.
Mazziotta, J.C., Phelps, M.E. and Carson, R.E. 1984. Tomographic map-
    ping of human cerebral metabolism: subcortical responses to audi-
    tory and visual stimulation. Neurology, 34, 825-828.
Pantano, P., Baron, J.C., Lebrun-Grandie, P., et al. 1984. Regional
    cerebral blood flow and oxygen consumption in human ageing.
    Stroke, 15, 635-641.
Phelps, M.E., Mazziotta, J.C., Kuhl, D.E., et al. 1981. Tomographic
    mapping of human cerebral metabolism: visual stimulation and de-
    privation. Neurology, 31, 517-529.
Reivich, M., Kuhl, D., Wolf, A., et al. 1979. The 18-F-fluorodeoxy-
    glucose method for the measurement of local cerebral glucose
    utilisation in man. Circ. Res., 44, 127-137.
Simard, D., Olesen, J., Paulson, O.B., et al. 1971. Regional cerebral
    blood flow and its regulation in dementia. Brain, 94, 273-288.
Sokoloff, L. 1981. Localisation of functional activity in the central
    nervous system by measurement of glucose utilisation with radio-
    active deoxyglucose. J. Cereb. Blood Flow Metab., 1, 7-36.
Sokoloff, L., Reivich, M., Kennedy, C., et al. 1977. The (C-14)-deoxy-
    glucose method for the measurement of local glucose utilisation:
    theory, procedure and normal values in the concious anaesthetised
    albino rat. J. Neurochem., 28, 897-916.
Tomlinson, B.E., Blessed, G. and Roth, M. 1970. Observations on the
    brains of demented old people. J. Neurol. Sci., 11, 205-242.
Wong, D.F., Wagner, H.N., Dannals, R.F., et al. 1984. Effects of age
    on dopamine and serotonin receptors measured by positron tomo-
    graphy in the living human brain. Science, 226, 1393-1396.

PET IN DEMENTIA AND GLIOMAS

P. Bustany, M. Moulin

Centre Hospitalier Régional et Universitaire de Caen
Laboratoire de Pharmacologie et des Explorations Fonctionelles B
Caën, Cedex, France

The widening of the clinical application field of PET in the near future depends on its ability to provide clinical or diagnostic information which, in the clinical context, can reduce morbidity or mortality and the risk of treatment, improve patient care, or help to control the cost of medical care (Phelps et al., 1985; Nilsson et al., 1985; Powers et al., 1985; Wagner, 1985). PET correlations with widely applied diagnostic methods or low-cost methods of clinical investigation routinely used in general hospitals must be explored and soon be firmly established so as to allow a significant spreading of any positive results of a therapeutic action studied by PET in a limited group of carefully selected patients. Besides, under certain circumstances, PET can provide invaluable information favoring a therapeutic decision, where the benefit/risk ratio is positive for the patient: the elimination of invasive or agressive tests that are very likely negative, or inefficient revascularization surgery by arterial by-passing on definitely necrotic or unviable brain or heart tissue.

In vivo pharmacology designed to define the toxicology or usefulness of new drugs and their specific indications remains one of the major fields of the clinical application of PET. Quantitative data provided by PET, based on sophisticated models and statistical correlations, or even a qualitative imaging of human brain diseases, are among the most important findings of modern neurology. Furthermore, PET, in some of its uses, is the most sensitive way to detect directly and atraumatically the very early and mild metabolic impairments in borderline or still unclassified diseases, such as senile dementia of the Alzheimer type (SDAT) versus multi-infarct dementia (MID) - see below -, incomplete resection of a brain tumor, or its extension versus radionecrosis, metabolic sequelae of a transient ischemic attack, etc. In the actual cost-containment climate of health care, it is possible for PET to hold a growing share of interest in a clinical environment by the rapid and widespread integration of the results obtained by well-found clinical studies of the efficacy of the therapeutic regimen used during routine medical care in any hospital.

SENILE DEMENTIA OF THE ALZHEIMER TYPE

A better understanding of the basic biochemical abnormalities leading to the clinical state of dementia was one of the first aims chosen worldwide by many PET groups. Ten years later, the most important findings obtained by PET on various cerebral metabolic pathways can be summarized as follows:

Cerebral blood flow

Using for instance the ^{15}O method, PET made it possible to quantatively measure CBF in slices of human brain, but compared with other techniques, PET requires stricter control of study conditions (Dhawan et al., 1986). In summary, the etiology of SDAT seems to be unrelated to CBF and CBV (Lammertsma and Frackowiak, 1985). Today, the global CBF decrease during normal aging that was first reported, is no longer considered a functional reality (see below discussion about glucose metabolism). Nevertheless, in SDAT and MID, a specific pattern of decrease in frontal and temporo-parietal regions occurs. In MID patients, CBF values begin to decline some 2 years before onset of symptoms, while in SDAT patients, CBF levels remain normal until symptoms of dementia appear and CBF declines rapidly (Rogers et al., 1986). PET also confirmed ^{133}Xe findings of a frontal hypoperfusion in Pick's disease, SDAT and other disorders (Risberg, 1986), and it clearly showed typical patterns of hypoperfusion in SDAT: -15% in frontal cortex, -20% in temporal cortex, -18% in occipital cortex, -12% in thalamus, etc. (Amano et al., 1982; Dastur, 1985). This hemodynamic pattern is quite typical and it involves non-specifically various metabolic processes as well, suggesting that a real coupling between blood supply and local metabolic demands persists through dementia. In 1975, Hachinski et al. used Xe-133 measurements of CBF to differentiate between primary degenerative dementia where CBF was not correlated with the clinical degree of dementia, and MID where CBF seemed to be inversely correlated. Obrist et al. (1970) and Sokoloff (1978) also reported significant brain hypoperfusion in SDAT and suggested its use for the differential diagnosis of dementias. PET studies confirmed that the CBF pattern characteristic of SDAT was largely non-focal at a level significantly below the mean of age-matched control groups. PET abnormalities can be (and often have been) used by clinicians to distinguish between MID,

SDAT, and affective disorders, but in these cases, assessment of CBF was usually performed by ^{133}Xe techniques or SPECT (Gustafson et al., 1981) rather than by PET.

Oxygen metabolism

This PET method validated by Grubb et al. in 1977 was used by Frackowiak et al. (1981) and Lammertsma and Frackowiak (1985) in comprehensive studies of SDAT and vascular dementia. Depending on the severity of clinical symptoms, a marked drop in $CMRO_2$ and CBF (by 20 to 30%) in the same typical frontal and temporal regions was reported, confirming the decrease in brain oxygen consumption detected by the Kety-Schmidt method (Lassen et al., 1959).

Glucose metabolism

Contrary to many previous and even recent PET reports on absolute regional values of CMRG, the glucose metabolism of mammalian brains is now considered to remain globally unchanged during normal aging, provided that some corrections for brain atrophy are made in the computation of regional volume activities measured by PET (Herscovitch et al. 1986). The increasing dendritic branching and sprouting in aging brain seems to compensate for neuronal cells loss. This plasticity was considered to be the basis of "crystallized" intelligence accompanied by a general shrinkage of cells (Cutler et al., 1985a). This could explain the relative hypodensity revealed by X-ray CT in aging brains and, as the individual surface and volume of neural cells increases, the age-invariance and sometimes even small increase in glucose metabolic rates calculated for some regions after correction (Kuhl et al., 1982; Duara et al., 1983; Smith, 1984; Dastur, 1985; Cutler et al., 1985a, 1985b; Rapoport et al., 1985). These results are in good agreement with data on CBF and $CMRO_2$ in aging, collected by Pantano et al. (1984).

In dementia, FDG-PET procedures provide a unique way to quantify and validate in humans the effects of some drug treatments since no adequate animal model of the disease is known. The tremendous problem of experimentation was the reason why significant efforts were devoted worldwide to PET in SDAT. The decrease in metabolic activity in SDAT (up to 50%) was highly correlated with psychometric measures of cognitive impairment (Ferris et al., 1980; Farkas et al., 1982; Foster et al., 1984). The threshold of obvious metabolic impairment is reached very late in the evolution of SDAT, and it is impossible to study the early phases of the disease with sufficient statistical confidence in PET values to base on them any therapeutic protocol for an individual patient. Because of specific technical problems, such as a coefficient of variation of 20 - 26% for model values, a decrease in local CMRG of 20 - 25% (Duara et al., 1983; Reivich et al., 1983) can not be considered a "useful early marker" of SDAT (Haxby et al., 1985; Foster and Chase, 1986). With the usual statistical limit of $\pm$ 1.96 SD, direct estimates of CMRG are of negligible clinical use. A much more sensitive way of analysis is required to compare the absolute patterns of CMRG recorded in SDAT and other brain diseases.

Regional intercorrelations of CMRG are very sensitive to the disease (Kuhl et al., 1983; Kuhl, 1984; Horwitz et al., 1984). Also, metabolic asymmetries seem to be a valuable marker of SDAT (Haxby et al., 1985; Duara et al., 1986). This method allowed to distinguish typical FDG patterns in stroke, to categorize depressed (subnormal images) or demented patients (frontal and parieto-temporal decreases, with caudate and thalamus quite often normal), MID cases studded with multiple metabolic defects, Huntington's disease (caudate markedly hypometabolic, even without atrophy, and mildly hypometabolic before the appearance of symptoms), partial epilepsy (interictally well-defined hypometabolic zones were sites of onset of seizures), etc. (Benson et al., 1983; Kuhl, 1984; Heiss et al., 1986). Qualitative patterns were used to distinguish SDAT from normal-pressure hydrocephalus, a common clinical dilemma (Jagust et al., 1985), and to follow the course of SDAT (Friedland et al., 1985). Metter et al. (1984) differentiated primarily cortical disorders, such as SDAT, and subcortical disorders, such as Huntington's or Parkinson's disease, by screening local CMRG. The clinical signs of apraxia in SDAT patients were related to the functional impairment of a brain region that was known to be functionally linked to apraxia if injured, and the authors proposed a clinical grading of the disease according to this apraxia to command and imitation, since this easily evaluated sign was directly related to the biochemical abnormalities of the brain (Foster et al., 1986, Foster and Chase, 1986). As an important step toward the elucidation of the complex situation encountered in aging, depression and dementia, Rapoport's group correlated the asymmetrical patterns found

in FDG-PET studies of beginning diseases with psychometric test results
(see Haxby et al., 1985). Nevertheless, a noticeable memory loss often
preceded any measurable reduction of CMRG in early SDAT, where a potentially beneficial drug treatment could still be installed before
the eventual tissue destruction. At later stages, typical depression
of parietal lobe metabolism may not be accompanied by any further
measurable neuropsychological deficits in the same patients (Cutler et
al., 1985a, 1985b). This uncoupling between the metabolic activity of
the brain and its psychological function severely limits the use of PET
for the detection of, say, the onset of SDAT, and therefore comprehensive psychometric testing remains the most efficient way of screening
for the prevalence of the disease in an at-risk group of patients with
early forms of still uncategorized dementias (Israel et al., 1984).
Great hopes continue to be placed on FDG studies of schizophrenia,
major affective and sleep disorders (Kuhl, 1983; Dastur, 1985; Heiss
et al., 1986).

Protein synthesis

In aging rats, a decrease in the brain protein synthesis rate (PSR)
of 20 - 25% was reported by Ingvar et al. (1984) using labelled leucine.
This value is similar to the estimate obtained with deoxyglucose in the
same condition. It probably reflects the structural effect of age on
cells and could also be corrected according to the rules used for CMRG
(Cutler et al., 1985a, 1985b; Herscovitch et al., 1986), thus confirming
fundamental in vitro data: in rats, considering the number of remaining
brain cells, protein synthesis does not decrease markedly with age. In a
human PET study with methionine, we also observed a reduction of PSR in
the frontal lobe and in the whole brain, up to approx. 55 years of age,
where the negative slope of this straight line increased slightly
(Bustany et al., 1985a, 1985b). It should be noted though, that we de-
liberately studied aged subjects considered as clinically and psycho-
metrically normal with respect to age, without selection of a "super-
normal" cohort which would have kept during aging the intellectual and
psychometric abilities of the youngest control groups. The decrease with
age in brain protein turnover, possibly concurrent with a maintained
glucose consumption rate, is not paradoxical because the flux of a

metabolite (glucose) through any biochemical pathway in the brain is generally unrelated to the renewal rate of the enzyme proteins involved in this function. In rats, we recently found by direct cortical sampling from brain slices, TCA separation and characterization of labelled proteins that a 30 - 35% decrease in PSR occurred in 26-month-old rats, a value very similar to the human change of PSR (Bustany et al., 1985b). The extra activity in PSR found in young subjects versus old ones, compared to CMRG values, may be explained by the fact that many neuronal cells are in a quiescent state in young brain (redundancy; Rapoport et al., 1985) and are responsible for a noticeable percentage of normal PSR without being involved in the active circuitry of neuronal transmission and, therefore, exhibit only minimal glucose consumption. Loss of cells during aging is then accompanied by a proportional decrease in overall PSR, while gobal CMRG is maintained at about the same level.

TABLE 1 ^{11}C-L-Methyionine metabolism in normal and demented subjects (whole cortex at level OM + 5 cm)

	Normal (n=20) Age 80.2 ± 9.4 years	Demented (n=25) 86.3 ± 6.0 years
Input (nmol/g/min)	0.46 ± 0.16	$*0.31 \pm 0.12$
Half-life (min)	8.1 ± 1.9	$°9.0 \pm 2.7$
Incorporation (nmol/g/min)	0.15 ± 0.05	$**0.09 \pm 0.05$
Extraction (%)	24.7 ± 9.4	$*14.9 \pm 5.7$

**: $P<0.01$; °: $P>0.6$: N.S.; *: $P<0.05$

In SDAT, frontal PSR seems to be decreased very early (Fig. 1; Bustany et al., 1983a, 1985a, 1985b) as can be seen from Tables 1 and 2.

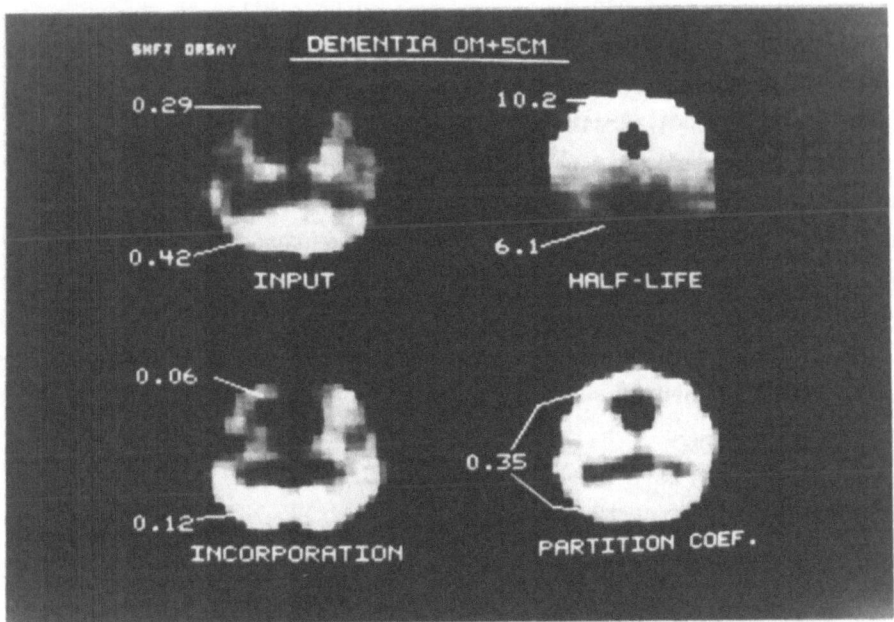

Fig. 1 Metabolic maps at 5 cm above orbitomeatal level in an Alz-heimer-type demented patient. Input and incorporation expressed as nmol/g brain/min (see Tables 1 and 2); half-life in min. Partition coefficient for methionine between brain spaces and blood remains very constant in all slices, reflecting the normal state of BBB. (Each image is scaled individually). No abnormalities were visible on the CT scan of this patient.

TABLE 2 Local brain protein synthesis
(L-methionine incorporation in nmol/g/min)

R.O.I.	Normal (n=20)	Demented (n=25)	Mild dementia (n=8)	Severe dementia (n=17)
Frontal	0.15 + 0.06	**0.09 + 0.03	0.13 + 0.03	***0.05 + 0.02
Occipital	0.16 + 0.06	°0.15 + 0.07	0.15 + 0.05	(*)0.10 + 0.04
F/O Ratio	0.96 + 0.11	**0.64 + 0.21	0.89 + 0.18	***0.52 + 0.13

°: $P < 0.10$: N.S.; (*): $P < 0.10$; **: $P < 0.01$; ***$P < 0.005$

The absolute degree of PSR impairment was quite similar to the respective CMRG changes and, likewise, could not be used without a complete statistical analysis for the purpose of early diagnostic classification. Like for CMRG in SDAT (Foster et al., 1984), at the clinical detection threshold of the dementia, where only transient or mild memory impairment could be demonstrated by the psychometric assessment of brain functions, a significant decrease in PSR was measured in the frontal lobes of young Alzheimer-type demented patients (-12 to -18%), when the partial correlation method was used (Horwitz et al., 1984). A poor correlation between frontal or other grey matter PSR and psychometric tests was also found in normal subjects (Fig. 2).

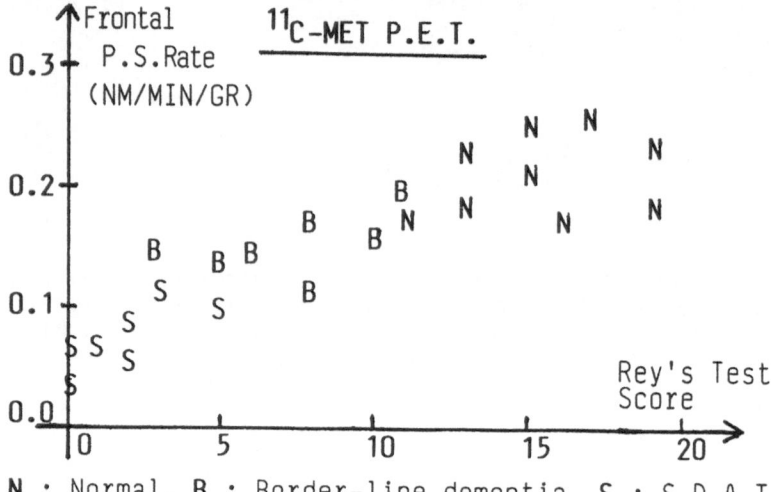

N : Normal, B : Border-line dementia, S : S.D.A.T

Fig. 2   Relationships between frontal cortex PSR and scores in Rey's test.

However, severely demented patients always exhibited a pronounced decrease in PSR, far below the CMRG values commonly reported for the same extreme clinical stage (up to -75% PSR versus up to -50% CMRG). The low PSR in SDAT can be related to similar decreases in numerous enzyme activities measured in brain samples by biochemical methods: up to -60% to -90% (Bowen et al., 1979; Perry et al., 1981; MacGeer, 1981; Rossor, 1982). This fact may not be an argument of sensitivity to detect SDAT in human with PSR, since many conditions are known to strongly decrease protein synthesis in normal rats, e.g., nicotine and tabacco smoking sleep abnormalities, transient hypoglycemia, and drugs (Felipo et al., 1986; Sershen et al., 1981; Ulovec et al., 1985). In demented patients, all these conditions are often superimposed on the disease itself.

Receptor studies

Too few data obtained by PET have been published about receptors in SDAT to review this newly opened field of research, which holds great promise for the study of the action of any potential drugs. Many PET centers currently devote much effort to receptor ligands, almost exclusively in the dopaminergic system (Wagner et al., 1983; Wong et al., 1985; Baron et al., 1985, 1986) with ^{11}C-3-methylspiperone or ^{76}Br-bromospiperone. Recently, interest arose in tracers of transmitter synthesis as are used for the quantitative autoradiography in animals: GBR-12935 (Janowsky et al., 1986) and dopamine uptake, ^{11}C-choline and Ach synthesis (Rosen et al., 1985). Modeling of the latter tracer method is easier than the analysis of the curves of ligand uptake in vivo, for which often a noticeable non-specific binding is a pitfall. Furthermore, many of the sophisticated and complex models do not have unique solutions. This problem can be solved only at the expense of additional biochemical assumptions, which seriously limits the number of clinically relevant parameters that can be estimated with labelled ligands and PET.

To conclude this review, it should be noted that, in strictly clinical diagnostic applications, single photon emission computed tomography (SPECT) recently offered new examination procedures, which were able to satisfy the physician's need to know about local CBF (Mathis et al., 1985) also in SDAT (Bonte et al., 1986). The same patterns of hypo-perfusion were found with SPECT and ^{123}I-isopropylamphetamine in SDAT, MID, Korsakoff's psychosis, and Huntington's chorea as with other metabolic variables studied by PET, while no characteristic abnormalities were observed with MRI (Sharp et al., 1986). SPECT was used successfully to distinguish SDAT from MID (Cohen et al., 1986), and a study of Ach receptors in SDAT was recently performed (Holman, 1986). The original part of the three complementary techniques, PET, MRI, and SPECT, was appreciated in clinical reviews by Ter-Pogossian (1985) and DeLeon (1985). From their remarks it is quite clear that, for a long time,

PET will remain the only method allowing to study _in vivo_ the metabolism
of a well-defined organ and to investigate local pharmacokinetics with
receptor ligands or labelled drugs (Paans et al., 1985).

BRAIN TUMORS

The metabolic grading of various brain tumors was attempted by
several investigators using ^{15}O, ^{18}FDG or ^{11}C-amino acids, but
the differences between grades III and IV often were of marginal significance and, therefore, did no influence therapeutic regimens. In
low-grade tumors, considerable variability was revealed with glucose
and its analogues, or with amino acids, around a mean quite similar to
control values (Fig. 3).

INCORPORATION OF ^{11}C-L.MET IN HUMAN BRAIN TUMORS

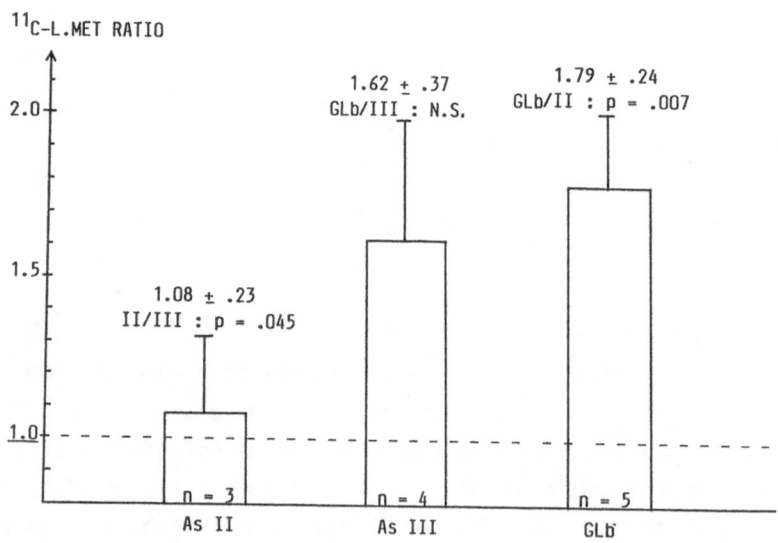

Fig. 3   Incorporation of 11-C-L-Methionine in human brain tumors

The hypermetabolism measured in tumors was generally less than twice
the control value, even for glioblastomas (Hubner et al., 1982; DiChiro
et al., 1982; Rhodes et al., 1983; Patronas et al., 1984; Brooks et
al., 1986; Bustany, 1986). Major clinical interest in PET scanning of
tumors arose from the fact that one could obtain with many tracers
a very reliable measure of the histological extension of the tumor
(Bergström et al., 1983; Ilsen et al., 1984; Hawkins et al., 1984;
Paul et al., 1985; Bustany et al., 1985b; Bustany, 1986) that could
not be visualized by X-ray CT. These merely qualitative images can
actually provide the rational basis for the indications of surgery; they
also allow to follow the evolution of a recurrence. Furthermore, the
therapeutic efficacy of treatment, e.g., standard radiotherapy with 60
Gy applied according to grading, was demonstrated objectively (Fig. 4;
Bustany, 1986).

EFFECT OF RADIOTHERAPY ON GLIOBLASTOMAS

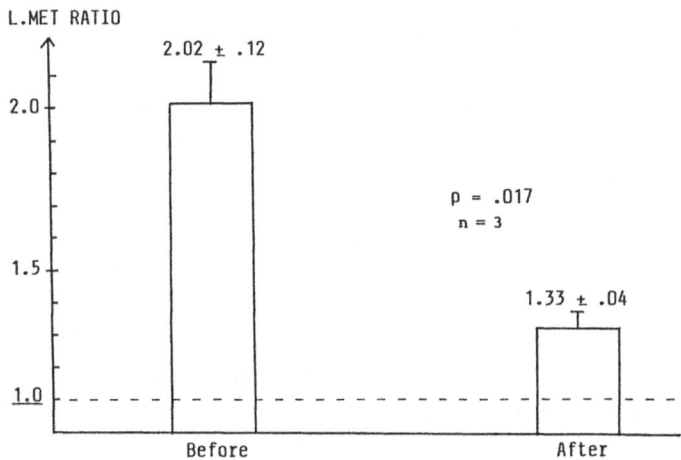

Fig. 4   Effect of radiotherapy on glioblastomas

The effect of brain compression and edema induced by a tumor (Ito et
al., 1982; Patronas et al., 1984), and the results of decompression
surgery were investigated (Beaney et al., 1985). The same studies
focussed on local intra-arterial chemotherapy of gliomas, using [11]C-
BCNU (Tyler et al., 1986).

PET in oncology is rapidly advancing and this is probably the field where PET results can directly influence clinical action. The possibility to perform a set of examinations in a group of patients, using a simplified qualitative imaging protocol, and the relative deficiencies of other diagnostic methods, lead to the central question of the inclusion of PET in the diagnosis of brain tumor extension, a key parameter of the patient's treatment.

CONCLUSION

PET will stay for a long time a means of monitoring new clinical treatments in carefully designed studies of selected pathologies. Both qualitative and quantitative PET examinations can be introduced in clinical trials. But PET will always lack the excellent anatomical resolution that many physicians are accustomed to from their experience with CT and MRI. The esoteric models often needed and the subsequent statistical analysis of individual results denies a certain "transparency" to PET examinations. The results can only be interpreted by a very small number of specialists, who would gain a lot by promoting and explaining the PET technique outside of their laboratories. Ford's editorial in 1983 ("Can Statistics Cause Brain Damage?") was at the core of the problem. In view of moderate metabolic or binding variations, numerous statistical methods have been employed to find demonstrable results that could be used to categorize patients or to clinical action (Horwitz et al., 1984; Clark et al., 1984, 1985; Soncrant et al., 1986; Ford, 1986). It is only by the generalization of these methods which require very efficient computers that, after a "wild period" of description during the 70's, PET will continue to be an essential tool of fundamental and clinical medical research.

REFERENCES

Amano, T., Meier, J.S., Okabe, T., et al. 1982. Stable Xenon CT cerebral blood flow measurements computed by a single compartment - double integration model in normal aging and dementia. J. Comput. Assist. Tomogr., 6, 923-932.

Baron, J.C., Samson, Y., Comar, D., et al. 1985. Etude in vivo des récepteurs sérotoninergiques centraux chez l'homme par tomographie a positons. Rev. Neurol. (Paris), 141, 537-545.

Baron, J.C., Maziere, B., Loc'h, C., et al. 1986. Loss of striatal (76-Br)-Bromospiperone binding sites demonstrated by positron tomography in progressive supranuclear palsy. J. Cereb. Blood Flow Metab., 6, 131-136.

Beaney, R.P., Brooks, D.J., Leenders, K.L., et al. 1985. Blood flow and
oxygen utilization in the contralateral cerebral cortex of
patients with untreated intracranial tumors as studied by
positron emission tomography, with observation on the effect of
decompressive surgery. J. Neurol., Neurosurg., Psychiat., 48, 310-
319.
Benson, D.F., Kuhl, D.E., Hawkins, R.A., et al. 1983. The fluorodeoxyglucose 18-F scan in Alzheimer's disease and multi-infarct
dementia. Arch. Neurol., 40, 711-714.
Bergström, M., Collins, V.P., Ehrin, E., et al. 1983. Discrepancies in
brain tumor extent as shown by computed tomography and positron
emission tomography using 68-Ga-EDTA, 11-C glucose, and 11-C
methionine. J. Comput. Assist. Tomogr., 7, 1062-1066.
Bonte, J.F., Ross, E.D., Chehabi, H.H., et al. 1986. SPECT study of
regional cerebral blood flow in Alzheimer's disease. J. Comput.
Assist. Tomogr., 10, 579-583.
Bowen, D.M., White, P., Spillane, J.A., et al. 1979. Accelerated ageing
or selective neuronal loss as an important course of dementia?
Lancet, 1, 11-14.
Brooks, D.J., Beaney, R.P., Lammertsma, A.A., et al. 1986. Glucose
transport across the blood brain barrier in normal human subjects
and patients with cerebral tumors studied using 11-C 3-0-Methyl-
D-glucose and positron emission tomography. J. Cereb. Blood Flow
Metab., 6, 230-239.
Bustany, P., et al. 1983a. In "Functional Radionuclide. Imaging of the
Brain" (Eds. P. Magistretti et al.). (Raven Press, New York).
pp. 319-326.
Bustany, P., Henry, J.F., Sargent, T., et al. 1983b. Local brain
protein metabolism in dementia and schizophrenia, in vivo studies
with 11-C-L-Methionine and Positron emission tomography. In
"Positron Emission Tomography of the Brain" (Eds. W.-D. Heiss,
M.E. Phelps). (Springer Verlag, Berlin). pp. 208-211.
Bustany, P., Henry, J.F., de Rotrou, J., et al. 1985a. Correlations
between clinical state and PET measurement of local brain protein
synthesis in Alzheimer's dementia, Parkinson's disease,
schizophrenia, and gliomas. In "The Metabolism of the Human Brain
Studied with Positron Emission Tomography" (Eds. T. Greitz et
al.). (Raven Press, New York). pp. 241-249.
Bustany, P., et al. 1985b. In "Positron Emission Tomography" (Eds.
M. Reivich et al.). (Alan R. Liss Inc., New York). pp. 183-201.
Bustany, P. 1986. Brain tumor protein-synthesis an histological grades:
A study by PET with 11-C-L-Methionine. J. Neurol. Oncol., 3, 397-
404.
Clark, C.M., Kessler, R., Buchsbaum, M.S., et al. 1984. Corre-
lational methods for determining regional coupling of cerebral
glucose metabolism: a pilot study. Biol. Psychiat., 19, 663-678.
Clark, C., Carson, R., Kessler, R., et al. 1985. Alternative
statistical models for the examination of clinical positron emission tomography/fluorodeoxyglucose data. J. Cereb. Blood Flow
Metab., 5, 142-150.
Cohen, M.B., Graham, L.S., Lake, R., et al. 1986. Diagnosis of Alzheimer's disease and multiple infarct dementia by tomographic
imaging of iodine 123-IMP. J. Nucl. Med., 27, 769-774.

188

Cutler, N.R., Haxby, J.V., Duara, R., et al. 1985a. Brain metabolism measured with positron emission tomography: serial assessment in patients with familial Alzheimer's disease. Neurology, 35, 1556-1561.

Cutler, N., et al. 1985b. In "Normal Aging, Alzheimer's Disease and Senile Dementia. Aspects on Etiology, Pathogenesis, Diagnosis and Treatment" (Ed. C.G. Gottfries). (Editions de l'Universite de Bruxelles, Bruxelles). pp. 181-198.

Dastur, D.K. 1985. Cerebral blood flow and metabolism in normal human aging, pathological aging, and senile dementia. J. Cereb. Blood Flow Metab., 5, 1-9.

DeLeon, M. 1984. In "Normal Aging, Alzheimer's Disease and Senile Dementia. Aspects on Etiology, Pathogenesis, Diagnosis and Treatment" (Ed. C.G. Gottfries). (Editions de l' Universite de Bruxelles, Bruxelles). pp. 199-202.

Dhawan, V., Conti, J., Mernyk, K.M., et al. 1986. Accuracy of PET RCBF measurements: effect of time shift between blood and brain radioactivity curves. Phys. Med. Biol., 31, 507-514.

DiChiro, G., DeLaPaz, R.L., Brooks, R.A., et al. 1982. Glucose utilization of cerebral gliomas measured by (18-F)fluorodeoxyglucose and positron emission tomography. Neurology, 32, 1323-1329.

Duara, R., Margolin, R.A., Robertson-Tchabo, E.A., et al. 1983. Cerebral glucose utilization, as measured with positron emission tomography in 21 resting healthy men between the ages of 21 and 83 years. Brain, 106, 761-775.

Duara, R., Grady, C., Haxby, J.V., et al. 1986. Positron emission tomography in Alzheimer's disease. Neurology, 36, 879-887.

Farkas, T., Ferris, S.H., Wolf, A.P., et al. 1982. 18-F-2-deoxy-2-fluoro-D-glucose as a tracer in the positron emission tomography study of senile dementia. Am. J. Psychiat., 139, 352-353.

Felipo, V., et al. 1986. Neurochem. Res., 11, 63-69.

Ferris, S., et al. 1980. In "Aging of the Brain" (Eds. S. Algeri et al.). (Raven Press, New York). pp. 123-133. (Raven Press

Ford, I. 1983. Can statistics cause brain damage? (Editorial). J. Cereb. Blood Flow Metab., 3, 259-262.

Ford, I. 1986. Confound correlations: Statistical limitations in the analysis of interregional relationships of cerebral metabolic activity. J. Cereb. Blood Flow Metab., 6, 385-388.

Foster, N.L., Chase, T.N., Mansi, L., et al. 1984. Cortical abnormalities in Alzheimer's disease. Ann. Neurol., 16, 649-654.

Foster, N.L and Chase, T.N. 1986. Cerebral metabolic rate of glucose and Alzheimer's disease. J. Cereb. Blood Flow Metab., 6, 125-127.

Foster, N.L., Chase, T.N., Patronas, N.J., et al. 1986. Cerebral mapping of aproxia in Alzheimer's disease by positron emission tomography. Ann. Neurol., 19, 139-143.

Frackowiak, R.S.J., Pozzilli, C., Legg, N.J., et al. 1981. Regional cerebral oxygen supply and utilization in dementia. A clinical and physiological study with oxygen-15 and positron tomography. Brain, 104, 753-778.

Friedland, R.P., Budinger, T.F., Koss, E., et al. 1985. Alzheimer's disease: Anterior-posterior and lateral hemispheric alteration in cortical glucose utilization. Neurosci. Letters, 53, 235-240.

Grubb, R.L., Raichle, M.E., Gado, M.H., et al. 1977. Cerebral blood flow, oxygen utilization and blood volume in dementia. Neurology, 27, 905-910.

Gustafson, L., et al. 1981. Adv. biol. Psychiat., 6, 109-116.

Hachinski, V.C., Iliff, L.D., Zilhka, E., et al. 1975. Cerebral blood flow in dementia. Arch. Neurol., 32, 632-637.

Hawkins, R.A., Phelps, M.E., Huang, S.C., et al. 1984. A kinetic evaluation of blood-brain barrier permeability in human brain tumors with 68-Ga-EDTA and positron computed tomography. J. Cereb. Blood Flow Metab., 4, 507-515.

Haxby, J.V., Duara, R., Grady, C.L., et al. 1985. Relation between neuropsychological and cerebral metabolic asymmetries in early Alzheimer's disease. J. Cereb. Blood Flow Metab., 5, 193-200.

Heiss, W.-D., Herholz, K., Pawlik, G., et al. 1986. Positron emission tomography in neuropsychology. Neuropsychologia, 24, 141-149.

Herscovitch, P., Auchus, A.P., Gado, M., et al. 1986. Correction of positron emission tomography data for cerebral atrophy. J. Cereb. Blood Flow Metab., 6, 120-124.

Holman, B.L. 1986. Perfusion and receptor SPECT in dementia - George Taplin Memorial Lecture. J. Nucl. Med., 27, 855-860.

Horwitz, B., Duara, R. and Rapoport, S.I. 1984. Intercorrelations of glucose metabolic rates between brain regions: Application to healthy males in a state of reduced sensory input. J. Cereb. Blood Flow Metab., 4, 484-499.

Hübner, K.F., Purvis, J.T., Mahaley, S.M., et al. 1982. Brain tumor imaging by positron emission computed tomography using 11-C-labeled amino acids. J. Comput. Assist. Tomogr., 6, 544-550.

Ilsen, H.W., Sato, M., Pawlik, G., et al. 1984. (68-Ga)-EDTA positron emission tomography in the diagnosis of brain tumors. Neuroradiology, 26, 393-398.

Ingvar, M.C., Maeder, P., Sokoloff, L., et al. 1984. The effects of aging on local rates of cerebral protein synthesis in rats. Monogr. Neurol. Sci., 11, 47-50.

Israel, L., et al. 1984. Source Book of Geriatric Assessment. Karger, New York.

Ito, M., Lammertsma, A.A., Wise, R.J.S., et al. 1982. Measurement of regional cerebral blood flow and oxygen utilisation in patients with cerebral tumours using 15-O and positron emission tomography: Analytical techniques and preliminary results. Neuroradiology, 23, 63-74.

Jagust, W.J., Friedland, R.P., Budinger, T.F., et al. 1985. Positron emission tomography with (F-18)Fluorodeoxyglucose differentiates normal pressure hydrocephalus from Alzheimer-type dementia. J. Neurol., Neurosurg., Psychiat., 48, 1091-1096.

Janowsky, A., Berger, P., Vocci, F., et al., 1986. Characterization of sodium-dependent (3-H)GBR-12935 binding in brain: A radioligand for selective dopamine transport complex. J. Neurochem., 46, 1272-1276.

Kuhl, D.E., Metter, E.J., Riege, W.H., et al. 1982. Effects of human aging on patterns of local cerebral glucose utilization determined by the (18-F)Fluorodeoxyglucose method. J. Cereb. Blood Flow Metab., 2, 163-171.

Kuhl, D.E. 1983. Mapping local cerebral glucose utilization in normal aging and in cerebrovascular, degenerative, and epileptic disorders. In "Positron Emission Tomography of the Brain" (Eds. W.-D. Heiss, M.E. Phelps). (Springer-Verlag, Berlin-Heidelberg-New York). pp. 128-138.

Kuhl, D.E. 1984. Imaging local brain function with emission computed tomography. Radiology, 150, 625-631.

Lammertsma, A.A. and Frackowiak, R.S. 1985. Positron Emission Tomography. CRC Crit. Rev. Biomed. Engineering, 13, 125-169.

Lassen, N.A., Munck, O., Tottey, E.R., et al. 1959. Mental function and cerebral oxygen consumption in organic dementia. Arch. Neurol., Psychiat., 77, 126-133.

McGeer, E. 1981. Neurotransmitter systems in aging and senile dementia. Prog. Neuropsychopharmacol., 5, 435-445.

Mathis, C.A., Sargent III, T, Shulgin, A.T., et al. 1985. Iodine-122-labeled amphetamine derivate with potential for PET brain flow studies. J. Nucl. Med., 26, 1295-1301.

Metter, E.J., Riege, W.H., Kuhl, D.E., et al. 1984. Cerebral metabolic relationships for selected brain regions in healthy adults. J. Cereb. Blood Flow Metab., 4, 500-506.

Nilsson, J., et al. 1985. In "New Methods in Drug Research" (Ed. A. Makriyannis). (Prous Pub., New York). pp. 69-82.

Obrist, W.D., Chivian, E., Cronquist, S., et al. 1970. Regional cerebral blood flow in senile and presenile dementia. Neurology, 20, 315-322.

Paans, A.M., Vaalburg, W., Woldring, M.G, et al. 1985. A comparison of the sensitivity of PET and NMR for invivo quantitative metabolic imaging. Eur. J. Nucl. Med., 11, 73-75.

Pantano, P., Baron, J.C., Lebrun-Grandie, P., et al. 1984. Regional cerebral blood flow and oxygen consumption in human aging. Stroke, 15, 635-641.

Patronas, N.J., DiChiro, G., Smith B.H., et al. 1984. Depressed cerebellar glucose metabolism in supratentorial tumors. Brain Res., 291, 93-101.

Paul, R., Johansson, R., Kellokumpu-Lehtinen, P.L., et al. 1985. Tumor localization with 18-FDG: comparative autoradiography, glucose 6-phosphatase histochemistry, and histology of renally implanted sarcoma of the rat. Res. Exp. Med., 185, 87-94.

Perry, E.K., Blessed, G., Tomlinson, B.E., et al. 1981. Neurochemical activities in human temporal lobe related to aging and Alzheimer-type changes. Neurobiol. Aging, 2, 251-256.

Phelps, M.E., Mazziotta, J.C., Schelbert, H.R., et al. 1985. Clinical PET: What are the issues?. J. Nucl. Med., 26, 1353-1358.

Powers, W.J., Raichle, M.E., Wagner, H.N., et al. 1985. PET: The new focus of nuclear medicine. J. Nucl. Med., 26, 1499-1500.

Rapoport, S.I., Duara, R., Grady, C.L., et al. 1985. Cerebral glucose utilization in relation to age in man. In "The Metabolism of the Human Brain Studies with Positron Emission Tomography" (Ed. T. Greitz). (Raven Press, New York). pp. 339-350.

Reivich, M. et al. 1983. In "CNS Regulation of Carbohydrates Metabolism - Advances in Metabolic Disorders" (Ed. A. Szabo). (Acad. Press 10, New York). 135-176.

Rhodes, C.G., Wise, R.J.S., Gibbs, J.M., et al. 1983. In vivo disturbances of the oxidative metabolism of glucose in human cerebral gliomas. Ann. Neurol., 14, 614-626.

Risberg, J. 1986. Regional cerebral blood flow in neuropsychology. Neuropsychologia, 24, 135-140.

Rogers, R.L., Meyer, J.S., Mortel, K.F., et al. 1986. Decreased cerebral blood flow precedes multi-infarct dementia, but follows senile dementia of Alzheimer type. Neurology, 36, 1-6.

Rosen, M.A., Reese, M.J., Yano, Y., et al. 1985. Carbon-11 choline: Synthesis, purification, and brain uptake inhibition by 2-dimethyl-aminoethanol. J. Nucl. Med., 26, 1424-1428.

Rossor, M.N. 1982. Neurotransmitter and CNS disease, dementia. Lancet, 2, 1200-1204.

Sershen, H., Reith, M.E., Gennaro, A., et al. 1981. Effects of cigarette-smoke on protein synthesis in brain and liver. Neuropharmacol., 20, 451-456.

Sharp, P., Gemmell, H., Cherrymann, G., et al. 1986. Application of iodine-123-labeled isopropylamphetamine imaging to the study of dementia. J. Nucl. Med., 27, 761-768.

Smith, C.B. 1984. Aging and changes in cerebral energy metabolism. Trends in Neuro-Sciences, 6, 203-208.

Sokoloff, L. 1978. Alzheimer's disease. In "Senile Dementia and Related Disorders, Aging Vol 7" (Eds. R. Katzman, R.D. Terry). (Raven Press, New York). pp. 197-202.

Soncrant, T.T., Horwitz, B., Holloway, W.H., et al. 1986. The pattern of functional coupling of brain regions in the awake rat. Brain Res., 369, 1-11.

Ter-Pogossian, M.M. 1985. PET, SPECT and NMRI: Competing or complementary disciplines? J. Nucl. Med., 26, 1487-1498.

Tyler, J.L., Yamamoto, Y.L., Diksic, M., et al. 1986. Pharmacokinetics of superselective intra-arterial and intravenous (11-C)BCNU evaluated by PET. J. Nucl. Med., 27, 775-780.

Ulovec, Z., Narancsik, P., Gamulin, S., et al. 1985. Effects of hypoglycemia on rat brain polyribosome sedimentation pattern. J. Neurochem., 45, 352-354.

Wagner, H.N.Jr., Burns, H.D., Dannals, R.F., et al. 1983. Imaging dopamine receptors in the human brain by positron tomography. Science, 221, 1264-1266.

Wagner, H.N.Jr. 1985. PET: The new focus of nuclear medicine. Reply. J. Nucl. Med., 26, 1500-1501.

Wong, D.F., Wagner, H.N.Jr., Dannals, R.F., et al. 1985. Effects of age on dopamine and serotonine receptors measured by positron tomography in living human brain. Science, 226, 1393-1396.

VALUE OF PET IN THE CLINICAL EVALUATION OF DEMENTIAS

M. Berger, Zentralinstitut für Seelische Gesundheit, Mannheim, FRG

Clinical relevance of research on dementia

Although during the last decades psychiatric research has widely neglected the issue of senile dementia the tide has recently turned decisively. This change is consequence of a new knowledge about the medical problems of aging. In the meantime it is like bringing coals to Newcastle to stress the tremendous importance of dementia for psychiatry and for health care as a whole. Due to the sharp increase of life expectancy particularly in highly developed countries it can be expected that the number of persons older than 65 years will increase from 250 million in 1980 to 403 million in the year 2000 and to 760 million in year 2035 (Hauser, 1986). In the highly developed countries, the number of people older then 65 years has already reached 11 %. The relevance of these data for medical and health care systems is illuminated when taking the prevalence of dementia into consideration. About 5 % of persons aged 65 years or older have a moderate or severe dementia and persons older than 80 are afflicted in even 20 % to 30 % (Katzman, 1976; Cooper, 1986; Henderson, 1986). This means, that presently about 12 million people suffer from dementia and the number will increase to more then 20 million within the next 1 1/2 decades. The overwhelming impact of dementia on organisational, economic, and medical fields becomes more and more obvious.

These problems can only be attenuated if relevant diagnostic and therapeutic approachs in regards to this insidious epidemic can be developed. This holds true particularly for the still present short-comings in the differential diagnosis of dementia and the lack of convincing preventative and therapeutic properties. Therefore, the clinicians' high expectations regarding PET studies in dementia are clearly understandable.

Diagnostic issues

As the psychopathological disturbances are unspecific for any form of dementia, an early and accurate diagnosis of the different subgroups using the PET would be of significant value, particularly in identifying presenile Alzheimer's disease (AD), senile dementia of the Alzheimer's type (SADT), multi-infarct dementia (MID), and mixed forms of AD/SDAT and MID. In regards to insidiously starting mild forms of the dement illness the diagnostic efforts should be extended to separate these mild forms from the normal consequences of aging. Concerning these questions recent studies give the impression that PET seems to be an effective aid of differential diagnosis (de Leon et al., 1983; Duara et al., 1986).

Although the current technique of PET does not allow to use this tool in clinical routine, it does show, however, that these differential diagnostic decisions can be done with quite a high degree of convidence. Whereas in recent years, the ability to diagnose Alzheimer's disease during the patients lifetime was only about 50 %, this improved to at least 80 % assurance by using imaging methods. Clinicians expect that the further development of a brouder range of radioactively labeled compounds like aminoacids, proteins and transmitter agonists and antagonists will allow qualitative imaging of processes such as metabolisation of various substrates, protein synthesis, function and distribution of different receptor types and the distribution of drugs throughout the brain (Heiss et al., 1986). This may contribute to a further clarification of diagnostic boundaries. Moreover the cholinergic system seems to offer a pathway, worthwile for further efforts.

In gerontopsychiatric research much attention has been focused on disturbances in the cholinergic system in dementia. Particularly because of possibilities of measuring ligand bindings on cholinergic receptors PET may contribute to the question of the relevance of cholinergic deficiencies in AD/SDAT. As was shown by different research groups, post-mortem studies in SDAT revealed a highly significant reduction of the activity of cholineacetyltransferase (CAT) and a loss of cholinergic neurons in the basal forebrain especially in the nucleus basalis of Meynert (overview see Coyle et al., 1983). In comparative investigations it was revealed that in presenile dementia this cholinergic impairment is additionally linked with significant disturbances in the catecholaminergic transmitter systems. This signifies among others a degeneration of the locus coeruleus (Carlsson, 1986). If these results could be confirmed by in vivo PET techniques this would support that presenil and senile dementia of the Alzheimer's type are two different disorders. It also could provide tools for differentiating AD/SDAT from MDI.

The most relevant differential diagnostic problem in geronto-psychiatry, however, is the differential diagnosis between dementia and depressive pseudodementia. Besides dementia depression is the dominant psychic disorder in the elderly. The prevalence of pervasive depression is about 12 to 16 % (overview see Henderson, 1986). Since Madden et al. (1952) realized that purely depressed patients may show reversable cognitive disturbances and therefore may simulate dementia, he created the term "depressive pseudodementia". In the meantime a lot of authors focused on this topic (overview see Grunhaus et al., 1983). Ten to 30 % of patients under evaluation for dementia have a reversible form of the syndrome and primary depression seems to be the most important contributor to these reversible clinical pictures. The differential diagnostic task is impeded by the fact that about 20 % of demented patients also show coexisting depressive mood disturbances (Reifler et al., 1982). In this respect PET studies may also contribute to a more precise distinction which will be of high prognostic and therapeutic relevance. Interestingly the model of depression, which currently possesses the best experimental evidence is that of a relative overactivity of the central cholinergic system in relation to the aminergic transmitters (Sitaram et al., 1984; Berger et al., 1986). Therefore, PET studies with adequate radioligands focusing on the activity of the cholinergic system may differentiate these diagnostic entities better than by measuring blood flow or the central metabolic rates of glucose, especially as depression has also been reported to be linked with hypometabolism.

Intervening variables

Considering the aim of improving the differential diagnostic process by PET some critical remarks should be made, however. During the last decade biological research in psychiatry especially in depression was dominated by the search for biological markers for nosological entities. This ambitious approach did not lead to the expected bio-logical classification of psychiatric disorders, but was a strong and sometimes painful educational process. Biological abnormalities, as the pathological dexamethasone supression test, a shortened REM latency, or an abnormal growth hormone response to insulin induced hypoglycemia, for example, were believed to be of diagnostic specificity. More extensive studies, however, revealed these abnormal test results to be a consequence of unspecific intervening variables (overview see Berger et al., 1982). Therefore, the extensive consideration of influencing factors independent of the psychopathological state have been recognized as important elements in the process of data interpretation. With regard to PET studies, only a few variables of possible relevance should be mentioned here: Cahill et al. (1966) demonstrated that under conditions of starvation, glucose becomes increasingly deficient so that finally 70 % of the brain's energy needs are supplied by ketone bodies. As many demented as well as depressed patients are in a situation of malnutrition, this factors may influence the results of PET studies on glucose metabolism. Kuhl et al. (1982) assumed the relation of glucose and ketone metabolism to be important for metabolic studies even in the process of normal aging. Differencies in food choices (for example avoidance of proteins) may be another relevant issue.

Some authors already stressed the possible influence of psycho-active drugs on PET data. From animal studies it is known, that chronic application of antidepressants lowers cerebral glucose metabolism (Gerber et al., 1983), neuroleptics may also change metabolic rates (Buchsbaum et al., 1982). Baxter mentioned the results of increased dose-dependent glucose metabolic rates by dopamin agonists and Soncrast et al. (in press) found an enhancement of cerebral glucose metabolism by application of the cholinomimetic drug arecoline in rats. These preliminary results stress the importance of studying unmedicated patients after sufficiently long wash-out periods.

Another intervening variable may be situational stress. The individual state of arousal, due to the test situation itself, may decisively influence the test results. There is no doubt, that the functional acitivity of the brain influences the glucose metabolism. In psychiatric patients the stress caused by the procedure of PET may be enhanced. Additionally, the psychiatric disorder itself may be linked with strong inner turmoil. It is of interest that in normal subjects sleep, when sensory stimuli from the outside are mainly reduced, leads to a decrease of metabolic rates between 10 to 20 %. If however the stimuli from inside increase, that means during dreaming metabolic rates may increase above the level of the waking state (Heiss et al., 1985). This interaction of current psychic arousal and metabolic rate may explain that repeated PET scans in normal subjects revealed differencies in metabolic values of in mean 12 % (Lenzi et al., 1983). It has to be proven whether trials to minimize the inter- and intraindividual differencies of strain by applying defined painful stimuli or psychological tasks during the PET procedure are successful (Buchsbaum et al., 1986, in press).

A further problem with regard to improvement of diagnosis is that of adequate control groups. Although the majority of about 90 % of dementias are of the Alzheimer's type or MID there exists another broad spectrum of possible etiological or pathophysiological causes, for example, infections, multiple sclerosis, mongolism, Wilson disease, hyperthyreosis, B-12-avitaminosis or chronic alcohol or/and drug abuse. To avoid assumptions of specificity of PET results for AD/SDAT the studies should be extended to these other forms of dementia and also to pseudodement diseases.

Therapeutic issues

For clinical practice improvement of the diagnostic properties gets relevant if it is linked with therapeutic approaches. Up to now we are in lack of adequate treatment propensities to prevent, cure, or at least to slow down the process of Alzheimer's disease and senile dementia of the Alzheimer's type. In MID at least risk factors like hypertension and diabetes can be treated adequately. In AD/SDAT however convincing therapeutic tools are missing. One difficulty of studies on this topic seems to be the lack of adequate and generally accepted methods for assessing the drug efficacy. Only recent approaches aim on multimodal assessments in which information from clinical rating systems, psychological performance tests and measures of physiological functions are combined. It seems necessary that clinicians agree to a standardization of these instruments to allow comparable studies on this field (Loew, 1986).

From PET studies a wide range of essential contributions to therapeutic efforts can be expected. Especially longitudinal studies will be fruitful to investigate the influence of different drugs not only on the spontaneous clinical course but also on different parameters like brain hemodynamics, metabolism, and chemistry. PET studies should help to clarify the controversy on the efficacy of psychogeriatric drugs of which vasodilation, activation of brain metabolism, or actions on synaptic transmission are believed to be their principal mode of action. It can be assumed that PET studies will allow not only to illuminate the pharmacokinetics of these drugs but will also elucidate their different central nervous activities. This again may lead to further clarification of the pathogenetic mechanisms of dementia.

As one example for possible strategies the cholinergic deficiency hypothesis can serve. Within the last ten years about 50 studies have been performed with cholinergic precursors, cholinesterase-blocker and direct acting cholinergic agonists to improve AD/SDAT. The majority of these trails only led to a therapeutic effect in a minority of patients (Kurz et al., 1986). This has been discussed in regard to diagnostic heterogeneity, different degrees of alterations of the cholinergic neurons and different degrees of disturbances in others, like the dopaminergic or noradrenergic transmitter systems. With regard to precursors it is still unclear whether they have any effect on the central nervous system at all. Progress in labeling techniques of new radioligands should contribute to decisive progress in this fields. A promising approach in the therapy of dementia seems urgently necessary, as up to now this topic is widely determined by lack of knowledge and prejudice.

REFERENCES

Berger, M., Doerr, P., Lund, R. et al. 1982. Neuroendocrinological and neurophysiological studies in major depressive disorders: Are there biological markers for the endogeneous subtype? Biol. Psychiatry, 17, 1217-1242.
Berger, M., Höchli, D., Krieg, C. et al. 1986. The diagnostic and therapeutic utility of cholinomimetics in affective disorders. Biol. Psychiatry, 273-275.
Buchsbaum, M.S., Ingvar, D.H., Kessler, R. et al. 1982. Cerebral glucography with positron tomography. Arch. Gen. Psychiatry, 39, 251-259.
Buchsbaum, M.S., Tang, S.W., Wu, J.C. et al. 1986. In Press. Effects of amoxapine and imipramine on cerebral glucose metabolism assessed by positron emission tomography. J. Clin. Psychiatry.
Cahill, G.F., Herrera, M.G., Morgan, A.P. et al. 1966. Hormone-fuel interrelationships during fasting. J. Clin. Invest., 45, 1751-1768.

Carlsson, A. 1986. Neurotransmitters in old age and dementia. In "Mental Health in the Elderly". (Eds. H. Häfner, G. Moschel, N. Sartorius). (Springer, Berlin, Heidelberg, New York, Tokyo). p. 154.

Cooper, B. 1986. Mental illness, disability and social conditions among old people in Mannheim. In "Mental Health in the Elderly". (Eds. H. Häfner, G. Moschel, N. Sartorius). (Springer, Berlin, Heidelberg, New York, Tokyo). p. 35.

Coyle, J.T., Price, D.L., DeLong, M.R. 1983. Alzheimer's disease: A disorder of cortical cholinergic innervation. Science, $\underline{219}$, 1184-1190.

Duara, R., Grady, C., Haxby, J. et al. 1986. Positron emission tomography in Alzheimer's disease. Neurology, 36, 879-887.

Gerber, J., Choki, J., Brunswick, D. et al. 1983. Effect of antidepressant drug on regional cerebral glucose utilization in the rat. Brain Res., $\underline{269}$, 319-325.

Grunhaus, L., Dilsaver, S., Greden, J.F. et al. 1983. Depressive pseudodementia: A suggested diagnostic profile. Biol. Psychiatry, $\underline{18}$, 215-225.

Hauser, P.M. 1986. Aging and increasing longevity of world population. In "Mental Health in the Elderly". (Eds. H. Häfner, G. Moschel, N. Sartorius). (Springer, Berlin, Heidelberg, New York, Tokyo). pp. 10-14.

Heiss, W.-D., Pawlik, G., Herholz, K. et al. 1985. Regional cerebral glucose metabolism during wakefulness, sleep, and dreaming. Brain Res., $\underline{327}$, 362-366.

Heiss, W.-D., Pawlik, G., Herholz, K. et al. 1986. Regional cerebral blood flow and glucose metabolism in old age and in dementia evaluated by PET. In "Mental Health in the Elderly". (Eds. H. Häfner, G. Moschel, N. Sartorius). (Springer, Berlin, Heidelberg, New York, Tokyo). pp. 140-145.

Henderson, A.S. 1986. Epidemiology of mental illness. In "Mental Health in the Elderly". (Eds. H. Häfner, G. Moschel, N. Sartorius). (Springer, Berlin, Heidelberg, New York, Tokyo). p. 29.

Katzman, R. 1976. The prevalence and malignancy of Alzheimer disease a major killer. Arch. Neurol., $\underline{33}$, 217-218.

Kuhl, D.E., Metter, E.J., Riege, W.H. et al. 1982. Effects of human aging on patterns of local cerebral glucose utilization determined by the (18F)fluorodeoxyglucose method. J. Cereb. Blood Flow Metabol., $\underline{2}$, 163-171.

Kurz, A., Rüster, P., Romero, B. et al. In Press. Cholinerge Behandlungsstrategien bei der Alzheimer'schen Krankheit. Nervenarzt.

Lenzi, G.L., Gibbs, J.M., Frackowiak, R.S.J. et al. 1983. Measurement of cerebral blood flow and oxygen metabolism by positron emission tomography and the 15-O steady-state technique: Aspects of methodology, reproducibility and clinical application. In "Functional Radionuclide Imaging of the Brain". (Ed. P.L. Magistretti). (Raven Press, New York). pp. 291-309.

Leon, M.J. de, Ferris, S.H. George, A.E. et al. 1983. Positron emission tomographic studies of aging and Alzheimer disease. Am. J. Neuroradiol., $\underline{4}$, 568-571.

Loew, D.M. 1986. Issues in geriatric psychopharmacology. In "Mental Health in the Elderly". (Eds. H. Häfner, G. Moschel, N. Sartorius). (Springer, Berlin, Heidelberg, New York, Tokyo). p. 166.

Madden, J.J., Luhan, J.A., Kaplan, L.A. et al. 1952. Nondementing
    psychosis in older persons. J. Am. Med. Assoc., 150, 1567-1570.
Reifler, B.V., Larson, E., Hanley, R. 1982. Coexistence of cognitive
    impairment and depression in geriatric outpatients. Am. J.
    Psychiat., 139, 623-626.
Sitaram, N., Gillin, J.C., Bunney, W.D. 1984. Cholinergic and catecho-
    laminergic receptor sensitivity in affective illness: strategy and
    theory. In "Neurobiology of Mood Disorders". (Eds. R.M. Post, J.C.
    Ballenger). (Baltimore, London). pp. 629-651.
Soncrast, T.T., Holloway, H.W., Rapoport, S.I. In Press. Arecoline-
    induced elevations of regional cerebral metabolism in the
    conscious rat. Brain Res.

B R A I N

Schizophrenia

REGIONAL BRAIN METABOLISM IN DRUGFREE SCHIZOPHRENIC PATIENTS
AS MEASURED BY POSITRON EMISSION TOMOGRAPHY

F.-A. Wiesel*, G. Wik*, I. Sjögren*, G. Blomqvist**, T. Greitz***,
S. Stone-Elander****

*Dept. of Psychiatry and Psychology
**Clinical Neurophysiology
***Neuroradiology
****Karolinska Pharmacy
Karolinska Hospital
Stockholm, Sweden

The development of positron emission tomography (PET) is of great interest in the study of psychiatric disorders. In comparison with other functional imaging techniques PET has a better resolution and makes it also possible to study both cortical and subcortical structures three dimensionally. Of the psychiatric disorders, schizophrenia has attracted the most interest. The main reason for this are the character of the disease like disturbed thinking, hallucinations, delusions and the development of social incapability and the number of neurobiological disturbances found in the patients.

In 1974 Ingvar and Franzen could demonstrate changes in the pattern of cortical blood flow in chronic and old schizophrenic patients. It seemed as if the frontal cortical areas were most affected and the concept of hypofrontality was put forward (Ingvar 1979). In later studies with PET in schizophrenic patients similar changes in the cortical glucose metabolism were found (Buchsbaum et al., 1982; Farkas et al., 1984). However, in more recent studies the concept of hypofrontality has not always been possible to confirm (Sheppard et al., 1983; Wolkin et al., 1985). Inconsistancy of PET results may be due to differences in patient materials (first episode psychotic patients or chronic old patients) drug treatment and the state of the patient at the investigation. Another important difference between groups of researchers is how the regions of interest are defined. In comparison of absolute metabolic levels the importance of the tracer and the model used in the calculations is obvious.

In the present study regional brain glucose metabolism was investigated in drugfree schizophrenic patients in an acute phase of the disease. Regions of interest were determined from the brain morphology of the individual subjects with the aid of computed tomography (CT).

METHODS

Twenty patients (15 men and 5 women, mean age 27 ± 6.5, range 19 - 41) with an acute psychosis of the schizophrenic type were selected for the study. The patients were somatically healthy and did not abuse alcohol or narcotics. The diagnosis of schizophrenia was made according to Research Diagnostic Criteria (Spitzer and Endicott, 1977) and DSM-III. Eight patients had their first psychotic episode and the remaining patients were subchronic or chronic with an acute exacerbation. Subtypes were hebephrenic (8), paranoid (10), and 2 undifferentiated cases. No patient had taken oral neuroleptics three weeks before the PET investigation. Depot neuroleptics had not been given 6 months prior to the study. The control group consisted of 10 somatically and psychiatrically healthy male volunteers (mean age 27 ± 6.8, range 22 - 41).

Measures of psychotic morbidity

Clinical morbidity was measured by using the Comprehensive Psychopathological Rating Scale (CPRS) (Asberg et al., 1978). The rating of the patients was made the day before or the same day as the PET investigation. Global rating of psychosis was made in order to determine the patient's over all degree of morbidity. Different subscales made from the CPRS items were constructed to measure depressive symptoms (Montgomery and Asberg, 1979), positive symptoms (Alfredsson et al., 1985) and autistic or negative symptoms. The last subscale consisted of the following items: inability to feel, lassitude, lack of appropriate emotion, withdrawal, reduced speech and slowness of movement.

Regions of interest

All subjects were examined by CT of the brain. Displayed CT images were used for marking brain regions of interest and the marked regions were transformed to the corresponding slice from the PET examination. To allow identical positioning in the CT and the PET scans, a special haed positioning device was used (Bergström et al., 1981). Frontal, two parietal and one temporal cortical regions were drawn on the CT images according to the Brodmann areas. The subcortical structures, the caudate nucleus, lentiform nucleus, thalamus, amygdala and hippocampus were drawn according to anatomical boundaries seen on the CT images.

PET procedure

The PET investigation was made with the subject in a resting condition with the eyes covered. A plastic mould covered the ears. Electroencephalographic recordings were made in order to check that the subjects were awake during the investigation. Between 150 and 400 MBq of ^{11}C-glucose was injected intravenously as a bolus (Nilsson et al., 1985). From the contralateral arm blood samples were taken during the investigation from an artery or from a distant vein (arterialized venous blood by warming the hand). The samples of blood or plasma were measured in a wellcounter. The content of unlabelled glucose was determined in plasma. The time course of the tracer uptake in the brain was measured with a four ring positron camera (PC-384-7B). PET images of ^{11}C activity were constructed and metabolic maps were obtained by fitting the rate constants pixel by pixel according to a three compartment kinetic model for ^{11}C glucose and using the algorithm developed by Blomqvist (1984). The observed ^{11}C activity was corrected for the cummulative loss of CO_2 (Blomqvist et al., 1985). Since this correction increases with time only data up to the first 15 minutes were used.

Absolute metabolic values are only reported in the subjects where arterial blood samples were obtained since the use of the model implies an accurate input function of plasma glucose to the brain. Relative metabolic values i.e. the ratio between the metabolism in one region and the whole brain, were calculated in all subjects.

RESULTS

The whole brain metabolism did not differ significantly between the healthy volunteers (22.5 $\pm$ 2.1 µmol/100g/min) and the schizophrenic patients (19.9 $\pm$ 6.3 µmol/100g/min) but the variance did (F = 9.24, p < 0.01). In general regional metabolic values were lower in the schizophrenic patients and reached significance in Brodmann areas 22 (superior temporal cortex), 32 (medial frontal cortex) and lentiform nucleus (Table 1).

TABLE 1   Comparison of regional brain glucose metabolism in healthy and drugfree schizophrenic subjects

Brain region	CMR (μmol/100g/min)	
	Controls (n = 9)	Patients (n = 15)
Brod. area 22		
Right	24.6 + 2.9	$21.3 + 6.6^{1/}$
Left	25.8 $\mp$ 2.8	$20.8 \mp 6.9^{1/}$*
Brod. area 32		
Right	26.5 + 3.0	$22.4 + 6.2^{1/}$*
Left	27.5 $\mp$ 2.4	$22.7 \mp 7.3^{2/}$*
Lentiform. nucl.		
Right	25.9 + 4.0	21.6 + 7.5
Left	25.8 $\mp$ 2.9	$21.5 \mp 7.0^{1/}$*

Mean values $\pm$ S.D. Two tailed t-test adopted for equal or unequal variances.
p-values for F-ratios

$^{1/}$p<0.05, $^{2/}$p<0.01,

p-value for t-values *p<0.05

The major difference between the controls and the patients was the increased variance in several of the regions. This is illustrated by the range of metabolic values for the whole brain which in the patients was 9.7 - 28.0 μmol/100g/min and in the healthy volunteers 19.5 - 26.0 μmol/100g/min. The relative metabolism was lower in the temporal area 22, the medial frontal area 32 and the parietal areas 39 + 40 (Table 2).

A similar tendency was obtained for the lentiform nucleus. The caudate nucleus was the only region where the patients had a higher relative metabolism. In order to investigate for a hypofrontal distribution of glucose metabolism, ratios between the frontal areas 6 and 9 and the posterior areas 22 and 39 + 40 were formed. The ratios demonstrated a hyperfrontal distribution in the patients in comparison with the controls (Fig. 1).

TABLE 2   Comparison of regional relative brain glucose metabolism in healthy and drugfree schizophrenic subjects

Brain region	Relative metabolism	
	Controls (n = 10)	Patients (n = 20)
Brod. area 22		
Right	1.09 + 0.019	1.09 + 0.022
Left	1.15 ∓ 0.016	1.06 ∓ 0.018**
Brod. area 32		
Right	1.18 + 0.032	1.16 + 0.021
Left	1.22 ∓ 0.012	1.12 ∓ 0.020***
Brod. area 39 + 40		
Right	1.17 + 0.018	1.12 + 0.016*
Left	1.16 ∓ 0.018	1.11 ∓ 0.016+
Caudate nucl.		
Right	0.96 + 0.011	0.98 + 0.021
Left	0.91 ∓ 0.016	1.00 ∓ 0.022**
Lentiform. nucl.		
Right	1.13 + 0.035	1.08 + 0.017
Left	1.13 ∓ 0.020	1.08 ∓ 0.016+

Mean values $\pm$ S.D. Two tailed t-test

+$p<0.1$; *$p<0.05$; **$p<0.01$; ***$p<0.001$

A significant interaction between controls, patients and right/left metabolism was found for the Brodmann areas 11 and 22 with a higher activity at the left side in the controls and the opposite in the patients (Table 3).

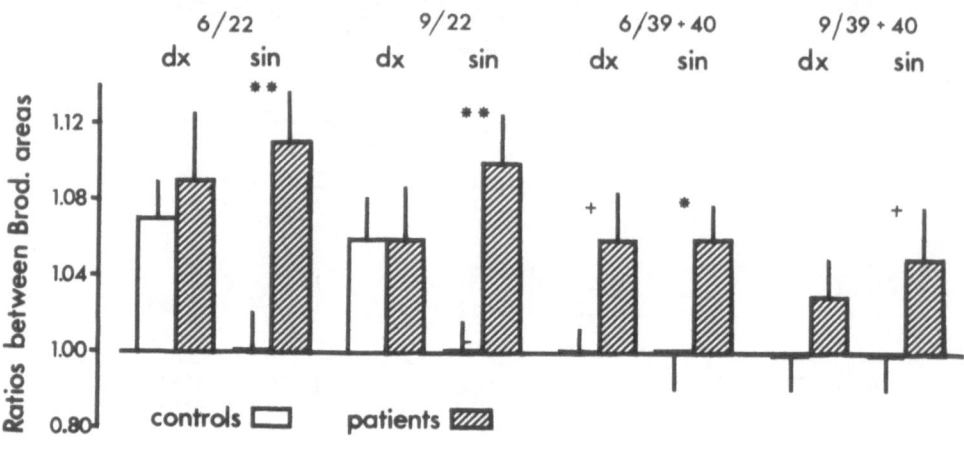

Fig. 1   Ratios between glucose metabolism in the frontal Brodmann areas 6 and 9 and the posterior areas 22 and 39 + 40 in healthy volunteers (n = 10) and drugfree schizophrenic patients (n = 20).

Two tailed t-test: [+]p<0.1; [*]p<0.05; [**]p<0.01

TABLE 3   Differences in regional left-right glucose metabolism between healthy volunteers and drugfree schizophrenic patients

Brain region	F-ratio Diagnose and laterality	Interpretation
Brod. area 11	5.18*	Controls (5): Left>right Patients (8): Left<right
Brod. area 22	6.24*	Controls (10): Left>right Patients (20): Left<right

There was also an imbalance between left-right activity for amygdala (left>right, F = 15.92, p<0.001) but the direction of the deviation was similar for the groups.
*p<0.05

Clinical symptoms were correlated to absolute regional metabolic values. No significant relationships were found between global morbidity, positive symptoms or depressive symptoms and metabolism. However, autistic or negative symptoms weresignificantly and negatively correlated to regional metabolism i.e. the lower the metabolism the higher the scores were in autistic or negative symptoms (Table 4).

TABLE 4   Correlation between regional brain glucose metabolism and clinical symptomatology in drugfree schizophrenic patients

| Brain region | Global morbidity | Subscales from the CPRS | | |
		Positive symptoms	Autism	Depressive symptoms
Brod. area 22				
Right	0.05	-0.20	-0.68**	-0.41
Left	-0.05	-0.28	-0.75**	-0.35
Brod. area 32				
Right	-0.01	-0.39	-0.65**	-0.43
Left	-0.03	-0.27	-0.70**	-0.25
Lentiform nucl.				
Right	-0.08	-0.34	-0.70**	-0.32
Left	-0.02	-0.36	-0.64**	-0.34

Product moment correlation coefficients
n = 15, **$p < 0.01$

DISCUSSION

The main difference between the healthy volunteers and the schizophrenic patients was the increased variance in the regional metabolism of the patients. This may also be one important factor explaining differences in results if small patient materials are used for comparison since selection errors may involve the risk of either exaggerate or underestimate differences between controls and patients.

Relative metabolic values and the ratios between frontal and posterior cortical areas indicated that the frontal areas were more preserved. However, this does not mean that the patients were hyperfrontal, in agreement with Wolkin et al. (1985) the frontal metabolism was lower in the patients, even if not significant due to the increased variance. The results rather illustrate the ambiguousness of the concept hypofrontality.

Most of the differences in the mean values between the controls and the patients were obtained at the left side. However, ANOVA demonstrated only significant interactions between groups and laterality for the Brodmann areas 11 and 22 with a higher left activity in the controls. This is in contrast with some previous findings indicating a higher oxygen metabolism in parts of the right hemisphere in controls or an increased blood flow of the left hemisphere in patients (Sheppard et al., 1983; Gur et al., 1985). Other investigators find no asymmetries. The disparate results may indicate differences in the attention of the subjects during the PET investigation.

By and large our results and those of others demonstrate that there are differences in the regional glucose metabolism in schizophrenic patients. However, the type of regional differences varies between investigators indicating that the cerebral dysfunction is not related to a specific region but probably a more general and fundamental disturbancy is operating resulting in various changes from one point in time to another.

A more consistent finding was the negative relationship between autistic or negative symptoms and metabolism. Such a relationship in cortical blood flow and autism was first reported by Ingvar and Franzen (1974) and has also been reported in glucose metabolism by Wolkin et al. (1985). Thus, flattened affect, lassitude, withdrawal, are probably not a secondary psychological phenomenon but is the result of a reduced brain energy metabolism.

ACKNOWLEDGEMENT

This study was supported by grants from the Sweden Tercentenary Bank Foundation of The Swedish Medical Research Council (B87-21P-07027- 03C), National Institute of Mental Health (MH 41205). Ms Birgit Lönn is gratefully acknowledged for preparing the manuscript.

REFERENCES

Alfredsson, G., Härnryd, C. and Wiesel, F.-A. 1985. Effects of sulpi-
     ride and chlorpromazine on autistic and positive psychotic sym-
     ptoms in schizophrenic patients - relationship to drug concentra-
     tion. Psychopharmacol., 85, 8-13.
Asberg, M., Montgomery, S., Perris, C., et al. 1978. CPRS- The psycho-
     pathological rating scale. Acta Psychiat. Scand., Suppl. 271,
     5-27.
Bergström, M., Boethius, J., Eriksson, L., et al. 1981. Head fixation
     device for reproducible position alignment in transmission CT and
     positron emission tomography. J. Comput. Assist. Tomogr., 5, 136-
     141.
Blomqvist, G. 1984. On the construction of functional maps in positron
     emission tomography. J. Cereb. Blood Flow Metab., 4, 629-632.
Blomqvist, G., Bergström, K., Bergström, M., et al. 1985. Models for
     11-C-glucose. In: "Metabolism of the Human Brain Studied with
     Positron Emission Tomography" (Eds. T. Greitz, D.H. Ingvar and
     L. Widen). (Raven Press, New York). pp. 185-194.
Buchsbaum, M.S., Ingvar, D.H., Kessle, R., et al. 1982. Cerebral
     glucography with positron tomography. Arch. Gen. Psychiat., 39,
     251-259.
Farkas, T., Wolf, A.O., Jaeger, J., et al. 1984. Regional brain
     glucose metabolism in chronic schizophrenia. Arch. Gen. Psychiat.,
     41, 293-300.
Gur, R.E., Gur, R.C., Skolnick, B.E., et al. 1985. Brain function in
     psychiatric disorders. Arch. Gen. Psychiat., 42, 329-334.
Ingvar, D.H. 1979. "Hyperfrontal" distribution of cerebral grey matter
     flow in resting wakefulness: On the functional anatomy of the
     conscious state. Acta Neurol. Scand., 60, 12-25.
Ingvar, D.H. and Franzen, G. 1974. Abnormalities of cerebral blood flow
     distribution in patients with chronic schizophrenia. Acta
     Psychiat. Scand., 50, 425-462.
Montgomery, S. and Asberg, M. 1979. A new depression scale designed to
     be sensitive to change. Br. J. Psychiat., 134, 382-389.
Nilsson, J.L.G., Stone-Elander, S., Ehrin, E., et al. 1985. 11-C-
     labelled compounds for the study of cerebral blood volume, blood
     flow and energy metabolism. In: "Metabolism of the Human Brain
     Studied with Positron Emission Tomography" (Eds. T. Greitz, D.H.
     Ingvar and L. Widen). (Raven Press, New York). pp. 107-112.
Sheppard, G., Manchanda, R., Gruzelier, J. et al. 1983. 15-0 positron
     emission tomographic scanning in predominantly never-treated acute
     schizophrenic Sheppard patients. Lancet, 24/31, 1448-1452.
Spitzer, R.L. and Endicott, J. 1977. Schedule for affective disorder
     and schizophrenia (SADS) 3rd edition. New York State Psychiatric
     Inst., Biometrics Res. New York.
Wolkin, A., Jaeger, J., Brodie, J.D., et al. 1985. Persistence of
     cerebral metabolic abnormalities in chronic schizophrenia as
     determined by positron emission tomography. Am. J. Psychiat., 142,
     564-571.

PET-DETERMINATION OF CENTRAL D1- AND D2-DOPAMINE RECEPTOR OCCUPANCY IN NEUROLEPTIC TREATED SCHIZOPHRENICS

L. Farde, F.A. Wiesel, C. Halldin, G. Sedvall
Department of Psychiatry and Psychology, Karolinska Hospital,
Stockholm, Sweden

Antipsychotic medication is of proved value in the treatment of schizophrenia. The individual response to drug treatment is however highly variable and in some patients severe extrapyramidal side effects have to be taken into account. The psychiatrist is constantly reminded of the need to minimise the risk of side effects without sacrificing the benefits of adequate dosage. For such reasons there is an urgent need for methods yielding useful measures to guide the dose-finding procedure.

During the last 20 years techniques have been available for the measurement of drug concentrations in serum (for references see Dahl, 1986). Despite a large number of published studies on the relationship between antipsychotic effect and serum drug concentrations, no generally accepted relationships have been demonstrated.

The current classification of central dopamine receptors postulates the existence of two subtypes, designated D1 and D2. The antipsychotic effect of neuroleptic drugs has been proposed to be mediated by a blockade of D2-dopamine receptors (Peroutka and Snyder, 1980). The effect of selective D1-antagonists on schizophrenic patients has not yet been examined.

The development of positron emission tomography (PET) has made it possible to study receptor binding in the living human brain (Sedvall et al., 1986). Using the 11C-labeled selective D2-dopamine receptor anta-gonist raclopride, we have developed a method for the quantitative measurement of drug interaction with central D2-dopamine receptors in neuroleptic treated schizophrenics (Farde et al., 1986). This measure is closer to the assumed target for antipsychotic drug action than serum concentration. We have also labeled the D1-dopamine receptor antagonist SCH-23390 with 11C and visualized D1-dopamine receptors in the living brain.

In this paper we present data from the determination of D1- and D2-

dopamine receptor occupancy in neuroleptic treated schizophrenic patients. We have also examined the relationship between central D2-dopamine receptor occupancy and serum drug concentrations of haloperidol and sulpiride.

METHODS

Four male chronic schizophrenic patients (DSM-III), age 25-51, were recruited. They were all outpatients and had responded well to treatment. Two of the patients were treated with conventional neuroleptics (haloperidol and flupenthixol), and two with unconventional neuroleptics (sulpiride and clozapine). One PET experiment with 11C-raclopride was made for the determination and calculation of D2-dopamine receptor occupancy on each patient. In the patients treated with flupenthixol and sulpiride a PET experiment with 11C-SCH-23390 was also made to obtain indications on drug interaction with D1-dopamine receptors at treatment with neuroleptics.

Another two male schizophrenic patients were recruited to study the relationship between serum drug concentration and receptor occupancy. One patient had been treated for seven weeks with sulpiride, 600 mg b.i.d. and a second patient had been on haloperidol, 6 mg b.i.d. for three months. After the morning dose on day one, treatment was withdrawn and three PET experiments were made in each patient during two to three days. Serum drug concentrations for haloperidol (Larsson et al., 1985) and sulpiride were followed simultaneously.

In a sulpiride treated patient the dose was reduced successively in four steps (800 mg, 600 mg, 400 mg, 200 mg, and 0 mg b.i.d.). Receptor occupancy and serum drug concentrations were determined during steady-state conditions at each dose level.

Calculation of receptor occupancy

Experiments with 11C-raclopride: Specific binding in the putamen was defined as the difference between radioactivity in the putamen and the cerebellum. The estimate of free radioligand concentration was obtained from the radioactivity in the cerebellum of each patient. Expected specific binding was then estimated from a hyperbolic curve calculated from average Bmax and Kd values obtained from healthy volunteers (Farde et al., 1986). The degree of D2-dopamine receptor blockade was defined as the difference between expected specific binding and measured specific binding. Receptor occupancy was expressed as percent reduction of expected specific binding.

Experiments with 11C-SCH-23390: Bmax and Kd values are not available for 11C-SCH-23390 binding. The ratio of specific binding in the putamen to free radioligand concentration in the cerebellum (B/F) was obtained from healthy volunteers. Receptor occupancy was expressed as percent reduction of the ratio B/F.

RESULTS

In the four patients treated with four chemically distinct antipsychotic drugs there was markedly less accumulation of radioactivity in the putamen when compared to healthy volunteers. The calculated D2-dopamine receptor occupancy varied between 73 and 90 % (Table 1).

TABLE 1 Effects of neuroleptic drug treatment on 11C-raclo-pride and 11C-SCH-23390 binding to dopamine receptors in the putamen of four male schizophrenic patients (A-D)

Subject	A	B	C	D
Age (years)	42	51	46	35
Drug	Haloperidol	Sulpiride	Flupenthixol decanoate	Clozapine
Dose (mg)	4 b.i.d.	400 b.i.d.	40 weekly	300 b.i.d.
Time after last administration (hrs)	6	5	30	6
D1-dopamine receptor occupancy (%)	-	0	20	-
D2-dopamine receptor occupancy (%)	90	84	87	73

After withdrawal from haloperidol 6 mg b.i.d. receptor occupancy and serum drug concentrations were followed for 53 hours. There was only a few percent reduction in D2-dopamine receptor occupancy in spite of a serveral fold reduction in the haloperidol serum concentration (Fig. 1)

216

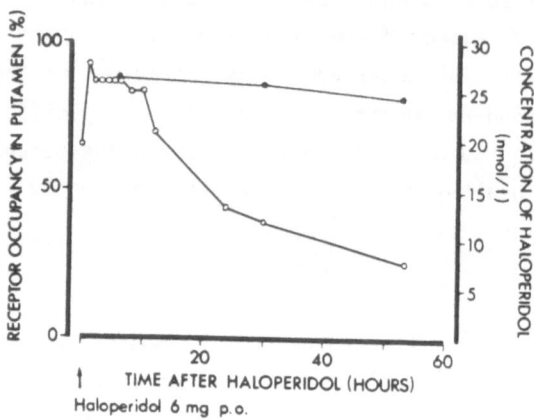

Fig. 1 Dopamine-D2 receptor occupancy in the putamen and haloperidol concentration in serum in a schizophrenic man. Solid dots = receptor occupancy, open dots = haloperidol concentration.

In the patient treated with sulpiride 600 mg b.i.d. receptor occupancy and serum drug concentrations were followed during 27 hours after withdrawal. Also in this patient the D2-dopamine receptor occupancy remained above 70 % in spite of a several fold reduction in serum concentration (Fig. 2).

In the patient treated with sulpiride 800 mg b.i.d. the dose was reduced stepwise. Nine days to three weeks elapsed between each dose reduction. In this patient D2-dopamine receptor occupancy was reduced following a curve with a hyperbolic shape (Fig. 3). The serum concentration of sulpiride was reduced following a curve with a linear shape.

217

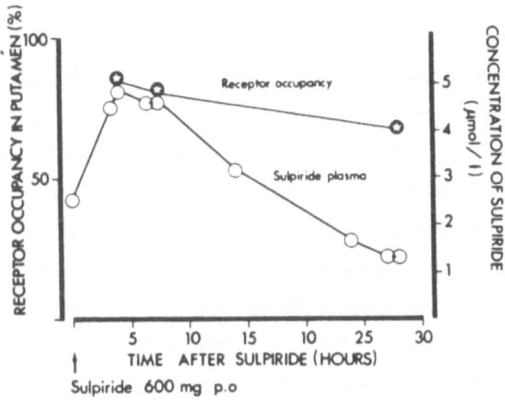

Fig. 2 Dopamine-D2 receptor occupancy in the putamen and sulpiride concentration in serum in a schizophrenic man.

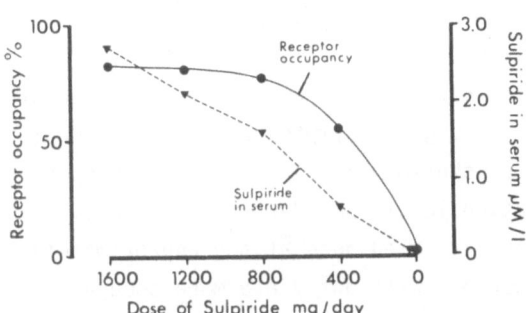

Fig. 3 D2-dopamine receptor occupancy in a sulpiride treated patient. The dose was successively reduced from 800 mg to 0 mg b.i.d.

DISCUSSION

This in vivo determination of receptor occupancy in neuroleptic treated patients demonstrated that conventional doses of 4 chemically distinct antipsychotic drugs induce a more than 70 % blockade of central D2-dopamine receptors. In the sulpiride treated patient there was no interaction with D1-dopamine receptors as measured with 11C-SCH-23390 binding. In the flupenthixol treated patient there was a 20 % reduction in specific binding when compared to normals. Sulpiride is a selective D2-dopamine receptor antagonist (Jenner et al., 1982) while flupenthixol is a mixed antagonist with a high affinity both for D1- and D2-receptors (Hyttel, 1983). The results indicate that antipsychotic drugs have a marked effect on D2-dopamine receptors but interact with D1-dopamine receptors to a much smaller extent.

The withdrawal experiments with haloperidol and sulpiride demonstrated that D2-dopamine receptor occupancy remained on a high level in spite of a substantial reduction in serum drug concentrations. In the experiment with the successive reduction of sulpiride the reduction in receptor occupancy followed a hyperbolic curve whereas the reduction in serum concentrations was linear. These results indicate a hyperbolic relationship between receptor occupancy and serum drug concentrations.

With PET and receptor ligands it is possible to relate receptor binding in the living human brain to physiological or pharmacological effects. In the seven patients of the present study 70 to 90 % of the striatal D2-dopamine receptors were blocked. In spite of the high blockade there was no sign or symptom of extrapyramidal side effects.

An equal antipsychotic effect has been reported on widely different dose and concentration levels (Marder et al., 1984). This fits to our present results. An increased dose at the approximately horizontal part of the binding hyperbola will not yield more occupancy at the already saturated D2-receptors. An increased dose will, on the other hand, place the patient at risk of unwanted side effects.

By relating receptor occupancy to the antipsychotic effect it might be possible to define a "threshold occupancy" above which an anti-psychotic effect is obtained. A low dose maintenance medication for schizophrenia has been proposed as an alternative to conventional doses (Manchanda and Hirsch, 1986). By PET it might be possible to define the

minimal individual dose giving enough occupancy to assure an antipsychotic effect but at the same time minimizing the risk of side
effects.

REFERENCES

Dahl, S. 1986. Plasma level monitoring of antipsychotic drugs clinical
     utility. Clin. Pharmacokin. 11, 36-61.
Farde, L., Hall, H., Ehrin, E. et al. 1986. Quantitative analysis of
     dopamine-D2 receptor binding in the living human brain by positron
     emission tomography. Science, 231, 258-261.
Hyttel, J. 1983. SCH-23390 - the first selective dopamine D1
     antagonist. Eur. J. Pharmacol., 91, 153-154.
Jenner, P., Testa, B., van de Waterbeemd et al. 1982. Interaction of
     substituted benzamide drugs with cerebral dopamine receptors. In
     "Special Aspects of Psychopharmacology". (Eds. M. Ackenheil, N.
     Matussek)
Larsson, M., Forsman, A., Öhman, R. 1985. Curr. Ther. Res. 34, 999-
     1008.
Marder, S.R., Van Putten, T., Mintz, J. et al. 1984. Costs and benefits
     of two doses of fluphenazine. Arch. Gen. Psych., 41, 1025-1029.
Manchanda, R., Hirsch, S. 1986. Low dose maintenance medication for
     schizophrenia. Br. Med. J., 293, 515-516.
Peroutka, S.J., Snyder, S.H. 1980. Relationship of neuroleptic drug
     effects at brain dopamine, serotonin, adrenergic and histamine
     receptors to clinical potency. Am. J. Psychiat., 137, 1518-1522.
Sedvall, G., Farde, L., Persson, A. et al. 1986. Imaging of
     neurotransmitter receptors in the living human brain. Arch. Gen.
     Psychiat., 43, 995-1005.

STRIATAL DOPAMINE RECEPTORS: DOSE-DEPENDENT OCCUPATION BY, AND RAPID WASHOUT OF, ORALLY GIVEN NEUROLEPTICS IN HUMANS

H. Cambon*, J.C. Baron*,**, J.P. Boulenger***, C. Loc'h*
E. Zarifian***, B. Maziere*

*Service Hospitalier Frédéric Joliot
CEA Département de Biologie, Orsay
**Clinique des Maladies du Système nerveux,
Hopital de la Salpétrière, Paris
***Centre Psychiatrique Esquirol
C.H.R.U. Cote de Nacre, Caën, France

Neuroleptic drugs are effective anti-psychotic agents, but the relationship between dosage and clinical response still is unclear (Curry,
1985). Likewise, the usefulness of maintenance therapy is debated
(Gaebel and Pietzcker, 1985). These uncertainties may reflect insufficient data regarding the access of neuroleptics to, and the rate of
elimination from, target structures in brain.

As the blockade of central dopamine receptors is considered to be
the main factor in the antipsychotic action of neuroleptics (Richelson
and Nelson, 1984), in vivo measurements using positron emission tomography (PET) of the actual rate of occupation of these receptors by
neuroleptics should provide an indirect but reliable estimate of effective neuroleptic tissue levels, in analogy with the radioreceptor
assay principle.

PATIENTS AND METHODS
Patients

Ten patients (three women, seven men) were studied (Table 1) after
informed consent. Their age ranged from 21 to 82 years (mean: 51.2). All
had been on chronic medication with oral neuroleptics for more than 3
months. Four patients were studied twice, first on treatment and then
after withdrawal. On the whole, there were six studies on treatment, and
eight off neuroleptics for periods from 1 to 12 days.

Each neuroleptic medication was expressed as weight-adjusted equivalent daily dose of chlorpromazine (CPZ) (Peroutka and Snyder, 1980).
When this was unavailable for a given neuroleptic, we calculated it from
its inhibition constant (Ki) for ^{3}H-haloperidol binding in vitro (Leysen, 1984), since a very good correlation between the average clinical
daily dose and the Ki for ^{3}H-haloperidol binding has been established

(Creese et al., 1976a, 1976b; Seeman et al., 1976).

PET studies

The method used has been described elsewhere (Maziere et al., 1984, 1985). About 1.3 mCi of (^{76}Br)-bromospiperone (^{76}Br-BSP) was injected i.v. as a bolus, with a specific activity of 330 $\pm$ 100 mCi/µmol. The amount of bromospiperone injected was 2.75 $\pm$ 1.26 µg.

PET studies were performed by means of the LETI time-of-flight positron camera. Seven slices were scanned simultaneously so that the cerebellum was studied at the lowest cut and the striatum at the third cut, 1 cm and 4 cm, respectively, above and in parallel with the orbito-meatal plane. A ^{68}Ge-^{68}Ga transmission scan was performed for accurate attenuation correction. A 30-minute ^{76}Br scan starting 4.5 h after injection was used for analysis (Baron et al., 1986; Maziere et al., 1985).

From these images, the striatal and cerebellar radioactivity concentrations were obtained by means of a standardized, previously validated method using regions of interest (ROIs) (Baron et al., 1986; Maziere et al., 1985).

Determination of the percentage of unoccupied binding sites

The cerebellum is virtually devoid of specific binding sites for neuroleptics (Martres et al., 1985). Therefore, the difference between ^{76}Br-BSP concentrations in striatum and in cerebellum represents the specifically bound ligand in striatum. The fraction f of dopamine sites occupied by the neuroleptic medication can thus be described by the following equation:

$$f = [(Sth - C) - (Sm - C)]/[Sth - C] \qquad (1)$$

where C is the radiocactivity concentration in the cerebellum, Sth the theoretical (expected) radioactivity concentration in the striatum, and Sm the one actually measured in the patient's striatum. By dividing each term by C, Eq. (1) becomes:

$$f = [(S/C)th - (S/C)m]/[(S/C)th - 1] \qquad (2)$$

where $(S/C)th$ and $(S/C)m$ are the expected and the measured striatum-to-cerebellum radioactivity concentration ratios, respectively.

The percentage of neuroleptic sites left unoccupied by the neuroleptic medication can be expressed as:

$$\% \text{ of unoccupied sites} = 100 \times (1 - f) \qquad (3)$$

which can be rewritten as:

$$\% \text{ of unoccupied sites} = 100 \times ([(S/C)m - 1]/[(S/C)th - 1]). \qquad (4)$$

Data analysis

From the radioactivity concentration values measured in the striatum and in the cerebellum, the $(S/C)m$ ratio was calculated for each subject.

To obtain the $(S/C)th$ value, data from 17 control subjects studied by the same procedure were used. However, it was necessary to adjust for age according to our findings in controls (Baron et al., 1986). Finally, using $(S/C)m$ and $(S/C)th$, the % of unoccupied sites was determined according to equation (4).

RESULTS

Studies during neuroleptic treatment

We found a clear-cut dose-dependent decrease in the $(S/C)m$ ratio, which ranged from 1.81 at the lowest dosage to 1.27 at the highest (Table 1).

The percentage unoccupied sites showed a striking dose-dependence (Fig. 1A), ranging from 93.7% to 26.8% for the lowest and highest doses, respectively (Table 1). The CPZ equivalent daily oral dose corresponding to 50% of unoccupied sites was about 6 µmol/kg.

TABLE 1   Clinical data and results

| Patient age/sex | Clinical diagnosis | Neuroleptic treatment (mg.kg^{-1}.day^{-1}) | (S/C)th[a] | Studies on treatment | | | Days off | Studies after withdrawal[e] | |
				CPZ eq. dose[b] (μmol.kg^{-1}.day^{-1})	(S/C)m[c]	p[d]		(S/C)m	p
1 - 62/M	Alzheimer's disease	Haloperidol (0.010)	1.86	1.4	1.81	93.7%	-	-	-
2 - 82/M	Senile dementia	Haloperidol (0.017)	1.69	2.4	1.64	92.2%	-	-	-
3 - 68/F	Chronic hallucinatory psychosis	Haloperidol (0.205)	1.81	-	-	-	1	1.90	111.6%
4 - 21/M	Schizophrenic disorder	Haloperidol (0.254) Levomepromazine (1.271)	2.21	94.3	1.33	27.3%	3	1.87	71.9%
5 - 50/M	Syphilitic dementia	Haloperidol (0.042) Levomepromazine (0.174)	1.96	13.9	1.40	41.1%	3	1.76	79.1%
6 - 43/F	Schizophrenia	Thioproperazine (1.429)	2.02	285.4	1.27	26.8%	3	2.31	127.8%
7 - 72/F	Post-stroke agitation	Haloperidol (0.027)	1.78	-	-	-	7	1.59	76.3%
8 - 21/M	Schizophrenic disorder	Haloperidol (0.031)	2.21	4.4	1.65	53.6%	7	2.17	96.9%
9 - 33/M	Alcoholism	Propericiazine (0.526)	2.11	-	-	-	10	2.15	103.6%
10 - 60/M	Vertigo	Thiethylperazine (0.375)	1.88	-	-	-	12	1.83	93.4%

(a) (S/C)th is the age-adjusted striatum/cerebellum theoretical ratio
(b) Neuroleptic daily dose expressed as chlorpromazine (CPZ) equivalent
(c) (S/C)m is the S/C ratio actually measured
(d) P is the percentage of unoccupied binding sites, calculated according to equation (4)

Studies after neuroleptic withdrawal

During withdrawal, there was a rapid trend for the (S/C)m ratio to return towards normal values (Table 1). This was strikingly demonstrated in the 4 patients who were studied on both occasions, and particularly in the 2 patients on high neuroleptic doses in whom the 4.5 h PET [76]Br-BSP image at basal ganglia level changed from a featureless pattern while on neuroleptics to the pattern of high striatal uptake, typical of normal subjects after only 3 days of withdrawal.

When the results were expressed as percentages of unoccupied sites (Fig. 1B), the majority of patients (6/8) followed a somewhat curvilinear recovery line apparently crossing the 100% level at 7 - 12 days after withdrawal. However, the extent of recovery seemed to depend on both the withdrawal interval and the % of unoccupied site during treatment; for the 3 repeated studies that followed this pattern, the mean percentage of recovery per day was 11.3% (range: 6.2 - 14.9%). The other two patients (patient 3 and 6) were somewhat atypical in that both not only reached, but even moved above the 100% level very early (112% and 128%, one and three days after neuroleptic withdrawal, respectively), including patient 6 whose percentage of unoccupied sited during treatment was very low (27%).

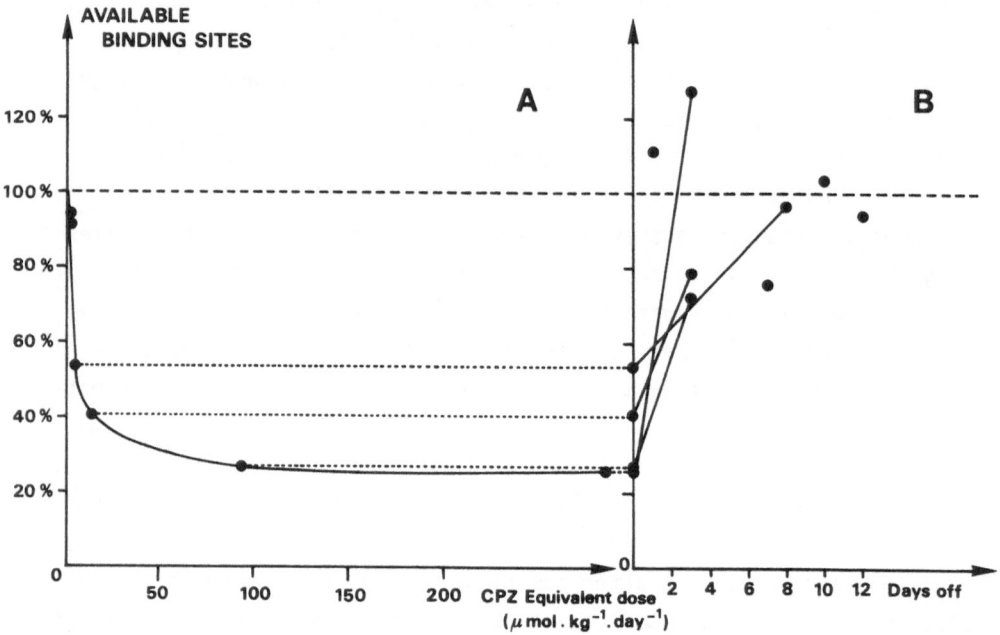

Fig. 1A   Available binding sites (equivalent to P, the percentage of unoccupied neuroleptic sites) in the six 76-Br-BSP studies performed during neuroleptic treatment, plotted against the weight-adjusted neuroleptic daily dose expressed as chlorpromazine (CE) equivalent. The data were fitted best by the bi-exponential line P = 98exp(-0.3 CE) + 34exp(-0.001 CE).

Fig. 1B   P values obtained in the 8 studies performed after neuroleptic withdrawal, plotted against the number of days off treatment. The lines connect the P values measured in 4 patients both <u>during</u> treatment and <u>following</u> withdrawal.
The <u>dotted lines</u> that link parts A and B of the graph connect the on-drug P values found in those 4 patients studied twice.

DISCUSSION

Extensive studies in animals and humans have demonstrated that [76]Br-BSP is a suitable ligand for the investigation of dopamine receptors in vivo (Baron et al., 1986; Crawley et al., 1983; Kulmala et al., 1981; Maziere et al., 1984; Owen et al., 1983). The purpose of the present study was to investigate whether this PET technique could be used to estimate in vivo the occupancy rate of neuroleptic binding sites in the striatum. Despite the limited number of studies available, the observed dose-dependent occupation (Fig. 1A) strongly supports the validity of our approach.

This seems to hold despite several potential limitations. For instance, the dopamine receptor density of our patients may have been affected not only by the neuroleptic treatment itself, but also by the underlying mental illness; the disease heterogeneity was deliberate in order to obtain a wide range of neuroleptic dosage. Patient comparability may have suffered from the variability in neuroleptic treatment duration and associated medication because both can result in variable drug metabolism (Rivera-Calimlim and Hershey, 1984) or dopamine receptor supersensitivity (Jenner and Marsden, 1983). Although based on well-established data, our method for estimating the CPZ equivalent dose may not be perfectly accurate. Similarly, the calculated fraction of unoccupied binding sites relies on an age-adjustement of the S/C ratio which is subject to small errors. Obviously, studying the patients both before and during treatment would provide more accurate estimates of occupation rates, but this poses considerable practical problems.

More importantly, the use of equations (1) and (2) for estimating the occupancy rate relies on the assumption that parameter C, the cerebellar [76]Br-BSP concentration at 4.5 h, which represents both free ligand and non-specific binding, is not affected by neuroleptic treatment: this assumption was verified (Table 2). Similarly, the initial cerebellar uptake, which was measured on an early PET scan systematically recorded between 5 and 20 min after radiotracer injection, and the blood concentration of [76]Br-BSP at 5 h were not affected by treatment (Table 2). These findings suggest an invariant a accessibility of the ligand to striatal binding sites. Errors in the estimated occupancy rates because of competition for binding between unlabeled neuroleptic and labeled bromospiperone are unlikely because the amount of bromospiperone injected was so small (5.8 ± 2.7 nmoles) as to theoretically occupy less than 1% of striatal receptors.

TABLE 2   76-Br-BSP relative radioactivity concentrations (mean ± SD).

76-BR-BSP concentration	Controls	On neuroleptics	Off neuroleptics	P
Cerebellum[a] t = 5 min	1.36+0.52 (N=11)	1.23+0.55 (N=6)	1.19+ ̄ ̄l (N= ̄	NS
Cerebellum[a] t = 4.5 h	1.41+0.41 (N=17)	1.42+0.27 (N=6)	1.42+0.20 (N=8)	NS
Blood[b] t = 5.0 h	0.47+0.19 (N=17)	0.50+0.19 (N=6)	0.50+0.12 (N=8)	NS

a: in units of % injected dose/l brain
b: in units of % injected dose/kg blood

Our results are the first to show a dose-dependent occupation of human striatal binding sites by orally given neuroleptics on chronic schedule. Using [76]Br-BSP or other radioligands, previous studies demonstrated full occupation of striatal neuroleptic binding sites by various neuroleptics in humans (Baron et al., 1983; Farde et al., 1986; Maziere et al., 1985), but none studied the full range of neuroleptic dosage.

The observation that, despite very high doses of neuroleptics, the striatum/cerebellum ratio did not reach unity (Table 1) may seem sur- prising, but it is consistent with previous findings (Maziere et al., 1984, 1985). We believe that there was indeed full receptor occupation, with the S/C ratio not reaching 1.0 because of higher non-specific uptake of [76]Br-BSP in striatum relative to cerebellum. This latter possibility is supported by results of animal experiments (Barone et al., 1985; Laduron et al., 1978).

By clearly showing a strictly dose-dependent occupation of the neuroleptic binding sites in the striatum (Fig. 1A), our data indicate that it should be possible to estimate the rate of dopamine receptor blockade from knowledge of the daily oral dose of neuroleptics, as well as the dose necessary to achieve full saturation of receptors, above which there may be no further therapeutic benefit. Although the

antipsychotic effect of the neuroleptics may be more related to
dopamine blockade in the mesolimbic system, there is little evidence to
suggest that mesolimbic and striatal receptors respond differently to
chronic neuroleptic treatment (Jenner and Marsden, 1983).

The studies performed after neuroleptic withdrawal showed return to
100% unoccupied sites within a few days (Fig. 1B), firmly establishing
that washout of neuroleptics from their striatal binding sites is a
rapid process. To date, it has been widely assumed that this washout is
much slower, based on clinical, behavioral and pharmacokinetic data
(Byck, 1975; Campbell et al., 1985; Hershon et al., 1972; Korpi et al.,
1984; Marsden et al., 1975). On the other hand, our results fully agree
with 1) the relatively short plasma half-life of most neuroleptics
(Byck, 1975; Itoh et al., 1984), 2) the pattern of haloperidol
elimination from rat brain after chronic treatment (Ohman et al., 1977),
and 3) three in vivo studies in rats (Ferrero et al., 1983; Owen et
al., 1983; Saelens et al., 1980). Our results may be important for the
design of improved treatment regimens. They also suggest that long-
lasting remissions of psychotic patients, following neuroleptic
withdrawal, are not due to persistent dopamine receptor occupation:
other explanations must be sought.

In two patients, the recovery rate was even faster, with levels
above 100% (supersensitivity?) at one and three days after neuroleptic
withdrawal, respectively. However, the intersubject variability in the
underlying mental disorder and in neuroleptic drug regimen may have
affected these recovery rates and should be controlled in future
studies.

REFERENCES

Baron, J.C., Comar, D., Zarifian, E., et al. 1983. An in vivo study of
the dopaminergic receptors in the brain of man using 11-C-pimozide
and positron emission tomography. In "Functional Radionuclide
Imaging of the Brain" (Ed. P.L. Magistretti). (Raven Press, New
York). pp. 337-345.
Baron, J.C., Maziere, B., Loc'h, C., et al. 1986. Loss of striatal
76-Br-bromospiperone binding sites demonstrated by positron tomography in progressive supranuclear palsy. J. Cereb. Blood Flow
Metab., 6, 131-136.
Barone, D., Luzzani, F., Assandri, A., et al. 1985. In vivo stereo-
specific 3-H-spiperone binding in rat brain: characteristics,
regional distribution, kinetics and pharmacological properties.
Eur. J. Pharmacol., 116, 63-74.

Byck, R. 1975. Drugs and the treatment of psychiatric disorders. In
" The Pharmacological Basis of Therapeutics" (Eds. L.S. Goodman
and A. Gilman). (MacMillan Publishing Co. Inc., New York).
pp. 156-200.

Campbell, A., Baldessarini, R.J., Teicher, M.H., et al. 1985. Prolonged
antidopaminergic actions of single doses of butyrophenones in the
rat. Psychopharmacol., 87, 161-166.

Crawley, J.C.W., Smith, T., Veall, N. et al. 1983. Dopamine receptors
displayed in living human brain with 77-Br-p-bromospiperone.
Lancet, 1, 975.

Creese, I., Burt, D.R. and Snyder, S.H. 1976a. Dopamine receptor
binding predicts clinical and pharmacological potencies of anti-
schizophrenic drugs. Science, 192, 481-483.

Creese, I., Burt, D.R. and Snyder, S.H. 1976b. Dopamine receptors and
average clinical doses. Science, 194, 546.

Curry, S.H. 1985. Commentary: the strategy and value of neuroleptic
drug monitoring. J. Clin. Psychopharmacol., 5, 263-271.

Farde, L., Hall, H., Ehrin, E., et al. 1986. Quantitative analysis of
D2 dopamine receptor binding in the living human brain by PET.
Science, 231, 258-261.

Ferrero, P., Vaccarino, F., Guidotti, A., et al. 1983. In vivo
modulation of brain dopamine recognition sites: a possible model
for emission computed tomography studies. Neuropharmacol., 22,
791-795.

Gaebel, W. and Pietzcker, A. 1985. Multidimensional study of the out-
come of schizophrenic patients 1 year after clinic discharge.
Predictors and influence of neuroleptic treatment. Eur. Arch.
Psychiat. and Neurol. Sciences, 235, 45-52.

Hershon, H.I., Kennedy, P.F. and McGuire, R.J. 1972. Persistence of
extra-pyramidal disorders and psychiatric relapse after withdrawal
of long-term phenothiazine therapy. Brit. J. Psychiat., 120, 41-
50.

Itoh, H., Yagi, G., Tateyama, M., et al. 1984. Monitoring of haloperidol serum levels and it's clinical significance. Progress in
Neuro-Psychopharmacol. and Biol. Psychiat., 8, 51-62.

Jenner, P. and Marsden, C.D. 1983. Neuroleptics and tardive dyskinesia.
In "Neuroleptics: Neurochemical, Behavioral and Clinical Per-
spectives" (Eds. J.T. Coyle and S.J. Enna). (Raven Press, New
York). pp. 223-253.

Korpi, E.R., Kleinman, J.E., Costakos, D.T., et al. 1984. Reduced
haloperidol in the post-mortem brains of haloperidol-treated
patients. Psychiat. Res., 11, 259-269.

Kulmala, H.K., Huang, C.C., Dinerstein, R.J., et al. 1981. Specific
in vivo binding of 77-Br-p-bromospiroperidol in rat brain: a
potential tool for gamma ray imaging. Life Sciences, 28, 1911-
1916.

Laduron, P.M., Janssen, P.F.M. and Leysen, J.E. 1978. Characterization
of specific in vivo binding of neuroleptic drugs in rat brain.
Life Sciences, 23, 581-586.

Leysen, J.E. 1984. Receptors for neuroleptic drugs. In "Advances in
Human Psychopharmacology, Vol. 3". (Eds. G.D. Burrows and J.S.
Werry). (JAI Press, Inc., Greenwich Conn.). pp. 315-356.

Marsden, C.D., Tarsy, D. and Baldessarini, R.J. 1975. Spontaneous
    and drug-induced movement disorders in psychotic patients. In
    "Psychiatric Aspects of Neurologic Disease" (Eds. D.F. Benson and
    D. Blumer). (Grune and Stratton, New York). pp. 219-265.
Martres, M.P., Bouthenet, M.L., Sales, N., et al. 1985. Widespread
    distribution of brain dopamine receptors evidenced with 125-I-
    iodosulpiride, a highly selective ligand. Science, 228, 752-755.
Maziere, B., Loc'h, C., Hantraye, P., et al. 1984. 76-Br-bromospiro-
    peridol: a new tool for quantitative in vivo imaging of neuro-
    leptic receptors. Life Sciences, 35, 1349-1356.
Maziere, B., Loc'h, C., Baron, J.C., et al. 1985. In vivo quantitative
    imaging of dopamine receptors in human brain using positron
    emission tomography and 76-Br-bromospiperone. Eur. J. Pharmacol.,
    114, 267-272.
Ohman, R., Larsson, M., Nilsson, I.M., et al. 1977. Neurometabolic and
    behavioural effects of haloperidol in relation to drug levels in
    serum and brain. Naunyn-Schmiedeberg's Archives of Pharmacology,
    299, 105-114.
Owen, F., Poulter, M., Mashal, R.D., et al. 1983. 77-Br-p-bromospi-
    perone: a ligand for in vivo labelling of dopamine receptors.
    Life Sciences, 33, 765-768.
Peroutka, S.J. and Snyder, S.H. 1980. Relationship of neuroleptic
    drug effects at brain dopamine, serotonin, adrenergic, and
    histamine receptors to clinical potency. Amer. J. Psychiat., 137,
    1518-1522.
Richelson, E. and Nelson, A. 1984. Antagonism by neuroleptics of neuro-
    transmitter receptors of normal human brain in vitro. Eur. J.
    Pharmacol., 103, 197-204.
Rivera-Calimlim, L. and Hershey, L. 1984. Neuroleptic concentrations
    and clinical response. Ann. Rev. Pharmacol. Toxicol., 24, 361-
    386.
Saelens, J.K., Simke, J.P., Neale, S.E., et al. 1980. Effects of halo-
    peridol and d-amphetamine on in vivo 3-H-spiroperidol binding in
    the rat forebrain. Arch. Int. Pharmacodyn., 246, 98-107.
Seeman, P., Lee, T., Chau-Wong, M., et al. 1976. Antipsychotic drug
    doses and neuroleptic/dopamine receptors. Nature, 261, 717-719.

SUMMARY of Discussion on Brain II

L. Widén, Dept. of Clinical Neurophysiology, Karolinska Institute, Stockholm, Sweden

Diseases of the brain are unique in the sense that they may "strike directly at the very heart of human nature" as someone has said. The two diseases or, rather, syndromes discussed during the second session of the workshop give rise to serious disturbances of intellectual and emotional functions. One of them, the heterogeneous group of dementias, is relentlessly progressive and there exists no therapy for it, whatsoever. The other, schizophrenia, may also be heterogeneous not only with regard to symptomatology but also to etiology and pathogenesis. Though some patients may recover completely, this seems unrelated to therapy which, at best, suppresses the positive symptoms but often with undesirable side effects.

It is unlikely that an efficient therapy will be found for these disease states unless we learn much more about their pathophysiology. The PET-technique enables us for the first time to perform local, quantitative biochemical measurements in the brain of living humans. This is a breakthrough in clinical brain research. Only a decade has passed since it was first introduced, but remarkable progress has been made during these few years in positron camera design, radiochemistry and tracer kinetic modeling, making a wide range of biological applications possible. Yet, we are still only in the very beginning of the PET era. This powerful technique will undoubtedly provide us with new information of fundamental importance for the understanding of cerebral physiology and pathophysiology, a necessary first step towards a rational therapy of the diseases of the brain. There is no goal for medical research in the developed countries that is more worthwhile.

The papers presented during the second session of the workshop demonstrate that PET has already given results of potential value for practical clinical work, e.g. new data concerning pathophysiological mechanisms of cerebral ischemia and stroke or regarding the neuropharmacology of antipsychotic treatment.

The first part of the session was devoted to the dementias. Very little, if anything, of significance could be added to Dr. Frackowiak's masterful presentation.

When PET-studies of the dementias began there were certainly hopes that specific metabolic patterns would be found for the various types of dementia. These expectations have only partially been fulfilled. It is somewhat disappointing that, according to Frackowiak et al. (1981), the two big groups of vascular and degenerative dementias cannot be distinguished by their patterns of rCMR-O2 or rCBF determined by PET. Other researchers claim that the "focal" hypometabolism of glucose in the temporal-parietal cortex is characteristic of Alzheimer's disease and is not found in multi-infarct dementia (Friedland et al., 1985a). It has been pointed out that the most pronounced histopathological findings are located in the same cortical area and that, judging from investigations in the primate brain (Mesulam et al., 1983), this is the cholinergic projection region of the posterior portion of the nucleus basalis of Meynert, which, hypothetically, may be early involved in the disease (Friedland et al., 1985b). However, the hypothesis of a selective vulnerability of a specific neurotransmitter system in Alzheimer's disease seems difficult to adhere to since it is evident that several neurochemical systems are involved (Rasool et al., 1986).

The only type of dementia that is responsive to treatment is the normal pressure hydrocephalus. It is not always easy to distinguish from Alzheimer's disease and failures of treatment have been ascribed to confusion of the two states. It therefore seems to be of definite practical value that the PET patterns of rCMR-Gl can be used to discriminate between them (Jagust et al., 1985).

Most studies of Alzheimer's disease and multi-infarct dementia have been concerned with energy metabolism, measuring either glucose or oxygen consumption. The Orsay group has also investigated the regional uptake of the amino acid methionine. Studies of other functional aspects of cerebral metabolism may in the future provide new information of diagnostic value. This is indicated e.g. by the preliminary result of the studies of neurotransmitter function in the dementias of Parkinson's and Huntington's disease and of progressive supranuclear palsy, cited by Dr. Frackowiak.

The first paper of the schizophrenia session dealt with the much debated topic of the pattern of regional glucose consumption (rCMR-Gl) in schizophrenia. No other brain disease has been the object of so many PET-studies with so varying results. The respondent, Dr. Murray, expressed his satisfaction with this state of affairs, since it agrees so well with his opinion that schizophrenia is not a disease entity but a disturbance of brain function that has many different causes. There are also other reasons for the inconsistency of the PET findings, as pointed out by Dr. Wiesel.

Though significant differences have been found between groups of schizophrenic and non-schizophrenic subjects, these differences are not profound enough or typical enough to permit the diagnosis of schizophrenia to be made on the basis of the PET findings.

The ambiguity of the concept of hypofrontality was clearly demonstrated in Dr. Wiesel's report: the patients were hypofrontal relative to the control subjects but the ratio of rCMR-Gl between frontal and temporo-parietal areas was well above 1.

The negative relationship between negative symptoms and rCMR-Gl demontrated by Wiesel is of particular interest. Is the reduced rCMR-Gl related to schizophrenia as such or to the phenomenon of "autism" regardless of its cause? It is an important question to be answered by future PET-studies.

One of the most intriguing and promising fields in PET research is the study of the neurotransmitter system, to which the last two papers of session 2 were devoted. Imaging of neurons containing neurotransmitters entails well-known difficulties and has so far only been applied successfully to dopamine neurons using 18F-DOPA as a tracer (Garnett et al., 1983). Instead a simpler approach is offered by the technique of radioligand binding to the neurotransmitter receptors, even though we have learned by experience that tracers fulfilling the requirements of a good radioligand are not easily found, as was pointed out in the discussion of the two papers.

It is well known that for each neurotransmitter there are generally several subtypes of receptors. Therefore the potential number of radioligands is great. At present, however, only two subtype receptor ligands have been introduced for PET-imaging, namely for D1 and D2-dopamine receptors as described in the paper by Farde.

That progress in physics, technology, radiochemistry and neuropharmacology has enabled us to visualize neurotransmitter receptor populations in the brains of living human subjects is of course in itself a tremendous intellectual thrill. It is, nevertheless, justified

to ask ourselves what kind of information related to CNS physiology or disease might be obtained by studies of neurotransmitter receptors, given the fact that with a suitable radioligand and an adequate quantitative model, the density of receptors can be estimated
(Farde et al., 1986). We know of some disease states associated with the
degeneration of specific neurotransmitter neurons but hardly any condition which has been demonstrated to be caused by changes in receptor
number. The well-known findings of increased density of dopamine receptors in postmortem brains of schizophrenic subjects have been ascribed to drug treatment rather than the disease process itself. However, recent PET-studies of schizophrenic subjects who had never been on
antipsychotic drugs indicate a significant increase in the density of
D2-dopamine receptors, imaged with the radioligand 11-C-methylspiperone
(Wong et al., 1987). The significance of these findings was discussed by
the respondent, Dr. Murray, who reemphasized that schizophrenia is not a
disease entity and stated that though certain cases may be associated
with changes of the D2-dopamine receptors, these changes may be "at some
distance from the cause of the disease" and that the therapeutic effect
of antidopaminergic drugs may not shed more light on the disease mechanisms than does the effect of diuretics on the cause of heart failure.
Nevertheless, the D2-dopamine receptor studies - like the PET measurements of rCMR-Gl - might provide a method for dividing schizophrenia
into different subgroups, e.g. hereditary and exogenous with possible
consequences for the choice of therapy.

Might alterations of physiological states - e.g. the level of activity of nerve cells - be mirrored in changes in receptor density?
Certain results of animal experiments indicate that this may indeed be
the case (see Snyder 1986 for a review (Snyder, in press). It seems,
therefore, to be important for future receptor studies to clarify the
rule of altered physiological states for phenomena like receptor de-
sensitization or active states of receptors. These may substantially influence the apparent density of receptors measured with PET or other
techniques.

At present the most rewarding application of the PET technique for
neurotransmitter receptor studies seems to be in the field of neuropharmacology as was so beautifully illustrated by the papers of Farde
and Baron. Among other things their results demonstrate the limited
value of blood plasma concentration determinations as an indicator of
the pharmacological effect of neuroleptics on the target organ, the
brain. To the extent that the therapeutic effect is due to blockade of
the D2-dopamine receptor it is of course essential to monitor the receptor occupancy and it is a significant accomplishment that PET now
enables us to do so. Indeed, every patient who is put on a neuroleptic
drug ought to have the therapy controlled by PET, if it were practically
feasible.

An observation of equally great pharmacological and clinical importance is the finding of Farde that antipsychotic drugs acting on D2-
dopamine receptors have only a negligible blocking effect on D1-dopamine
receptors. Thus, these two receptor subtypes seem to have different
roles in mediating the antipsychotic drug effect.

In mice there are large numbers of dopamine receptors widely scattered in the frontal lobes and the antipsychotic effect of neuroleptic
drugs has been ascribed to blockade of receptors localized in limbic
structures of the frontal lobes. However, PET imaging of D2- dopamine
receptors has not revealed any specific binding sites outside the
caudate-putamen, not even with the sensitive technique of Farde, in

236

which the image obtained with the biologically inactive optic
isomer of raclopride - showing the amount of free and unspecifically
bound ligand - is subtracted from that acquired with the active form.
It was pointed out in the discussion that these findings illstrate the
importance of being cautious when drawing conclusions from one species
to another.

We have only taken the first steps in the PET-analysis of neurotransmitter systems of the human brain. What can we expect after this?
Of course, a number of postsynaptic receptors and subtypes of receptors
remain to be studied with the radioligand binding technique. On the
other hand, the precursor strategy for imaging of neurotransmitter
producing neurons still seems very difficult to apply. However, as
pointed out by Salomon Snyder in a thought-provoking essay (1986) there
is a possibility for PET studies of these neurons using ligands to label
their uptake receptors. This certainly ought to be tried. Furthermore,
imaging of second messenger proteins is "within the grasp of presently
existing technology" (Snyder loc. cit.). This seems an extremely
interesting possibility since it would enable us to map synaptic systems
that use different kinds of messengers.

REFERENCES

Farde, L., Hall, H., Ehrin, E. et al. 1986. Quantitative analysis of
    D2 dopamine receptor binding in the living human brain by PET.
    Science, 231, 258-261.
Frackowiak, R.S.J., Pozzilli, C., Legg, N.J. et al. 1981. Regional
    cerebral oxygen supply and utilization in dementia. Brain, 104,
    753-778.
Friedland, R.P., Budinger, T.F., Koss, E. et al. 1985a. Alzheimer's
    disease: anterior-posterior and lateral hemispheric alterations
    in cortical glucose utilization. Neurosci. Letters, 53, 235-240.
Friedland, R.P., Brun, A., Budinger, T.F. 1985b. Pathological and
    positron emission tomographic correlations in Alzheimer's disease.
    Lancet, 1, 228.
Garnett, E.S., Firnau, G., Nahmias, C. 1983. Dopamine visualised in
    the basal ganglia of living man. Nature, 305, 137-138.
Jagust, W.J., Friedland, R.P., Budinger, T.F. 1985. Positron emission
    tomography with (18F) fluorodeoxyglucose differentiates normal
    pressure hydrocephalus from Alzheimer type dementia. J. Neurol.
    Neurosurg. Psychiat., 48, 1091-1096.
Mesulam, M.-M., Mufson, E.J., Levey, A.I. et al. 1983. Cholinergic
    innervation of cortex by the basal forebrain: cytochemistry and
    cortical connections of the septal area, diagonal band nuclei,
    nucleus basalis (substantia innominata), and hypothalamus in the
    Rhesus monkey. J. Comp. Neurol., 214, 170-197.
Rasool, C.G., Svendsen, C.N., Selkoe, D.J. 1986. Neurofibrillary degene-
    ration of cholinergic and noncholinergic neurons of the basal fore-
    brain in Alzheimer's disease. Ann. Neurol., 20, 482-488.
Snyder, S.H. Basic research strategies for imaging neurotransmitter
    systems. NIDA Monograph. In press.
Wong, D.F., Wagner, Jr.H.N., Tune, L.E. et al. 1987. Positron emission
    tomography reveals elevated D2 dopamine receptors in drug-naive
    schizophrenics. Science, 234, 1558-1563.

H E A R T

Angina Pectoris

APPLICATION OF POSITRON EMISSION TOMOGRAPHY
TO THE STUDY OF ISCHEMIC HEART DISEASE

A. Maseri
Royal Postgraduate Medical School,
Hammersmith Hospital, London, U.K.

As the purpose of this seminar is to attempt to establish the state of the art in PET scanning and the lines of research for the near future, I am going to summarize the areas which in my opinion will benefit more immediately from the advent of multislice, high resolution tomography and from the development of new radiopharmaceuticals.

I will list the most immediate problems of clinical research which, although apparently simple, still do not have an adequate solution.

PET applied research in the field of ischemic heart disease should develop along two lines: pathophysiological and clinical.

For pathophysiological research the unique capabilities of PET are applied to the understanding of human pathophysiology as animal models of disease are an inadequate representation of conditions still poorly understood. Pathophysiological research should be developed both by exploring in greater detail already established avenues and by tackling problems that cannot otherwise be studied in patients.

For clinical research the potential of PET should be used on the one hand to establish the correlation of PET obtained measurements with those obtained by more generally available technqiues, and on the other to establish the cost benefit of information for clinical practice obtainable by PET scanning.

Pathophysiological Research

1. The assessment of myocardial blood flow (MBF) in quantitative, regional terms remains a fundamental problem in ischemic heart disease. It would be desirable to: a) obtain the regional distribution of MBF for the entire ventricular myocardium, possibly with a resolution adequate to distinguish subendocardial from subepicardial perfusion; b) express the flow values in ml/min/g of viable myocardium; and c) perform repeated measurements at frequent time intervals in order to study transients of the order of minutes, when this is required.

Measurement of flow per unit volume of viable myocardium is a prerequisite to interpret comprehensively measurements of any other myocardial, metabolic of functional feature.

2. The spatial detection of myocardial ischemia, the definition of the time course of ischemic episodes and of their effect on cardiac metabolism and on the rate of development of necrosis, are other fields which require investigation in patients, as animal models may not necessarily reflect all the complex events that occur in patients.

3. The study of receptor density and activity in the coronary vasculature, and in the heart is a new domain for which PET studies are uniquely suited. Indeed the only other alternative for patient studies is cardiac biopsy. At the present time it is difficult to anticipate the potential benefit of these studies for the understanding of human diseases, but there is experimental evidence that both ischemia and failure can profoundly effect receptor behaviour. Whether altered behaviour of vascular receptors in coronary vessels contributes to ischemic syndromes is unknown, but it can only be established by studies in patients.

Clinical Research

There is information of considerable practical value that PET could offer if the entire ventricular myocardium could be enclosed in the counting field with adequate resolution, once the appropriate measurements are appropriately validated. The measurements produced by PET would not only be useful on their own but also as a standard of reference for other techniques more widely available.

The major areas of potential practical interest that I can see are twofold:

1. The accurate detection of regional coronary flow reserve for assessing the functional severity of coronary artery obstructions remains a major goal. This also requires the definition of the mass of myocardium with reduced coronary flow reserve that is at risk,

2. the accurate detection of the location and extension of areas of ischemic but still viable myocardium represents another field of great potential clinical interest. This information would best be expressed both in grams of ischemic myocardium per unit volume and per gram of viable myocardium.

CONCLUSIONS

These considerations are intended to outline the main areas of interest in the field of ischemic heart disease for clinical research and clinical practice to non-clinical investigations and to set the stage for general discussion.

Technical limitations certainly do not allow perfect answers to the problems outlined above. For clinical research, compromises can be accepted as long as PET studies provide additional understanding of the problem under study. For clinical practice, approximations can be accepted as long as they still allow us to obtain information which is of proven value for a better management of the patient in relation to other procedures and to its cost.

PET IN THE STUDY OF ANGINA PECTORIS

P. Camici* and L. Araujo**
*C.N.R. Institute of Clinical Physiology and
Instituto di Patologia Medica
University of Pisa, Italy
**MRC Cyclotron and Cardiovascular Units,
Hammersmith Hospital, London, U.K.

Important metabolic changes take place in the myocardium during conditions of recuded oxygen supply. The oxidation of free fatty acids (FFA) is impaired, and a greater percentage of FFA is converted into tissue lipids, while myocardial glucose consumption is enhanced due to a faster rate of anaerobic glycolysis (Neely and Morgan, 1974; Rovetto et al., 1972, 1975).

However, in the isolated perfused rat heart, major differences in both exogenous glucose utilization and total glycolytic flux have been described between hypoxia or anoxia, and ischemia (Rovetto et al., 1972). In severely ischemic myocardium, the utilization of exogenous glucose is not accelerated, unlike in the anoxic perfused heart, and total glycolysis decreases after glycogen stores in the tissue are depleted. The accumulation of lactate and the reduction of pH in the ischemic tissue are responsible for the inhibition of glycolysis which seems to be proportional to the degree of restriction of coronary flow (Rovetto et al., 1975).

Anoxia and hypoxia, however, are only rarely responsible for reduced myocardial oxygen supply in man. Ischemia, due to either a primary reduction of coronary flow (primary ischemia) or to an imbalance between oxygen supply and demand (secondary ischemia), is the most common cause of reduced myocardial oxygen supply in man (Maseri et al., 1978). Moreover, myocardial ischemia in man is usually a regional phenomenon and has a differential transmural severity (i.e., it is more severe in the inner than in the outer myocardial layers of the left ventricle (Maseri et al., 1978).

In the clinical setting, myocardial ischemia can be either transient and reversible (angina pectoris) or prolonged and irreversible, i.e., associated with permanent tissue damage (myocardial infarction). Between these two extremes (angina and infarction), many situations can be found in which varying proportions of viable and necrotic tissue coexist (jeopardized myocardium).

In summary, the metabolic basis of human heart disease differs from most experimental animal models because of the interplay of essentially four factors: (a) ischemia rather than anoxia is the mechanism of reduced oxygen supply; (b) ischemia in man is a regional phenomenon both along the heart walls and across them; (c) it can be primary or secondary; (d) the duration and severity of flow reduction have important consequences of their own.

The recent availability of positron emission tomography (PET) renders possible the non-invasive evaluation or regional myocardial perfusion and metabolism in man (Phelps, 1977).

In this paper, the preliminary data obtained by PET in patients with coronary artery disease and stable or unstable angina pectoris are reported.

STABLE ANGINA

In patients with angiographically proven coronary artery disease and severe stable angina pectoris, regional myocardial perfusion and glucose utilization were assessed with PET using the cation Rubidium-82 (Selwyn et al., 1982) and (^{18}F)-2-fluoro-2-deoxyglucose (FDG) (Gallagher et al., 1977; Phelps et al., 1978), respectively. Studies were carried out in the absence of medical treatment and after overnight fasting (Camici et al., 1985, 1986a).

In patients at rest, myocardial glucose utilization was comparable to that found in normal volunteers studied in the same condition (Fig. 1). As expected, when cardiac work and blood insulin levels were low, the utilization of exogenous glucose in the myocardium was minimal, and FDG matched the regional distribution of perfusion.

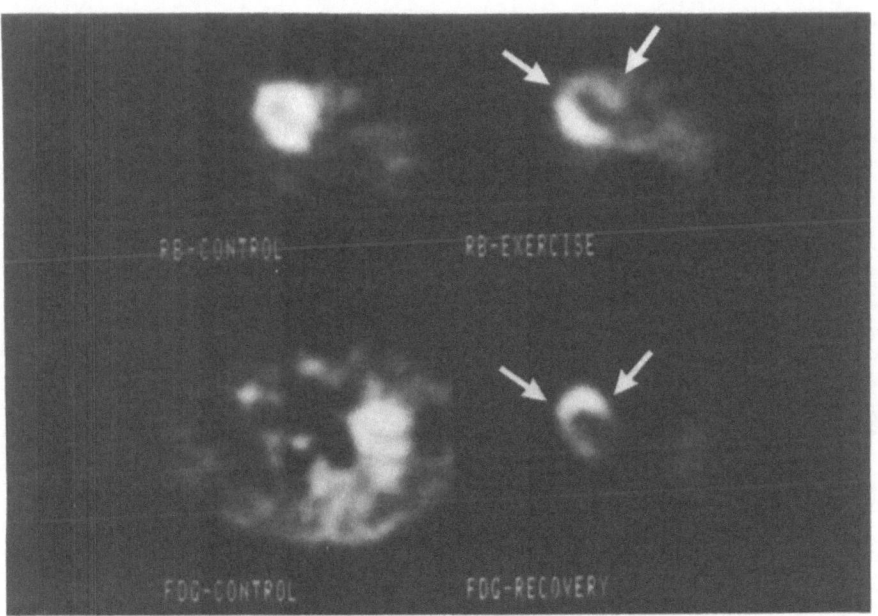

Fig. 1   Positron tomographic images of the chest of a patient with stable angina. In each image, the left ventricle free wall is in the 6 to 10 o'clock position, the anterior wall and septum are in the 10 to 3 o'clock position, and the remaining open area is the plane of the mitral valve.
Myocardial uptake of Rb at rest (top left) is homogeneous, while during exercise (top right), cation uptake is severely reduced in the anterior wall (arrows). When FDG was injected at rest (bottom left) after overnight fasting, myocardial tracer uptake was very low, the heart profile being barely detectable. In this patient, FDG was also injected during the recovery from the stress test, when all the signs of ischemia had disappeared. Under these conditions (bottom right), the region of previous ischemia was clearly identifiable (arrows), tracer uptake in the anterior wall being 1.75 times higher than in non-ischemic myocardium.

Patients were also studied following a maximal bicycle ergometer test performed in the supine position, with the subject inside the positron camera. Owing to the very short half-life of the potassium analogue Rubidium-82 (78 seconds), repeated measurements of myocardial perfusion were performed in the same patient under different experimental conditions (i.e., before the stress test, at its peak, and in the recovery phase).

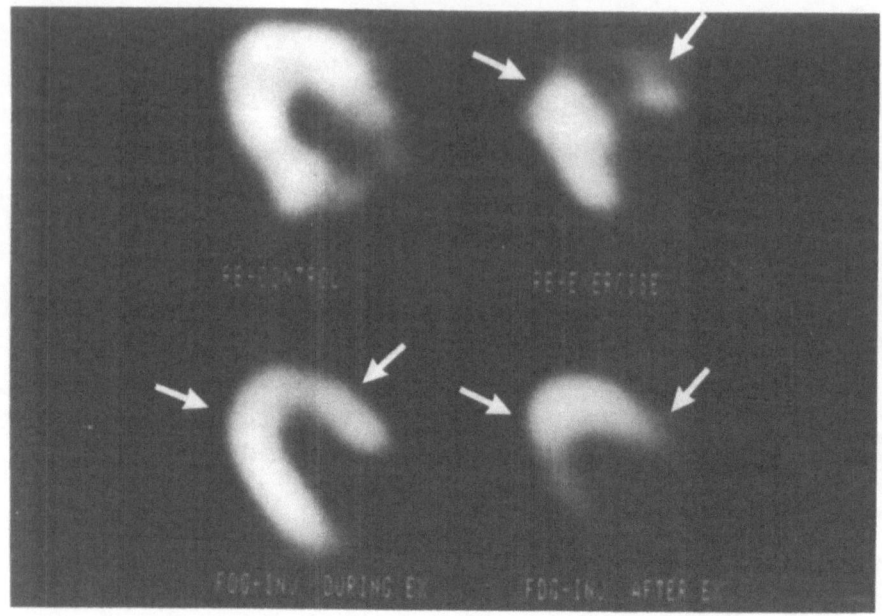

Fig. 2   Positron computed tomographic images of the heart of a patient with stable exertional angina, obtained with Rubidium-82 (Rb) and F-18-deoxyglucose (FDG). The Rb scan at rest (Rb control) shows homogenous perfusion in all cardiac walls. At peak exercise (Rb-exercise), severely reduced cation uptake is evident in the anterior wall of the left ventricle (arrows). When FDG was injected during exercise (FDG-Inj. during ex.), tracer concentration in the ischemic region (arrows) was 0.75 times lower than that in non-ischemic myocardium. The FDG scan obtained in the recovery phase (FDG-Inj. after ex.), when all the symptoms and signs of ischemia had disappeared, demonstrates a 1.8 times higher tracer concentration in the previously ischemic region as compared with non-ischemic tissue. For image orientation see legend to Fig. 1.

In all the patients studied, the exercise test induced typical chest pain and ischemic changes of the electrocardiogram that were accompanied by regional abnormalities of Rubidium-82 myocardial uptake (Fig. 1, 2). A significant increase in myocardial glucose utilization was observed, when FDG was administered during the stress test. This increase, however, was not regionally homogenous: glucose utilization in the non-ischemic areas (i.e., the ones showing a normal increase in Rubidium-82 uptake during exercise) increased more than in the ischemic regions (i.e., the ones where an abnormal Rubidium-82 uptake was demonstrated during exercise).

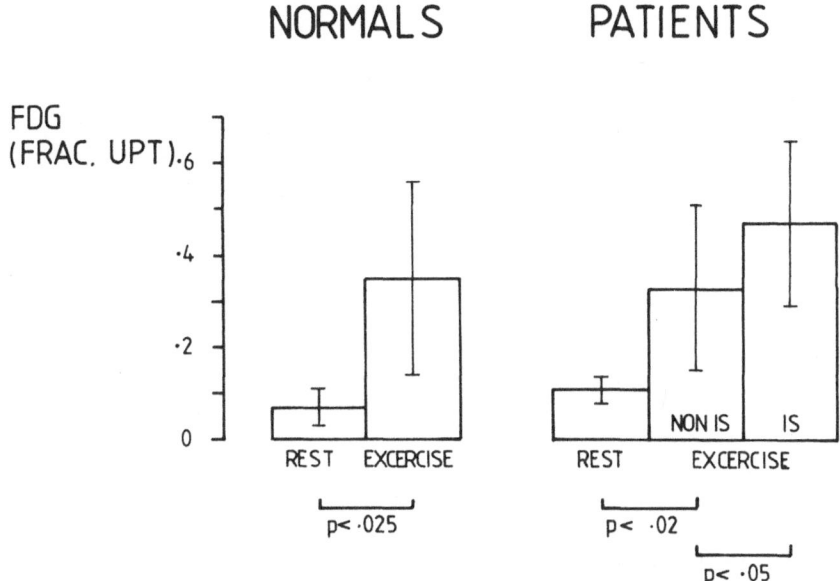

NORMALS   PATIENTS

Fig. 3   Fractional uptake of FDG (FRAC. UPT.) in the myocardium of normals and patients with stable angina at rest and following exercise. FDG uptake in non-ischemic (NON IS) myocardium is comparable to that in normals following exercise, while post-ischemic (IS) myocardium shows a persistently higher FDG uptake in the recovery phase.

In contrast, during recovery from exercise, when all the indices of ischemia including myocardial Rubidium-82 uptake had normalized, a significantly greater glucose utilization could be demonstrated in the regions that were ischemic during exercise (Fig. 1, 2, 3). This persistently high glucose utilization in the postischemic myocardium is suggestive of a greater glycolytic flux and/or an increased rate of glycogen synthesis due to the depletion of this polysaccharide induced by ischemia as suggested by preliminary animal experiments (Camici and Bailey, 1984) (Fig. 4).

248

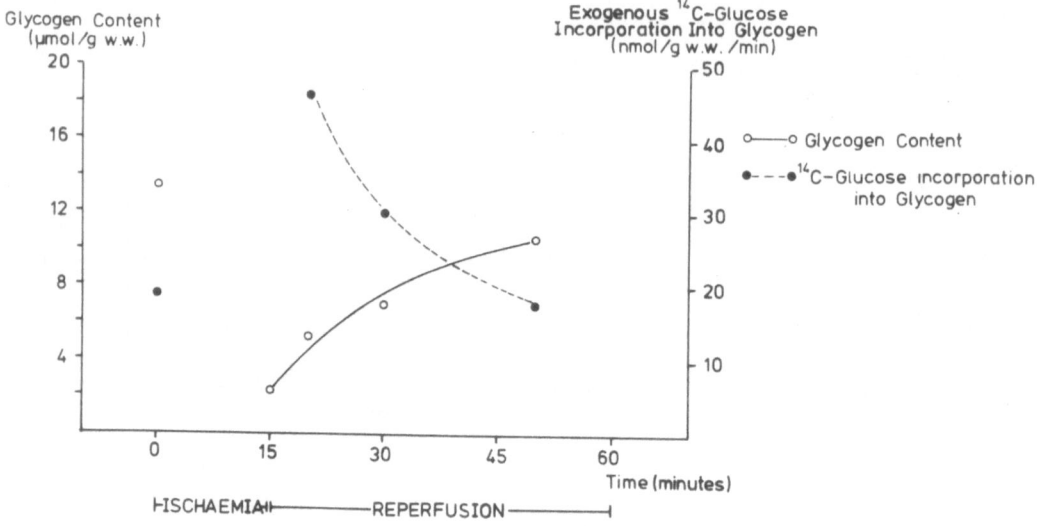

Fig. 4   Content of myocardial glycogen (open circles) measured in
the isolated perfused working rat heart together with the rate of
incorporation of 14-C-glucose into glycogen pool (closed circles).
The content of glycogen following 15 minutes of global ischemia is
reduced to less than 20% of the control value. During reperfusion,
glycogen is re-synthetized at the expense of exogenous glucose as
indicated by the higher rate of incorporation of 14-C-glucose into
the glycogen pool.

UNSTABLE ANGINA

Regional myocardial perfusion and glucose utilization were assessed
using Rubidium-82 and FDG, respectively, with PET in patients with
severe coronary artery disease and repeated episodes of spontaneous
depression of the ST segment of the electrocardiogram, without evidence
of acute myocardial infarction (Camici et al., 1984, 1986b). Studies
were carried out at rest, after overnight fasting, off therapy, and in
the absence of symptoms or ECG signs of acute ischemia.

Myocardial glucose utilization in patients with unstable angina was
significantly different from that observed in normal volunteers and in
patients with stable angina at rest.

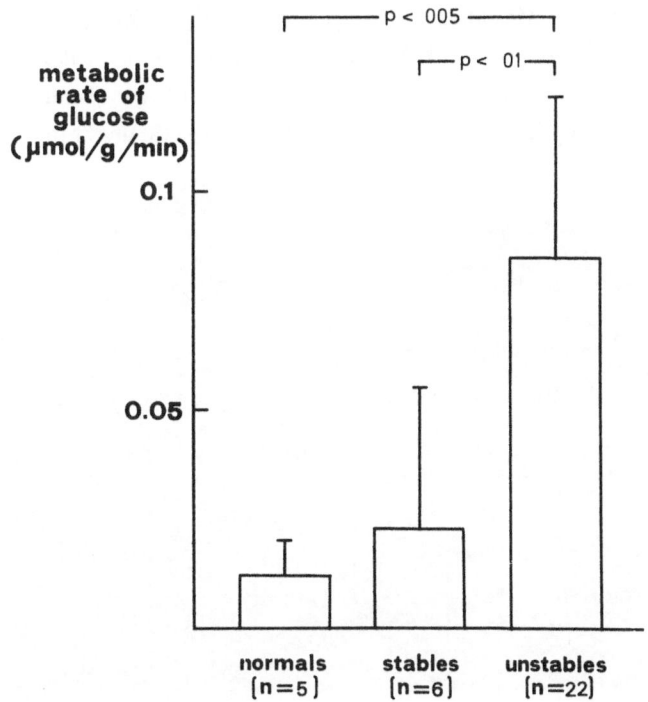

Fig. 5   The metabolic rate of glucose measured in patients with
unstable angina during resting condition is significantly higher
than that measured in normal volunteers and patients with stable
exertional angina at rest.

In fact, in patients with unstable angina, myocardial glucose utilization was found to be regionally or globally increased already at rest as compared to that in normal volunteers and patients with stable angina (Fig. 5). This occurred in the absence of symptoms and electrocardiographic signs of ischemia at the time of the study and most often in the absence of clearly detectable abnormalities of Rubidium-82 myocardial uptake.

A significant reduction of myocardial glucose utilization, which however remained higher than in normals and in patients with stable angina, was observed in some of these patients who were restudied during i.v. infusion of nitrates, starting 24 hours before the study (Fig. 6). Finally, normal glucose utilization (comparable to that found at rest in normals and in patients with stable angina was found in patient, who had successfully undergone aortocoronary bypass grafting (Fig. 6).

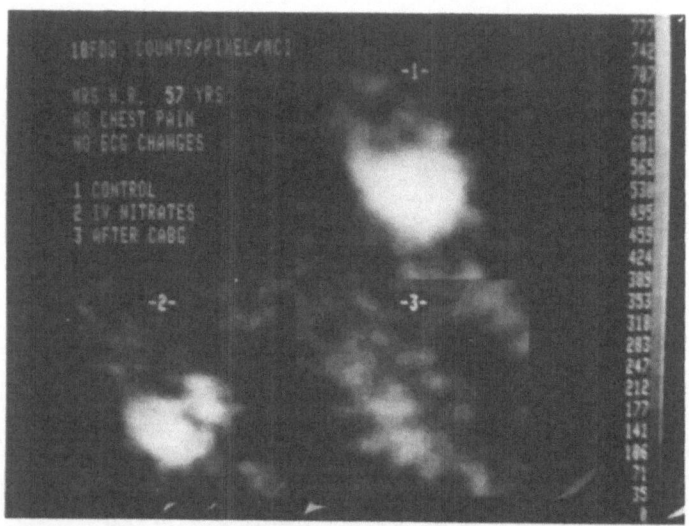

Fig. 6   Positron computed tomographic images of the heart of a patient with unstable angina, who had angiographically proven severe coronary artery disease and repeated episodes of spontaneous ST depression but no evidence of acute infarction. At the time of the study, however, the patient did not show any symptom or electrocardiographic sign of acute ischemia. The control FDG scan (1) shows a large area of significantly greater glucose utilization at the level of the inferior wall of the left ventricle as compared to the other cardiac walls. The FDG scan obtained 1 week later, during i.v. infusion of nitrates (2), shows a reduction of FDG uptake in the inferior wall that, however, is still hotter than the remaining myocardium. The FDG scan obtained 4 months after a successful bypass graft (3) is normalized. For image orientation see legend to Fig. 1.

The significance of the described findings in patients with unstable angina remains to be elucidated. The metabolic alterations in patients with chronic ischemic heart disease may suggest a more efficent glyco-lytic production of high-energy phosphate due to adaptive biochemical changes associated with long-lasting hypoperfusion.

REFERENCES

Camici, P. and Bailey, I. 1984. Time course of myocardial glycogen repletion following acute myocardial ischemia. Circulation, 70, II-85.
Camici, P. Araujo, L., Spinks, T. 1984. Persistent chronic metabolic abnormalities in patients with unstable angina pectoris. Circulation, 70, II-249.
Camici, P., Kaski, J.C., Shea, M.J., et al. 1985. Selective increase of glucose utilisation in the postischemic myocardium of patients with stable angina. In "Hammersmith Cardiology Workshop Series, Vol. 2" (Ed. A. Maseri). (Raven Press, New York). pp. 81.
Camici, P., Araujo, L., Spinks, T., et al. 1986a. Increased uptake of 18-F-fluorodeoxyglucose in postischemic myocardium of patients with exercise-induced angina. Circulation, 74, 81.
Camici, P., Araujo, L. Spinks, T., et al. 1986b. Myocardial blood flow and glucose metabolism in exercise induced and spontaneous ischemia. Eur. J. Nucl. Med., 12, 549.
Gallagher, B.M., Ansari, A., Atkins, H., et al. 1977. Radiopharmaceutic-als XXVII. 18-F-labelled 2-deoxy-2-fluoro-D-glucose as a radio-pharmaceutical for measuring regional myocardial glucose metabolism in vivo: tissue distribution and imaging studies in animals. J. Nucl. Med., 18, 990.
Maseri, A., Klassen, G.A., Lesch, M. 1978. Primary and Secondary Angina Pectoris. (Grune & Stratton Inc., New York-San Francisco-London).
Neely, J.R. and Morgan, H.E. 1974. Substrate and energy metabolism of heart. In "Annual Reviews of Physiology" (Ed. J.H. Conroe Jr.) Palo Alto, Ca., 36, 413.
Phelps, M.E. 1977. Emission computed tomography. Seminars of Nuclear Medicine, 7, 337.
Phelps, M.E., Hoffman, E.J., Selin, E., et al. 1978. Investigation of (18-F) 2-fluoro-2-deoxyglucose for the measurement of myocardial glucose metabolism. J. Nucl. Med., 19, 1311
Rovetto, M.J., Whitman, J.T., Neely, J.R. 1972. Comparison of the effects of anoxia and whole heart ischemia on carbohydrate utili-zation in isolated working rat hearts. Circ. Res., 32, 699.
Rovetto, M.J., Lamberton, W.F., Neely, J.R. 1975. Mechanisms of glyco-lytic inhibition in ischemic rat hearts. Circ. Res., 37, 742.
Selwyn, A.P., Allan, R.M., L'Abbate, A., et al. 1982. Relation between regional myocardial uptake of Rubidium-82 and perfusion: absolute reduction of cation uptake in ischemia. Am. J. Cardiol., 50, 112.

INVESTIGATION OF MYOCARDIAL RECEPTORS
BY PET IN HEART DISEASES

A. Syrota
Service Hospitalier Frédéric Joliot
Département de Biologie du Commissariat à l'Energie Atomique
Orsay, France

Changes in number and/or affinity of cardiac neurotransmitter receptors have been associated with myocardial ischemia and infarction, congestive heart failure, cardiomyopathy, as well as diabetes or thyroid-induced heart muscle disease. These alterations of cardiac receptors have been demonstrated in vitro on membrane homogenates from samples collected mainly during surgery or post mortem. The disadvantage of these in vitro binding techniques is that receptors loose their natural environment and their relationships with the other components of the tissue. With the advent of positron emission tomography (PET) it is now possible to obtain noninvasively quantitative determination of regional biochemical processes in the heart.

The feasibility of characterizing muscarinic acetylcholine receptors, beta-adrenergic receptors and alpha$_1$-adrenergic receptors has been shown in animals and in man (Syrota, 1986). The receptor PET technique begins to be applied to clinical investigations.

A. Criteria for identification of ligand-receptor interaction in the
   myocardium by PET

Receptor-mediated localization of a ligand in the myocardium must be validated in vivo by the same criteria as those for in vitro binding studies (Laduron, 1984).

1. Saturability of the ligand-receptor complex can be demonstrated by two kinds of experiments. In the displacement experiments an excess of cold agonist or antagonist is intravenously injected some time after injection of the labeled ligand. The radioactive concentration then rapidly decreases with time because of the competitive inhibition between the tracer and the excess of unlabeled ligand.

The receptor sites can also be blocked by an excess of unlabeled ligand injected prior to the radioligand. In this case the tracer radioactive concentration in the tissue is lower than that measured in the absence of injection of the cold molecule.

2. Stereoselectivity is a powerful proof for receptor binding. If two stereoisomers are available, one with and the other without pharmacologic activity, the displacement must be obtained only with the active isomer. The stereospecificity of the binding of the muscarinic antagonist ^{11}C-MQNB was proved: only the pharmacologically active isomer of benzetimide (dexetimide) could displace ^{11}C-MQNB, the inactive isomer (levetimide) being ineffective (Mazière et al., 1981).

3. Correlation between the binding and a biological effect is essential for distinguishing between a displaceable binding site with no signal transmission and a receptor binding site which is related to physiological responses. A correlation between receptor binding and biological effect was shown with ^{11}C-pindolol, ^{11}C-CGP 12177 and ^{11}C-MQNB. The percentage of ^{11}C-MQNB or ^{11}C-CGP 12177 displaced by various amounts of unlabeled atropine or propranolol was proportional to the decrease or increase in heart rate.

4. Complementary criteria must also be validated such as the specific regional distribution of the receptors and the high affinity of receptor sites for the radioligand.

B. Characterization of cardiac adrenergic receptors by PET

Catecholamines, acting through alpha- and beta-adrenergic receptors, modulate a variety of physiological responses in the heart, the most important being an increase in the rate and force of cardiac contraction. The two types of adrenergic receptors, alpha and beta, can be classified into two subtypes termed alpha$_1$, alpha$_2$ and beta$_1$, beta$_2$ using both pharmacological and anatomical criteria (Motulsky and Insel, 1982; Stiles and Lefkowitz, 1984).

1. In vivo demonstration of beta-adrenergic receptors

Both beta$_1$- and beta$_2$-adrenergic receptors are present in the mammalian heart. Basically, beta$_2$-receptors exhibit equal affinity for both epinephrine and norepinephrine, whereas beta$_2$-receptors exhibit a higher affinity for epinephrine than for norepinephrine (Molinoff, 1984). Beta$_1$-adrenergic receptors are the predominant beta-adrenergic receptors (Stiles et al., 1983). However, a relatively high proportion of beta$_2$-receptors, up to 50 %, is found in the human heart, especially in the atria (Robberecht et al., 1983).

2. PET

Four antagonists, propranolol, practolol, pindolol, and CGP 12177 have been labeled with ^{11}C. They differ for affinity, liposolubility and subtype-selectivity. ^{11}C-propranolol a lipophilic, nonselective antagonist cannot be used for studying the beta-adrenergic receptor with PET because it accumulates in the lungs after i.v.injection during the time of PET scanning. ^{11}C-practolol is a hydrophilic molecule that binds on homogenates to beta$_1$-receptor. A few minutes after i.v. injection in man the heart was well visualized but the tracer con- centration decreased rapidly with time even when ^{11}C-practolol was injected at very high specific activity (Dormont et al., 1983). The percentage of bound tracer that could be displaced by injection of an excess of unlabeled antagonist (practolol, propranolol, atenolol, pindolol) 20 min later was also low. Both results can be explained by the relatively low affinity of practolol (high K_D).

^{11}C-pindolol and ^{11}C-CGP 12177 have in common a high affinity (low K_D) and a low lipophilicity. ^{11}C-CGP 12177 presents the greatest advantages. It is a very potent hydrophilic nonselective betablocker which shows little nonspecific binding on membranes and little cellular uptake (Steahelin and Hertel, 1983). It must be noted that CGP-12177 also has a slight partial agonist effect. This hydro- philic beta-adrenergic ligand that is not taken up by cells is therefore an ideal probe to specifically measure in vivo the cell surface receptors, that is the "functionally active" beta receptor.

A high myocardial uptake was measured after ^{11}C-pindolol or ^{11}C-CGP 12177 injection and a displacement of both bound tracers was obtained after injection of an excess of cold pindolol (Seto et al., 1986). Saturation of the beta-adrenergic receptor was also demonstrated by a preinjection of an unlabeled betablocker a few minutes before the

injection of ^{11}C-CGP. The preinjection reduced the number of unoccupied receptor sites available for the binding of radiotracer.
Compared to the control curve, the radioactive concentration measured in
the ventricular myocardium was therefore lower. A correlation was
observed between the tracer displacement and the decrease in heart rate
induced by the displacing agent. The validation of this important
criterium is a strong indication that receptor sites and not only
binding sites are visualized. Myocardial beta-adrenergic receptor
density has been found to differ among species: B_{max} = 152, 150 and
311 fmol/mg protein in rat, rabbit and dog respectively using ^{3}H-DHA as
ligand (Mukherjee et al., 1983). Beta-adrenoceptor density has been also
measured in biopsies of human left ventricle and found to vary between
30 fmol.mg^{-1} and 79 fmol.mg^{-1} using ^{125}I-cyanopindolol (Stiles et
al., 1983). Beta-adrenergic receptor density has been measured in the
dog ventricular myocardium by PET. B_{max} was found to be 113 pmol/g of
tissue (unpublished data). The presence of beta-adrenergic receptors in
the ventricles of all studied species is consistent with the findings
that sympathetic nerve fibers innervate all regions of the heart.

3. In vivo study of alpha-adrenergic receptors
Alpha-adrenergic receptors have been also classified into two
subtypes, alpha$_1$ and alpha$_2$ (Motulsky and Insel, 1982; Stiles and
Lefkowitz, 1984; Stiles et al., 1983). The alpha$_1$ receptors are the
classical postsynaptic alpha receptors mediating smooth muscle
contraction. Alpha$_2$ receptors are found in several locations,
particularly on presynaptic nerve terminals, where they mediate feedback
inhibition of norepinephrine release. The alpha$_1$- and alpha$_2$-
receptors can be distinguished pharmacologically by their relative
affinities for various agonists and antagonists. Prazosin, a selective
alpha$_1$-adrenergic blocker was labeled with ^{11}C and injected to dogs
(Ehrin et al., in press). PET scans showed a high and homogeneous
myocardial uptake with a much lower pulmonary uptake. However, the
validation of criteria needed for the characterization of receptors
could not be achieved probably because of to high nonspecific binding
(unpublished data).

C. Characterization of cardiac muscarinic acetylcholine receptors by PET
The neurotransmitters acetylcholine and norepinephrine exert their

chronotropic and inotropic effects on the heart by an opposite coupling
of the cholinergic and beta-adrenergic receptors to adenylate cyclase;
beta-adrenoceptors activate adenylate cyclase whereas muscarinic
cholinergic receptors inhibit it. The cholinergic receptor was
historically the first receptor in which subtypes were clearly
delineated. However, many classifications have been proposed
(Hirschowitz et al., 1984). Currently, the accepted scheme is that
muscarinic receptors exist in two subtypes. The M_1 class is defined as
those receptors exhibiting a high affinity towards the antagonist
pirenzepine, whilst the M_2 subclass is defined as those receptors
exhibiting a low affinity towards pirenzepine. The high affinity (M_1)
sites are thought to be primarily located in the central nervous system
whilst the low affinity (M_2) sites are thought to be mainly located on
peripheral effector organs. However, binding studies and functional
assays indicate heterogeneity for muscarinic receptors in myocardium
(Watson et al., 1986). Binding experiments with pirenzepine indicate
that there is a population of muscarinic receptors in myocardium that
could well be designated M_1 receptors. Chick myocardium has even a
predominance of M_1 receptors in contrast to rat heart (Brown et al.,
1985).

The most commonly used radiolabeled muscarinic antagonists, ³H-QNB
(quinuclidinyl benzylate) and ³H-NMS (N-methylscopolamine) appear to
recognize identical populations of muscarinic receptors. The presence of
a population of specific, saturable, high affinity acetylcholine
receptors in the mammalian heart was identified by the use of ³H-QNB
(Fields et al., 1978). However, when the same ligand was used to label
intact cells instead of membrane preparations a higher nonspecific
binding suggested a trapping of the ligand within the cells presumably
into the lysosomes.

These findings strengthen the choice of labeling MQNB with ^{11}C to
study the muscarinic acetylcholine receptor in vivo by PET (Mazière et
al., 1981). MQNB is a hydrophilic antagonist that is not extracted by
the lungs and that displays a high affinity for the cholinergic
receptors in rat heart homogenates. All the criteria needed to
characterize the muscarinic receptor were validated in the baboon and in
man with ^{11}C-MQNB. The ventricular septum and the left ventricle
contained high concentrations of ^{11}C-MQNB, the radioactivity in the
right ventricle was very low and the atria were never visualized.

Saturation experiments showed that the highest concentrations were found in the septum (98 pmol/g of heart) and in the left ventricle (89 pmol/g) (Syrota et al., 1985). It is reasonable to think that, although the receptor concentration could be higher in atria than in ventricles (Fields et al., 1978), because of their weight, ventricle and septum contain a higher percentage of acetylcholine receptors than atria. Although the existence of an abundant parasympathetic innervation of the atria is well known, that of the ventricles has been a subject of controversy. In the past decade numerous data, both chemical and physiological, have proved the existence of a direct parasympathetic innervation of the mammalian ventricle (see ref. Levy and Martin, 1981, for review). The localisation of these receptors and their precise role in the modulation of biochemical and electrophysiological events at the cellular level remains a subject of considerable interest. Saturability of the binding was demonstrated by saturation experiments. After a bolus injection of ^{11}C-MQNB at a high specific activity, the ^{11}C-MQNB blood concentration fell very rapidly to a negligible value a few minutes after i.v.injection. In contrast, the ^{11}C-MQNB concentration increased rapidly in the myocardium to reach a maximum in 1-5 min and then remained constant for 70 min. The rapid i.v.injection of unlabeled atropine led to a rapid decrease (lasting a few minutes) in the septal ^{11}C-MQNB concentration. This binding was stereospecific since dexetimide (the pharmacologically active isomer) but not levetimide could displace ^{11}C-MQNB from its binding sites (Mazière et al., 1981). A correlation between receptor occupancy and a physiological effect has also been demonstrated (Syrota et al., 1985). A relationship between the percentage of MQNB found in 1 cm³ of septum after rapid i.v. injection in 12 subjects injected with comparable amounts of MQNB and the heart rate value recorded at the time of injection was observed. For a given subject, the MQNB concentration in the ventricular septum was higher when the heart rate was lower. A low frequency is related to a predominant vagal influence. The greater ^{11}C-MQNB binding in the septum linked to vagal stimulation could be explained by an increase in either the number or the affinity of antagonist binding sites. In the physiologically active state, the agonist is released from the receptor in a low-affinity form, and more sites are available for ^{11}C-MQNB binding (Burgisser et al., 1982). These findings suggest that PET allows the identification of the physiologically active conformation of the muscarinic receptor under sympathetic and parasympathetic physiological control (Syrota et al., 1985).

D. Characterization of the peripheral-type benzodiazepine receptor

Specific high-affinity benzodiazepine binding sites have been demonstrated in several peripheral organs including the heart (Davies and Huston, 1981; Taniguchi et al., 1982). The ligand specificity and affinity for the peripheral-type binding site is completely different from that of the central-type site (Trifiletti et al., 1984). The demonstration of peripheral-type benzodiazepine binding sites was first made in vitro with ^{3}H-diazepam (Davies and Huston, 1981). New ligands which only bind to peripheral-type site and not to the classical central-type have been synthetized. RO 5-4864 and PK 11195 are almost inactive in binding inhibition of ^{3}H-diazepam on its sites in the brain but have a very high affinity for peripheral sites (Le Fur et al., 1983). In vitro the PK 11195 binding sites in rat cardiac membranes are specific, saturable with a K_D of 1.41 nM and a B_{max} of 2250 pmol/g of protein (Le Fur et al., 1983). PK 11195 was labeled with carbon 11 at very high specific activity and injected intravenously in dogs and humans. An initial uptake of ^{11}C PK 11195 was seen in the lung, followed by a high uptake in the heart. Benzodiazepine binding sites were uniformly distributed (Charbonneau et al., 1986). The amount of PK 11195 found in the heart was proportional to the quantity injected at values below 40 nmol/kg. Above 40 nmol/kg, however, the curve showed a plateau due to saturation of the benzodiazepine binding sites. This result agrees with the mathematical model of a ligand-receptor interaction studied in vivo (Syrota et al., 1984). A similar curve was also obtained when studying the muscarinic acetylcholine receptor (Syrota et al., 1985). From the PK 11195 concentration values, the number of benzodiazepine binding sites in the dog ventricular myocardium (B_{max}) was found to be around 6,000 pmol/cm^3 of heart. Other criteria needed for identification of a ligand receptor interaction by PET were validated. Saturability was demonstrated by coinjection or displacement experiments with unlabeled PK 11195 and other ligands which compete for peripheral-type sites such as RO 5-4864 and diazepam. Ligands that only bind to brain-type sites such as RO 15-1788 and clonazepam were ineffective (Charbonneau et al., 1986). PK 11195 antagonizes the effects of several calcium channel blockers and of a calcium channel agonist in a guinea pig papillary muscle preparation. It also inhibits arrythmias induced by ischemia and abnormalities after reperfusion in the dog heart (Mestre et al., 1985). A PET study of these receptors in man could thus be interesting in clinical situations.

E. Future implications

PET has only recently begun to be applied to the study of cardiac physiology and disease. It is the only methodology able to demonstrate the physiological regulation of receptors (Motulsky and Insel, 1982). Treatment of cells or animals with agonists or antagonists influence receptor number. Agonist treatment leads to down-regulation (decrease in receptor density) and antagonist treatment leads to up-regulation. Many cardiovascular drugs influence synaptic mechanisms to elicit their therapeutic effects. Treatment with beta blocking agents causes up-regulation of human myocardial beta receptor density. Among these agents, pindolol, a drug with intrinsic sympathomimetic activity, seems to favour up-regulation (Golf and Hansson, 1986). Dysopyramide and quinidine exercise their anticholinergic effects by blocking cardiac muscarinic receptors in canine ventricular myocardium (Mirro et al., 1980). PET is thus a unique tool for studying the mechanisms of action of drugs in clinical pharmacology. PET could also be able to investigate changes in receptor number and/or affinity in cardiac diseases. Experimental studies have shown that coronary occlusion for 30 min to 1 hour is associated with an increase in the density of alpha-and beta-adrenoceptors (Mukherjee et al., 1982). Beta-adrenergic receptor density increases during relatively early stages of injury in metabolically impaired myocytes and decreases subsequently (Buja et al., 1985). However, the mechanism mediating this up-regulation of receptors is unknown. During myocardial ischemia, beta-adrenergic receptors could be redistributed from intracellular vesicles to sarcolemnal membranes (Maisel et al., 1985).

$beta_1$- and $beta_2$-receptor subtypes have been studied in congestive heart failure. Failing human ventricular myocardium shows a decrease in the $beta_1$ proportion and an increase in the $beta_2$ proportion due to selective down-regulation of $beta_1$-receptors (Bristow et al., 1986).

PET is thus able to provide noninvasively information not only on cardiac receptor density and affinity but also on the physiologically active form of the receptor under physiological regulation in man. It shows the interactions between drugs acting on the heart and myocardial receptors. One can therefore anticipate its interest for the investigation of cardiac ischemia and cardiomyopathy in man.

REFERENCES

Bristow, M.R. et al. 1986. Beta-1- and beta-2-adrenergic receptor subpopulations in nonfailing and failing human ventricular myocardium: coupling of both receptor subtypes to muscle contraction and selective beta-1-receptor down-regulation in heart failure. Circ. Res., 59, 297-309.

Brown, J.H., Goldstein, D., Masters, S.H. 1985. The putative M1 muscarinic receptor does not regulate phosphoinositide hydrolysis: studies with pirenzepine and McN A 343 in chick heart and astrocytoma cells. Mol. Pharmacol., 27, 525-531.

Buja, L.M. et al. 1985. Characterization of a potentially reversible increase in beta-adrenergic receptors in isolated, neonatal rat cardial myocytes with impaired energy metabolism. Circ. Res., 57, 640-645.

Burgisser, E., De Lean, A., Lefkowitz, R.J. 1982. Reciprocal modulation of agonist and antagonist binding to muscarinic cholinergic receptor by guanine nucleotide. Proc. Natl. Acad. Sci. (USA), 79, 1732-1736.

Charbonneau, P. et al. 1986. Peripheral-type benzodiazepine receptors in the living heart characterized by positron emission tomography. Circulation, 73, 476-483.

Davies, L.P., Huston, V. 1981. Peripheral benzodiazepine binding sites in heart and their interaction with dipyridamole. Eur. J. Pharmacol., 73, 209-211.

Dormont, D. et al. 1983. C11 ligand binding to adrenergic and muscarinic receptors in the human heart studied in vivo by PET. J. Nucl. Med., 24, P 20.

Ehrin, E. et al. In press. Preparation of carbon-11 labeled prazosin, a potent and selective alpha-1-adrenoreceptor antagonist. Int. J. Appl. Rad. Isot.

Fields, J.Z. et al. 1978. Cardiac muscarinic cholinergic receptors. Biochemical identification and characterization. J. Biol. Chem., 253, 3251-3258.

Golf, S., Hansson, V. 1986. Effects of beta blocking agents on the density of beta-adrenoceptors and adenylate cyclase response in human myocardium: intrinsic sympathomimetic activity favours receptor regulation. Cardiovasc. Res., 20, 637-644.

Hirschowitz, B.I. et al. 1984. Subtypes of Muscarinic Receptors. Trends in Pharmacological Sciences. Suppl. Elsevier, Amsterdam.

Laduron, P.M. 1984. Criteria for receptor sites in binding studies. Bichochem. Pharmacol., 33, 833-839.

Le Fur, G. et al. 1983. Peripheral benzodiazepine binding sites: effect of PK 11195, 1-(2-chlorophenyl)-N-methyl-N-(1-methylpropyl)-3-isoquinolinecarboxamide. I. In vitro studies. Life Sic., 32, 1839-1847.

Levy, M.N., Martin, P.J. 1981. Neural regulation of the heart beat. Ann. Rev. Physiol., 43, 443-453.

Maisel, A.S., Motulsky, H.J., Insel, P.A. 1985. Externalization of beta-adrenergic receptors promoted by myocardial ischemia. Science, 230, 183-186.

Mazière, M. et al. 1981. In vivo characterization of myocardium muscarinic receptors by positron emission tomography. Life Sci., 29, 2391-2397.

Mestre, M. et al. 1985. PK 11195, an antagonist of peripheral benzodiazepine receptors, reduces ventricular arrhythmias during myocardial ischemia and reperfusion in the dog. Eur. J. Pharmacol., 112, 257-260.

Mirro, J.M. et al. 1980. Anticholinergic effects of disopyramide and quinidine on guinea pig myocardium mediation by direct muscarinic receptor blockade. Circ. Res., 47, 855-865.

Molinoff, P.B. 1984. Alpha- and beta-adrenergic receptor subtypes properties, distribution and regulation. Drugs, 28, (Suppl. 2), 1-15.

Motulsky, H.J., Insel, P.A. 1982. Adrenergic receptors in man. Direct identification, physiologic regulation and clinical alterations. New Engl. J. Med., 307, 18-28.

Mukherjee, A. et al. 1983. Differences in myocardial alpha- and beta-adrenergic receptor numbers in different species. Am. J. Physiol., 245, (Heart Circ. Physiol., 14), H957-H961.

Mukherjee, A. et al. 1982. Relationship between beta-adrenergic receptor numbers and physiological responses during experimental canine myocardial ischemia. Circ. Res., 50, 735-741.

Robberecht, P. et al. 1983. The human heart beta-adrenergic receptors. I. Heterogeneity of the binding sites: Presence of 50 % beta-1- and 50 % beta-2-adrenergic receptors. Mol. Pharmacol., 24, 169-173.

Seto, M. et al. 1986. Beta-adrenergic receptors in the dog heart characterized by 11C-CGP 12177 and PET. J. Nucl. Med., 27, 949.

Syrota, A. 1986. In vivo study of receptors for neuromediators with PET. Int. J. Nucl. Med. Biol., 13, 127-134.

Syrota, A. et al. 1985. Muscarinic cholinergic receptor in the human heart evidenced under physiological conditions by positron emission tomography. Proc. Natl. Acad. Sci. (USA), 82, 584-588.

Syrota, A. et al. 1984. Kinetics of in vivo binding of antagonist to muscarinic cholinergic receptor in the human heart studied by positron emission tomography. Life Sci., 35, 937-945.

Staehelin, M., Hertel, C. 1983. (3H)CGP-12177, a beta-adrenergic ligand suitable for measuring cell surface receptors. J. Rec. Res., 3, 35-43.

Stiles, G.L., Lefkowitz, R.J. 1984. Cardiac adrenergic receptors. Ann. Rev. Med., 35, 149-164.

Stiles, G.L., Taylor, S., Lefkowitz, R.J. 1983. Human cardiac beta-adrenergic receptors: subtype heterogeneity delineated by direct ligand binding. Life Sic., 33, 467-473.

Taniguchi, T., Wang, J.K.T., Spector, S. 1982. 3(H)diazepam binding sites on rat heart and kidney. Biochem. Pharmacol., 31, 589-590.

Trifiletti, R.R., Lo, M.M.S., Snyder, S.H. 1984. Kinetic differences between type I and type II benzodiazepine receptors. Mol. Pharmacol., 26, 228-240.

Watson, M., Yamamura, H.I., Roeske, W.R. 1986. (3H)pirenzepine and
(-)-(3H)-quinuclidinyl benzilate binding to rat cerebral cortical
and cardiac muscarinic cholinergic sites. I. Characterization and
regulation of agonist binding to putative muscarinic subtypes. J.
Pharmacol. Exp. Ther., 237, 411-418.

HEART

Infarction

POSSIBLE CLINICAL EFFICACY OF POSITRON EMISSION TOMOGRAPHY
IN MYOCARDIAL INFARCTION

B. Lösse

Dept. of Cardiology, Pneumology and Angiology,
Univ. of Düsseldorf, FRG

If the clinical cardiologist is asked for his expectations from the
new method of positron emission tomography (PET) in myocardial infarction, one has to consider 1) the problems of myocardial infarction in
its different clinical stages, 2) how they are currently faced in
clinical practice, and 3) where the clinician feels urgent need of
extension of his diagnostic tools in favour of greater accuracy of his
diagnostic and therapeutic decisions.

In clinical terms we have to distinguish the acute phase of the
first few hours after onset of complaints, which is followed by the
postacute phase lasting until discharge of the patient from hospital
after 2 to 3 weeks. This is followed by the chronic phase (Table 1).

The acute phase is governed by attempts to ascertain the definite
diagnosis of myocardial infarction, which is made by physical
examination and ECG, and urgent attempts to establish early reperfusion
of the jeopardized myocardium, which is made by thrombolysis and/or
mechanical procedures, e.g., thrombus perforation or percutaneous
transluminal coronary angioplasty (PTCA). These attempts have to begin
as early as possible. Once the infarction is accomplished, they are
useless and expose the patient to further risks. Unfortunately, there
are at present no clinical methods to judge exactly the temporal
evolution of the definite infarction in the individual patient: time
varies between 60 min and several hours, depending on residual flow,
collateral flow, and myocardial oxygen demand (Maroko et al., 1971;
Müller et al., 1980; Schaper and Pasyk, 1976; Klein and Kreuzer, 1986).
If PET measurements could solve this dilemma and provide an accurate
distinction between irreversibly damaged and viable tissue, they would
be deeply appreciated. But, since from ethical reasons no time delay is
allowed to attempt restoration of blood flow in promising cases, these
methods had to be quickly applicable close to the coronary care unit and
accessible around the clock. From this standpoint it appears improbable

that PET measurements will get importance in the clinical setting of
acute myocardial infarction.

TABLE 1   Risk stratification after myocardial infarction
(one-year mortality)

	low <5 %	intermediate 5-20 %	high > 20 %
Left ventricular function	EF > 50 %	EF 35-50 %	EF < 35 %
Ischemia	not present at rest and exercise	severe during exercise	severe at rest
Ventricular arrhythmias	VEB < 10/h	VEB 10-30/h	VEB > 30/h recurrent VT

EF = ejection fraction, VEB = ventricular ectopic beats, VT =
ventricular tachycardia

The postacute and chronic phase of myocardial infarction are
governed by gradual remobilization and rehabilitation depending on
proper estimation of fatal risks, especially the risk of reinfarction
and sudden death due to arrhythmias. The risks of future coronary
morbidity and mortality decline with the temporal distance from acute
infarction. Clinical experience, supported by a number of well performed
studies, indicates that poor left ventricular function, persistent
ischemia and frequent ventricular ectopic beats are associated with a
high risk of early coronary mortality, whereas well preserved left
ventricular function, non-existence of ischemia and rare ventricular
arrhythmias identify low-risk patients (DeBusk et al., 1986; Esterbrooks
et al., 1983; The Multicenter Postinfarction Research Group, 1983;
Bigger et al., 1981; Fioretti et al., 1984). Between these two extremes
a group of patients with an intermediate early mortality risk can be
identified with moderately depressed left ventricular function, ischemic
symptoms only during stress, and moderately increased incidence of
ventricular arrhythmias (Table 2).

TABLE 2 Myocardial infarction

	Problems	Methods
Acute phase	diagnosis, acute therapy, limitation of infarct size	ECG, enzymes, angiography, thrombolysis, PTCA
Postacute phase	risk stratification (ventricular function, ischemia, arrhythmias), mobilization or urgent aggressive therapy (surgery or PTCA)	ECG, Holter monitoring, echocardiography, radio-nuclide ventriculography, submaximal exercise testing (ECG, radionucli-des), angiography, hemo-dynmaic measurements, electrophysiologic studies
Chronic phase	risk stratification, definite therapy (medical, PTCA, surgical), rehabilitation, risk factor modification	as in postacute phase, but maximal exercise testing

Risk stratification according to these criteria has to start as early as possible after infarction to identify patients in need of urgent aggressive interventional therapy including PTCA and surgery in order to prevent early reinfarction and early death. Risk stratification has to be continued throughout the chronic phase to decide on definite therapy (medical, PTCA or surgical).

A broad spectrum of methods is currently in use to fit this purpose (Table 1) and must be combined to meet the different aspects of prognosis. The traditional cardiological equipment including ECG and angiography is often not able to discriminate correctly between reversibly and irreversibly damaged myocardium in infarcted regions and to determine the functional significance of coronary artery stenoses related to infarcted and non-infarcted regions. Clarification of these questions is, however, mandatory for the decision about suitability for coronary revascularization or aneurysmectomy. Currently available radionuclide methods like 201-thallium myocardial scintigraphy and gated blood pool imaging have considerably enlarged the diagnostic spectrum especially with respect to the assessment of left ventricular function and myocardial ischemia (Rozanski et al., 1981, 1982; Gibson et al., 1983; Pohost et al., 1977).

In an own study (Lösse et al., 1983) we were able to show that thallium scintigraphy improved the accuracy of detection of surgically proved myocardial scars as compared to contrast ventriculography and ECG, especially in the anterior wall. This was mainly due to a reduction of false positive results in cases with angiographically akinetic or dyskinetic wall regions. Recent studies indicate that PET with fluorine-18-deoxyglucose (FDG), a tracer of exogeneous glucose uptake, might be even more accurate in predicting potential reversibility of cardiac wall motion abnormalities (Tillisch et al., 1986).

There is general agreement that thallium scintigraphy improves detection of myocardial ischemia by about 10-20 % as compared to exercise ECG (Botvinick et al., 1978; Lenaers et al., 1977; Ritchie et al., 1977; Trobaugh et al., 1978; Turner et al., 1978; Verani et al., 1978; Lösse et al., 1979). To gain maximal information, vigorous exercise is mandatory. This is, however, not possible in the early phase after acute myocardial infarction and, later on, in patients with severe regional or diffuse myocardial dysfunction. Therefore, a correct estimation of the functional significance of coronary stenoses in non-infarct-related regions may be difficult or impossible. There is need of a method which solves this problem even at low exercise levels or at rest. Preliminary work indicates that PET studies of alterations of myocardial metabolism (Schelbert et al., 1982) may be useful for this purpose. The question is raised whether and to what extent PET can contribute in this difficult field of clinical practice.

Finally I like to summarize a number of relevant questions that are open in the field of myocardial infarction and should be discussed with regard to the possibilities of PET: Problems in need of further clarification in the acute phase of myocardial infarction include 1) the time course of infarct evolution, 2) the early characterization of viable myocardial tissue which can be salvaged from irreversible injury,

3) the evolution of myocardial infarction in the case of angiographically normal coronary arteries. Problems related to the postacute and chronic phase of myocardial infarction include 1) the discrimination between reversible and irreversible damage in infarcted regions, 2) the detection of ischemia in infarct-related myocardial areas, 3) the detection of ischemia in non-infarct-related areas, 4) the pathogenesis and origin of complex ventricular arrhythmias after myocardial infarction. Whereas the application of PET in the acute phase appears to be restricted to animal experiments, its application during the postacute and acute phase of myocardial infarction bears lesser problems and should be forwarded, since preliminary studies indicate its potential benefit for clinically relevant diagnostic and therapeutic decisions.

REFERENCES

Bigger, J.T.Jr., Weld, F.M., Rolnitzky, L.M. 1981. Prevalence, characteristics and significance of ventricular tachycardia (three or more complexes) detected with ambulatory electrocardiographic recording in late hospital phase of acute myocardial infarction. Am. J. Cadiol., 48, 815.
Botvinick, E.H., Taradash, M.H., Shames, D.M. et al. 1978. Thallium-201 myocardial perfusion scintigraphy for the clinical clarification of normal, abnormal and equivocal electrocardiographic stress tests. Am. J. Cardiol., 41, 43.
DeBusk, R.F., Blomqvist, C.G., Kouchoukos, N.T. et al. 1986. Identification and treatment of low-risk patients after acute myocardial infarction and coronary-artery bypass graft surgery. N. Engl. J. Med., 314, 161.
Esterbrooks, D.J., Kiefer, S., Weatherbee, T. et al. 1983. After myocardial infarction: How to determine future risk and what to do then. Postgrad. Med., 73, 219.
Fioretti, P., Browner, R.W., Simoons, M.L. et al. 1984. Prediction of mortality in hospital survivors of myocardial infarction: Comparison of predischarge exercise testing and radionuclide ventriculography at rest. Br. Heart J., 52, 292.
Gibson, R.S., Watson, D.D., Taylor, G.J. et al. 1983. Prospective assessment of regional myocardial perfusion before and after coronary revascularization surgery by quantitative thallium-201 scintigraphy. J. Am. Coll. Cardiol., 1, 804.
Klein, H.H., Kreuzer, H. 1986. Neue Aspekte zum zeitlichen Verlauf der Myokardinfarktentwicklung. Dtsch. Med. Wschr., 111, 270.
Lenaers, A., Block, P., van Thiel, E. et al. 1977. Segmental analysis of Tl-201 stress myocardial scintigraphy. J. Nucl. Med., 18, 509.
Lösse, B., Baaken, U., Bircks, W. et al. 1983. Diagnostic value of thallium myocardial imaging in the recognition of left ventricular aneurysm - comparison with ECG and left ventricular angiography. 21th Internat. Ann. Meet. of the Soc. of Nucl. Med.-Europe.

Lösse, B., Krönert, H., Rafflenbeul, D. et al. 1979. Sensitivity and accuracy of thallium-201 myocardial scintigraphy in the detection of coronary artery and myocardial disease. Z. Kardiol., 68, 429.

Maroko, P.R., Kjeksus, J.K., Sobel, B.E. et al. 1971. Factors influencing infarct size following experimental coronary artery occlusion. Circulation, 43, 67.

Müller, K.D., Klein, H., Schaper, W. 1980. Changes in myocardial oxygen consumption 45 min after experimental coronary occlusion do not alter infarct size. Cardiovasc. Res., 14, 710.

Pohost, G.M., Zir, L.M., Moore, R.H. et al. 1977. Differentiation of transiently ischemic from infarcted myocardium by serial imaging after a single dose of thallium-201. Circulation, 55, 294.

Ritchie, J.L., Trobaugh, G.B., Hamilton, G.W. et al. 1977. Myocardial imaging with thallium-201 at rest and during exercise: Comparison with coronary arteriography and resting and stress electrocardiography. Circulation, 56, 66.

Rozanski, A., Berman, D., Gray, R. et al. 1982. Preoperative prediction of reversible myocardial asynergy by postexercise radionuclide ventriculography. N. Engl. J. Med., 307, 212.

Rozanski, A., Berman, D., Gray, R. et al. 1981. Use of thallium-201 redistribution scintigraphy in the preoperative differentiation of reversible and nonreversible myocardial asynergy. Circulation, 64, 936.

Schaper, W., Pasyk, S. 1976. Influence of collateral flow on the ischemic tolerance of the heart following acute and subacute coronary occlusion. Circulation, 53, Suppl. 1, 57.

Schelbert, H.R., Henze, E., Phelps, M.E. et al. 1982. Assessment of regional myocardial ischemia by positron-emission computed tomography. Am. Heart J., 103, 588.

The Multicenter Postinfarction Research Group. 1983. Risk stratification and survival after myocardial infarction. N. Engl. J. Med., 309, 331.

Tillisch, J., Brunken, R., Marshall, R. et al. 1986. Reversibility of cardiac wall motion abnormalities predicted by positron tomography. N. Engl. J. Med., 314, 884.

Trobaugh, G.B., Hamilton, G.W., Ritchie, J.L. et al. 1978. Usefulness and limitations of thallium-201 for detection of coronary artery disease based on Bayes theorem. Am. J. Cardiol., 41, 441.

Turner, D.A., Battle, W.E., Deshmukh, H. et al. 1978. The predictive value of myocardial perfusion scintigraphy after stress in patients without previous myocardial infarction. J. Nucl. Med., 19, 249.

Verani, M.S., Marcus, M.L., Razzak, M.A. et al. 1978. Sensitivity and specificity of thallium-201 perfusion scintigrams under exercise in the diagnosis of coronary artery disease. J. Nucl. Med., 19, 773.

THE ROLE OF PET IN THE CHARACTERIZATION OF MYOCARDIAL NECROSIS: CLINICAL PROBLEMS RELATED TO THE NON-Q-WAVE INFARCTION

O. Parodi
CNR Institute of Clinical Physiology
Pisa, Italy

In the past few years, selection of patients with myocardial infarction for many clinical and follow-up studies has been based on the ECG criteria of presence or absence of the Q wave (Santiago et al., 1983; Hutter et al., 1981). However, anatomo-pathological observations demonstrated that the development of transmural and non-transmural scars is poorly correlated with electrocardiographic signs of necrosis (Raunio et al., 1979). The inconclusive results of short and long-term prognosis (Madigan et al., 1976; Nicholson et al., 1983) may be related to the lack of consistent definition as well as inappropriate interpretation of the ECG findings which characterize the syndrome defined as "subendocardial infarction".

In order to obtain an "in vivo" characterization of perfusion abnormalities in this syndrome and to correlate this abnormalities with the ECG changes, a large population has been extensively studied by multiparametric approach since 1980.

Study protocol

A reasonable mean to assess the transmural extent of myocardial necrosis should be represented by evaluation of regional coronary blood flow. To overcome the limits of thallium scintigraphy (poor definition of perfusion defects, low heart to background activity ratio, blurring effect), we used human albumin labeled microspheres (HAM) as a flow marker (Parodi et al., 1982). With this technique the acquisition of intramyocardial HAM radioactivity is synchronized with patient electrocardiogram, such as for equilibrium blood pool scans. High contrast systolic and diastolic images can be obtained, which provide detection of small perfusion defects and information on residual wall motion of the ischemic/necrotic tissue. The HAM technique has been applied to 20 patients with persistent (2 days) post-anginal ST-T changes without newly developed Q waves or previous myocardial infarction (Marzullo et al., 1985).

Positron emission tomography (PET) has made possible correct information on regional myocardial blood flow (Schelbert et al., 1982) and viability (Marshall et al., 1983). Among the available flow tracers, rubidium-82 is easy to use because its production is cyclotron-independent; however, absolute measurements of regional blood flow distribution with this cation are hampered by the peculiar kinetics of the tracer and by the not proportional extraction with flow. N13-ammonia provides a more accurate quantification of myocardial blood flow by PET, although a slight underestimation versus the microspheres technique has been observed (Shah et al., 1985). We applied PET and N13-ammonia in a separate group of 15 patients with clinical and electrocardiographic findings superimposable to the group of patients studied by microspheres.

Clinical and radioisotopic results
    In these two groups of patients, the following results have been obtained:
- the ECG change do not predict location and extension of perfusion defects; normalization of the ECG does not imply normalization of flow;
- regional wall motion can be normal or markedly impaired; patients with isolated T wave changes show a higher global ejection fraction and a lower incidence of dyssynergies when compared to patients with ST changes;
- coronary anatomy can show subocclusive or occlusive disease, evidence of collateral circulation in all the occluded vessels, prevalence of isolated left descending artery disease in patients with T wave changes and of double or triple vessels disease in patients with ST changes. Thus, electrocardiogram, myocardial function and coronary anatomy do not provide specific findings to characterize this syndrome.

    HAM scintigraphy showed non-transmural (reduced end-diastolic activity or reduction of systolic thickening) perfusion defects in all patients, and in 85 % of those transmural defects (absence of detectable activity) were also detected. Thus, although the syndrome is better characterized by perfusion studies, quantification and extent of myocardial damage as well as the functional state of residual tissue still need to be assessed.

PET provides quantitative information on myocardial blood flow and a non-invasive evaluation of myocardial viability. The tomographic and quantitative approach obtained by PET and N13-ammonia confirmed the co-existence of transmural and non-transmural defects of perfusion in patients with "designated" subendocardial infarction by ECG criteria (Parodi et al., 1984).

Although N13-ammonia and PET allow better quantitative definition of regional blood flow impairment, the metabolic condition of hypo-perfused areas is not known. As a matter of fact, the two different perfusion patterns observed in the affected areas, namely 1) absent or very low flow, and 2) residual flow need to be characterized with respect to metabolism.

Metabolic approaches

F18-fluorodeoxyglucose (FDG) and PET allow identification of potentially reversible ischemic tissue from infarction (Marshall et al., 1983). In the very low-flow condition (regional coronary flow close to 0) FDG uptake indicates the presence of viable tissue, while the absence of FDG uptake confirms the presence of necrotic tissue. In the condition of some residual flow, FDG uptake indicates the presence of ischemic tissue while its absence will indicate the absence of a glycolytic pathway in these regions. Does this last condition mean a normal oxydative metabolism? The study of labeled free fatty acid distribution and kinetics (C11-palmitate) by PET would allow recognition of a moderate oxygen deprivation and hence the presence of myocardium with impaired metabolism.

A schematic flow-chart of the clinical recognition of non-transmural myocardial infarction is drawn in Table 1.

Collateral clinical problems in non-Q-wave infarction

The following clinical problems need to be focussed in patients with recent or previous non-Q-wave myocardial infarction:
1) normalization of negative T waves during resting angina (Parodi et al., 1981);

2) normalization of negative T waves during stress test;
3) normalization of negative T waves in the follow-up period.

Conventional diagnostic tools are not always able to solve these problems. Metabolic tracers and PET will provide a correct assessment of the clinical meaning of these electrocardiographic changes.

TABLE I : Clinical flow-chart in the assessment of non Q - wave infarction.

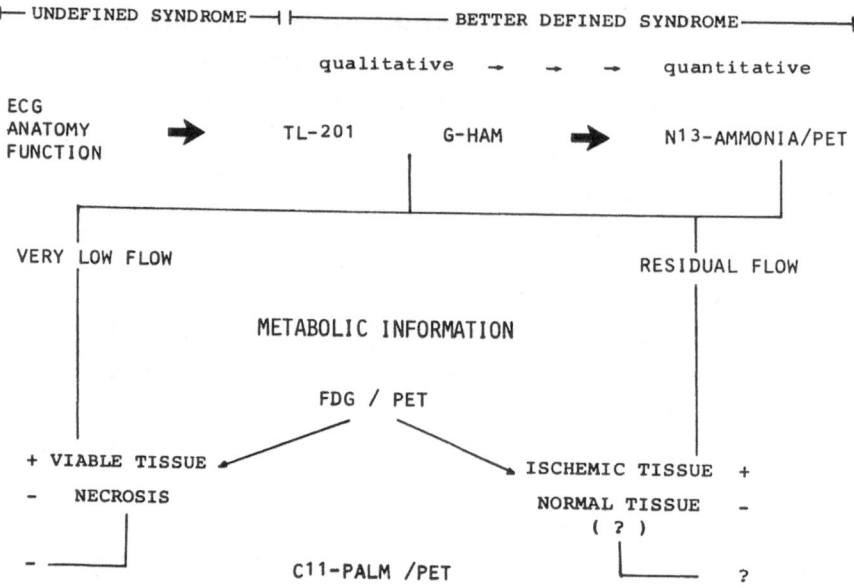

CONCLUSION

These findings justify that clinicians now attack this syndrome by the use of appropriate tests and techniques. Since the conventional clinical findings cannot predict the presence and extent of necrosis and its precise location, follow-up studies should be based on the appropriate characterization of perfusion and metabolic abnormalities. These studies will direct medical or surgical interventions to jeopardized myocardium under risk of necrotic transformation.

277

REFERENCES

Hutter, A.M., De Sanctis, R.W., Flynn, T. et al. 1981. Non-transmural myocardial infarction: a comparison of hospital and late clinical course of patients with that of matched patients with transmural anterior and transmural inferior myocardial infarction. Am. J. Cardiol., 48, 595.

Madigan, N., Rutheford, B., Frye, R. 1976. The clinical course, early prognosis and coronary anatomy of subendocardial infarction. Am. J. Med., 60, 634.

Marshall, R.C., Tillish, J.H., Phelps, M.E. et al. 1983. Identification and differentiation of resting myocardial ischemia and infarction in man with positron computed tomography, F18-labeled fluorodeoxyglucose and N13-ammonia. Circulation, 67, 766.

Marzullo, P., Carpeggiani, C., Parodi, O. et al. 1985 (in press). Scintigraphic assessment of myocardial infarction in absence of ECG Q waves. Proc. 7th Eur. Congr. Nucl. Med., Helsinki 1984.

Nicholson, M.R., Roubin, G.S., Bernstein, L. et al. 1983. Prognosis after an initial non Q wave myocardial infarction related to coronary arterial anatomy. Am. J. Cardiol., 52, 462.

Parodi, O., Marzullo, P., Bencivelli, W. et al. 1982. Microspheres in the assessment of both myocardial contractility and perfusion. In "Proceedings of III World Congr. Nucl. Med. Biol.". (Ed. C. Raynaud). (Pergamon Press, Paris). p. 3053.

Parodi, O., Schwaiger, M., Krivokapich, J. et al. 1984. Regional myocardial blood flow and wall motion study in patients with designated acute "subendocardial infarction". J.A.C.C., 3, 52.

Parodi, O., Uthurralt, N., Severi, S. et al. 1981. Transient reduction of regional myocardial perfusion during angina at rest with ST-segment depression or normalization of negative T waves. Circulation, 63, 1238.

Raunio, M., Rissanen, V., Ramppanen, T. et al., 1979. Changes in QRS complex and ST segment in transmural and non-transmural myocardial infarctions. A clinico-pathologic study. Am. H. J., 98, 176.

Santiago, C., Castaner, A., Gines, S. et al. 1983. Prevalence and prognosis after a first non-transmural myocardial infarction. Am. J. Cardiol., 51, 1584.

Schelbert, H.R., Wisenberg, G., Phelps, M.E. et al. 1982. Noninvasive assessment of coronary stenoses by myocardial imaging during pharmacologic vasodilation. VI. Detection of coronary artery disease in man with intravenous N13-ammonia and positron computed tomography. Am. J. Cardiol., 49, 1197.

Shah, A., Schelbert, H.R., Schwaiger, M. et al. 1985. Measurement of regional myocardial blood flow with N13-ammonia and positron emission tomography in intact dogs. J.A.C.C., 5, 92.

INVESTIGATION OF MYOCARDIAL VIABILITY AFTER AN ACUTE MYOCARDIAL INFARCTION USING POSITRON EMISSION TOMOGRAPHY

C. De Landsheere, D. Raets, L. Pierard, C. Lemaire
C. Berthe, G. Del Fiore, D. Lamotte, H.E. Kulbertus, P. Rigo
Cyclotron Research Center and Malvoz Institute
University of Liège, Belgium

Assessment of myocardial viability after an acute myocardial infarction is needed because the prognosis after the acute phase of a coronary event and the indication for revascularization therapy by percutaneous coronary angioplasty or coronary artery bypass grafting are linked to the amount of residual viable and contractile myocardium. Among noninvasive techniques of investigation, positron emission tomography can evaluate the myocardial viability by comparing the regional study of myocardial metabolism to flow.

In regional ischemia, oxygen uptake is reduced approximately to the same extent as the delivery of oxygen. The delivery of substrates is also decreased but not completely abolished. The removal of CO_2, H^+ and lactate is diminished (Opie, 1976). During oxygen deficiency, heart fatty acid beta-oxidation is not only depressed but also incomplete. Beta-hydroxyl fatty acyl intermediates accumulate and contribute to the increased fatty acid content characteristic of ischemic myocardium (Moore et al., 1980).

Applying these findings, Lerch et al. (1981) demonstrated with positron emission tomography (PET) and 11C-palmitate that the ischemic but still viable myocardium can still extract fatty acids but the rate of their metabolization is reduced. Regional clearance of 11C-palmitate was assessed by sequential PET in two groups of anesthetized dogs. The first was a control group of 7 dogs without coronary stenosis in which the myocardial clearance of 11C-palmitate was consistently monoexponential and homogeneous from 5 to 15 minutes after administration of the labeled fatty acid. The mean rate constant of the monoexponential palmitate clearance (k) averaged -0.060 ± 0.005 min^{-1} corresponding to a half-time of 11.6 minutes. This was calculated from 3 to 8 regions of interest, in each dog, with repeated one-minute emission scans using the positron-emission transaxial tomograph PETT V. The second group was composed of 5 dogs with a left circumflex (LCX) stenosis higher than 70 % (range 70-93 %) susceptible to produce regional ischemia in the free wall of the left ventricle. The absence of infarcted myocardium in the area supplied by the LCX was checked postmortem by histologic criteria. Emission scans did not show any detectable defect in the uptake of 11C-palmitate. Compared with normal dogs, considerably less homogeneity of palmitate clearance was evident: in each of the 5 dogs with significant LCX stenosis, the coefficient of variation of the clearance rate constant was high: 28.1 $\pm$ 5.5 % (compared to 11.1 $\pm$ 5.5 % in control dogs). Comparing the mean clearance rate of 11C-palmitate regions supplied by the stenotic LCX to the clearance in the left anterior descending artery (LAD) territory not affected by any stenosis, Lerch et al. (1981) found a clearance reduction by 31 %. K was -0.064 $\pm$ 0.011 min^{-1} in the LAD territory whereas it was -0.044 $\pm$ 0.011 min^{-1} in the region supplied by the stenotic LCX. The difference was accentuated by tachycardia induced by left arterial pacing. Therefore, ischemic but still viable myocardium can be identified by a reduction in the clearance rate of fatty acids such as 11C-palmitate.

The same group of St. Louis (Washington University) using 11C-palmitate studied the distribution of the long-chain fatty acid before and after the intracoronary administration of tissue-type plasminogen activator or streptokinase in 19 patients (Sobel et al., 1984). If the lysis was successful, myocardial accumulation of 11C-palmitate improved by an average of 29 % in the postintervention observation compared to the pretreatment data. This suggests that more cardiac cells are able to utilize fatty acids (in the presence of oxygen) when thrombolytic therapy is applied. Nevertheless, the authors observed a modest or absent improvement of regional left ventricular performance; global left ventricular ejection fraction in patients where the lysis was achieved did not change significantly (50.9 $\pm$ 3.6 % before and 51.4 $\pm$ 4.1 % after thrombolysis) although the trend was favorable. Therefore, thrombolysis seems to improve the regional myocardial viability but the effect on left ventricular contractility assessed soon (48 to 72 hours) after intracoronary administration of streptokinase or tissue-type plasminogen activator is variable.

The main and first adaptation of myocardial metabolism in response to oxygen deprivation is an increase in glycolytic flux that results

primarily from the breakdown of glycogen. Measurements of glycolytic
intermediates show an initial burst of accelerated glycolytic flux
lasting less than 1 min after coronary artery ligation (Opie, 1976). In
addition, the extraction of glucose by the ischemic but still viable
myocardium is increased as shown by Opie (1976) and Vary et al. (1981).
Applying these observations, the UCLA group and ours studied the
regional uptake of glucose in comparison to flow. In patients studies,
Marshall et al. (1983) were able to differentiate myocardial ischemia
from infarction using 13N-ammonia and 18F-deoxyglucose (18FDG) with
positron emission tomography. They investigated regional blood flow and
metabolism in 15 patients and 10 normal volunteers. Myocardial
infarction was transmural in 12 cases and non-transmural in 3 cases. The
delay betwen the infarction and the PET study varied from 2 days to 13
weeks. No patient was studied during the hyperacute stage of infarction.
Electrocardiographic evidence of postinfarction ischemia was considered
to be present if there was transient ST-T segment depression of more
than 1 mm or if T waves during chest pain were suspect for acute
myocardial ischemia. No patient experienced chest pain during the PET
study. Tomographic imaging was initiated 1-2 hours after a carbohydrate-
containing breakfast and additional oral glucose (40-50 g) was given 60-
90 min before administration of FDG to allow better evaluation of non-
ischemic myocardium by increasing the ratio of glucose to fatty acids
utilization in normal regions of the myocardium. All transmural
infarctions except 2 (inferiorly located) were identified by a parallel
reduction of perfusion and FDG uptake in an area corresponding to the
localization of infarction on the ECG. Eleven patients had symptoms of
ischemia either at rest or during mild exertional angina. A disproportionately high FDG uptake in a region of decreased perfusion was
observed in 10 cases, of whom 9 suffered from angina. Therefore, only
one false-positive signal of PET abnormality was noticed in this group.
The authors concluded that the presence of ischemia or angina is
correlated with a disproportionate increase of glucose relative to
perfusion.

Our group in Liège (Belgium) used a similar approach (De Landsheere
et al., 1985a,b; Rigo et al., 1985). The regional myocardial uptake of
18F-deoxyglucose was compared to the regional distribution of 13N-
ammonia or potassium-38 (38K) as flow indicators. Three groups of acute

myocardial infarct patients were studied within 10 days after the coronary event: the first group did not receive any thrombolytic drug, the second received intravenous streptokinase and the third group was submitted to streptokinase followed by transluminal percutaneous angioplasty. This procedure was applied at the acute phase of infarction, immediately following the coronary angiography (performed in order to check the reopening of the vessel after thrombolytic therapy and in order to analyse the number of diseased vessels). The present study aimes to investigate whether the extent of myocardial viability can be related to the mode of therapy.

Regional myocardial perfusion and glucose utilization were studied at rest in 5 control subjects and in 36 patients. The population of patients was composed of 9, 22, and 5 subjects in the first, second, and third group, respectively.

Coronarography and ventriculography were performed in all patients. In the first group, 7 patients had a left anterior descending (LAD) lesion, proximally located in 1 case, 1 patient circumflex (LCX), and 1 patient right coronary artery (RCA) proximal lesion. In the second group, the artery responsible for the infarction was the LAD in 18 cases, the LCX in 2 cases, and the RCA in 2 cases, respectively; a proximal lesion was observed in 10 LAD and in 1 RCA location respectively. In the third group, LAD was stenosed in all cases with proximal lesions in 2 cases. One patient only, belonging to group 1 had 3-vessel disease. There was a similar proportion of single and 2-vessel disease in the first two groups; in group 3, 4 patients suffered a single vessel and one patient a 2-vessel disease. In summary, in most of the cases, the infarction was anteriorly located (LAD disease in 30 out of 36); 1- or 2-vessel disease was observed in 35 out of 36 patients. In group 1, the vessel responsible for the infarction was obstructed in 8 out of 9 cases. Residual stenosis after streptokinase administration in group 2 was higher or equal to 90 % in 13 out of 22 cases, between 70 and 90 % in 6 cases and less than 70 % in 3 cases, only. In group 3, the stenosis was higher than 90 % in 4 patients and higher than 80 % in one case before PTCA. After the angioplasty, the residual stenosis was less than 30 % in 4 cases and in the order of 50 % in the patient with the initial stenosis of 80 %.

Contractility was analysed in all patients on biplane ventriculography: left and right anterior obliques. Global left ventricular ejection fraction was 44.3 $\pm$ 13.9, 50.0 $\pm$ 14.0, and 66.0 $\pm$ 7.7 (mean $\pm$ SD) in groups 1, 2, and 3, respectively. Regional contractility was qualitatively assessed and a score was calculated as follows: 1 for moderate hypokinesia, 2 for severe hypokinesia, 3 for akinesia, and 4 for dyskinesia, in each segment. Then, the scores calculated in the area supplied by the vessel responsible for the infarction were added. A mean score of 5.4 $\pm$ 3.4 was obtained in group 1, of 6.7 $\pm$ 3.3 in group 2, and of 1.8 $\pm$ 1.8 in group 3.

Enzymes detecting cardiac necrosis were systematically measured every 4 hours during 72 hours. For total creatine kinase, the peak value was 1334 $\pm$ 1118 U/L, 2032 $\pm$ 1314 U/L, and 1270 $\pm$ 1049 U/L in groups 1, 2, and 3, respectively. This peak value was reached 14.3 $\pm$ 7.3, 12.7 $\pm$ 4.6, and 9 $\pm$ 2 hours respectively after admission to the coronary care unit. For the myocardial fraction of creatine kinase (CK-MB), values measured in the same 3 groups were 124.7 $\pm$ 83.8 U/L, 236 $\pm$ 150 U/L, and 110 $\pm$ 123 U/L at 16.7 $\pm$ 8.9, 13.1 $\pm$ 5.5, and 9.3 $\pm$ 6.1 hours.

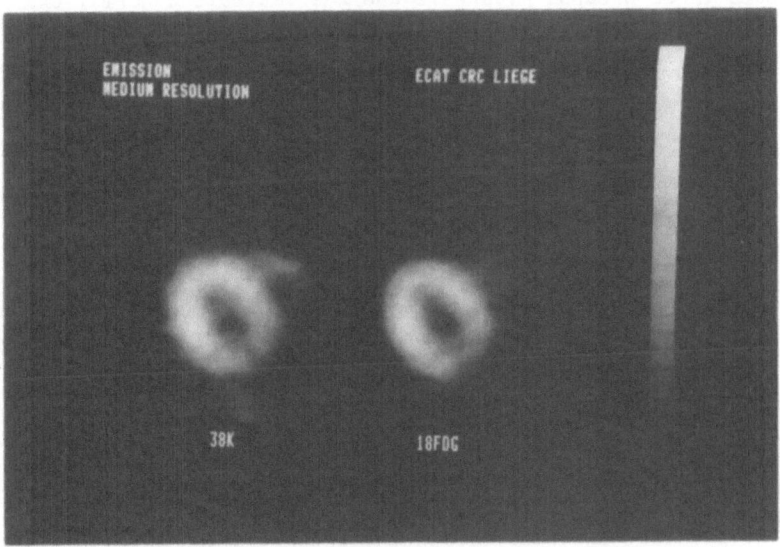

Fig. 1 Positron emission tomograms obtained after the successive intravenous injection of potassium-38 and 18F-deoxy-glucose (left and right panel, respectively) in a young normal volunteer. The distribution of both tracers is homogeneous and no region of the myocardium shows a high FDG uptake relative to flow.

Positron emission tomograms were recorded at rest, in 3 planes from the apex to the base of the left ventricle, with a single-slice machine (ECAT-II, Ortec Corp.). Blank attenuation and transmission scans were used for attenuation correction of the emission scan acquired thereafter. Transmission over blank ratio smoothing was applied using a five point transverse filter. Data were normalized to the peak activity (100 %) in each scan. A ratio of 18FDG over 38K or 13N-ammonia normalized activity was then calculated in each selected region of interest. In the upper plane, 3 regions were chosen: one in the free wall, one in the anterior wall, and one in the septum after a circumferential profile was drawn. In the 2 lower planes (mid-left ventricular and apical), 5 regions of interest were chosen: 2 in the free wall, 1 in the anterior wall, and 2 in the septum. From data obtained in 5 volunteers, the FDG over flow (DG:F) ratio was considered as abnormal if higher than 1.5. Evaluation of flow with cationic tracers showed a reduction to 32.5 $\pm$ 14.8 %, 39.5 $\pm$ 13.7 %, and 46.3 $\pm$ 16.0 % in the area of infarction, in the first, second, and third group, respectively. In this same area, DG:F ratio was 1.42 $\pm$ 0.25, 1.96 $\pm$ 0.21, and 1.85 $\pm$ 0.54 in the same three groups. Figures 1 and 2 illustrate a normal example of 38 K and 18FDG studies in a normal volunteer aged 22 years. Distributions of both tracers are homogeneous and similar in a mid-left ventricular transverse slice of the myocardium.

Among patients of group 1, 2 out of 9 had a DG:F ratio higher than 1.5. In the former case with an anterior myocardial infarction, a 95 % stenosis of the LAD was observed possibly related to a spontaneous fibrinolysis. The latter case who suffered a non-transmural lateral infarction had LCX obstruction but excellent collateral circulation and normal ventriculography. In group 2, 15 out of 22 patients had a DG:F ratio higher than 1.5.

The investigation represented in the figures 3 and 4 was recorded in a patient submitted to intravenous thombolytic therapy within 3 hours after the onset of symptoms. Coronary anatomy showed a residual stenosis of 99 % of the left anterior descending artery, after the first diagonal branch. The left circumflex and right coronary arteries were normal. Ventriculography and 2D-echocardiography showed a large zone of anteroapical akinesia. The PET study showed a profound reduction of perfusion in the anterior wall of 33.9 % in comparison to normal regions of the myocardium.

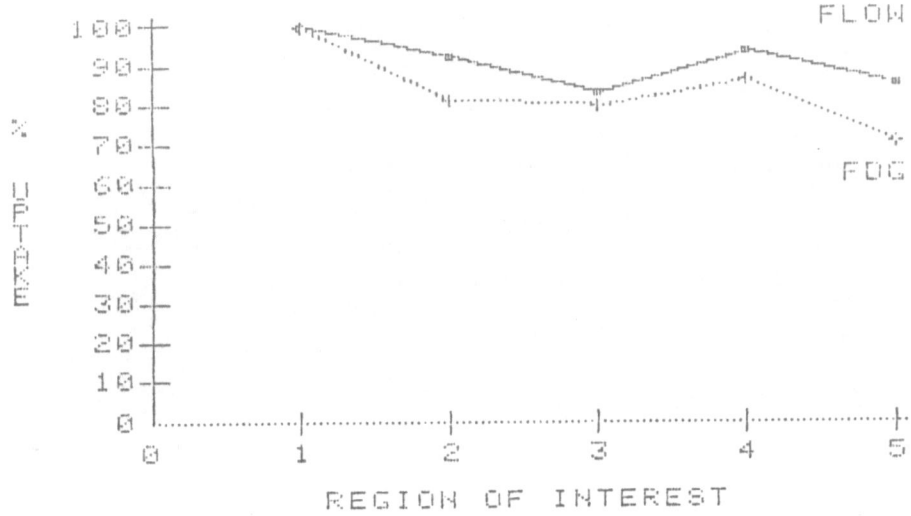

Fig. 2 Normalized uptake of potassium-38, indicating flow and
18F-deoxyglucose in same patient as Fig. 1. The uptake is represented in 5 regions of interest in the left ventricle: 1 for the
posterior part of the free wall, 2 for the anterior part of the
same wall, 3 for the anterior wall, 4 for the anterior part of the
septum, and 5 for the posterior part of the same region.

The uptake of FDG was similarly decreased in the affected territory
suggesting the absence of viable cells in this area. On the contrary, in
another patient of the same second group who received intravenous
streptokinase, a region of viable myocardium could be demonstrated by a
disproportionate increase of FDG uptake relative to perfusion (Figs. 5
and 6), leading to a DG:F ratio of 2.90 in the anterior wall, which was
the site of the acute myocardial infarction. This area was supplied by
the LAD with a stenosis of 80 % after the first diagonal branch.

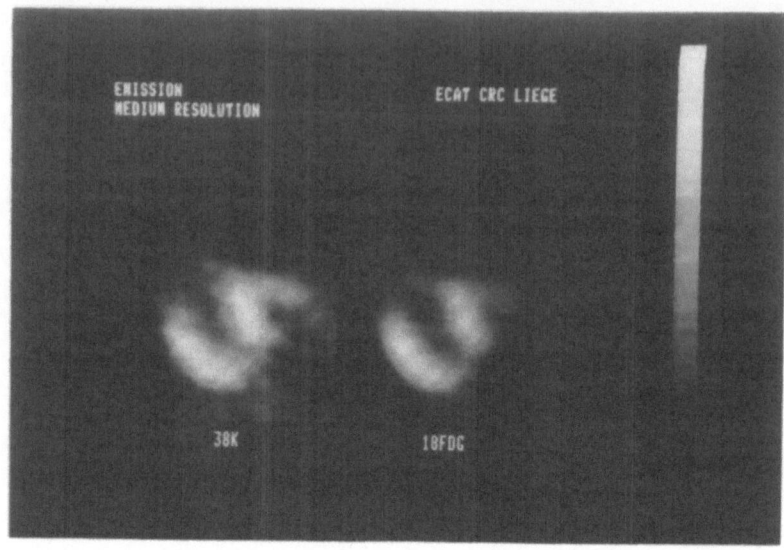

Fig. 3 Positron emission tomograms recorded in an apical
slice of the myocardium, after the successive injection of
potassium-38 and 18F-deoxyglucose (left and right panel,
respectively) in a patient submitted to thrombolytic intervention.
Coronary angiography showed a residual stenosis of 95 % on the left
anterior descending artery, after the first diagonal branch. In
this case, no significant uptake of any tracer can be detected in
the anterior wall (site of infarction) suggesting the absence of
myocardial viability in this affected area.

Ventriculography showed severe hypokinesia of anterolateral and apical

segments. No significant lesions was observed in the LCX territory

whereas the right coronary artery was proximally completely obstructed.

This patients was operated on with improvement of flow and disappearance

of the disproportion between glucose uptake and regional corresponding

perfusion.

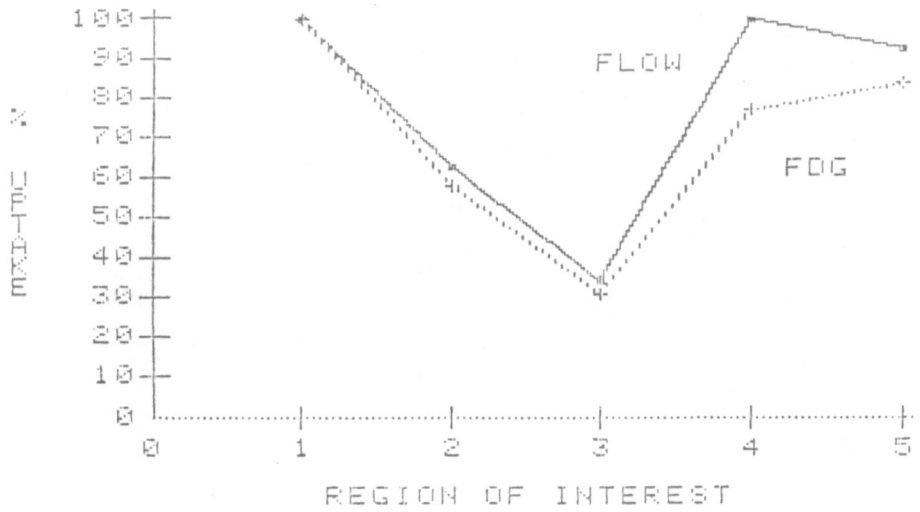

Fig. 4 Normalized uptake of potassium-38 and 18F-deoxy-
glucose in same patient as Fig. 3. The uptake is represented
in 5 regions of interest from the posterior part of the free wall
to the posterior part of the septum. Both tracers show a similarly
decreased uptake in the anterior wall (region 3); no disproportionately high FDG uptake relative to flow is obtained.

Myocardial viability can be identified both in the infarcted
territory and at a distance; this study is focussed on the former
possibility. In most of the patients submitted to thrombolytic therapy,
coronary angiography showed patency of the vessel responsible for the
infarction but a high grade residual stenosis was usually persisting.
Severe reduction of regional perfusion was initially demonstrated by
positron emission tomography in the area of infarction for the majority
of patients. Whether the perfusion of this area will improve with time
is presently unknown.

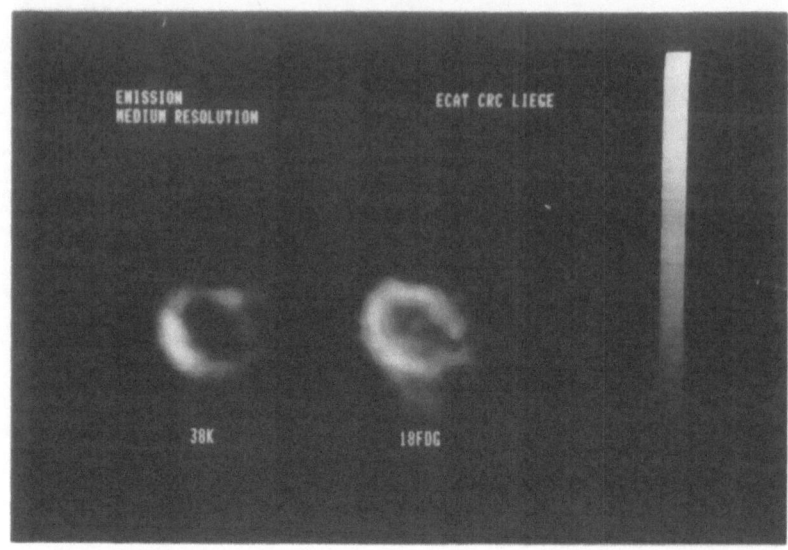

Fig. 5 Positron emission tomograms obtained after the injection of potassium-38 and 18F-deoxyglucose (left and right panel, respectively) in another patient who received intravenous streptokinase. Coronary angiography showed a 80 % LAD stenosis after the origin of the first diagonal branch. The FDG uptake is high with respect to flow in the anterior wall and in the septum (located to the right part of the right panel).

Viable myocardium was more frequently observed in the group treated with streptokinase than in the absence of thrombolytic therapy but it remains to be demonstrated in which proportion the utilization of substrates in the area of infarction will persist in a long-term follow-up.

Some patients submitted to fibrinolytic therapy did not preserve any significant myocardial viability in the infarcted territory. The explanation for this observation is not easy because the factors responsible for the salvage and persistence of viable cells are multiple (e.g., time interval between onset of symptoms and clot lysis, severity of residual stenosis, reocclusion of the affected vessel).

Among the patients who did not receive streptokinase, viable myocardium has been observed in 2 cases only. This finding can be related to spontaneous fibrinolysis or efficient collateral circulation.

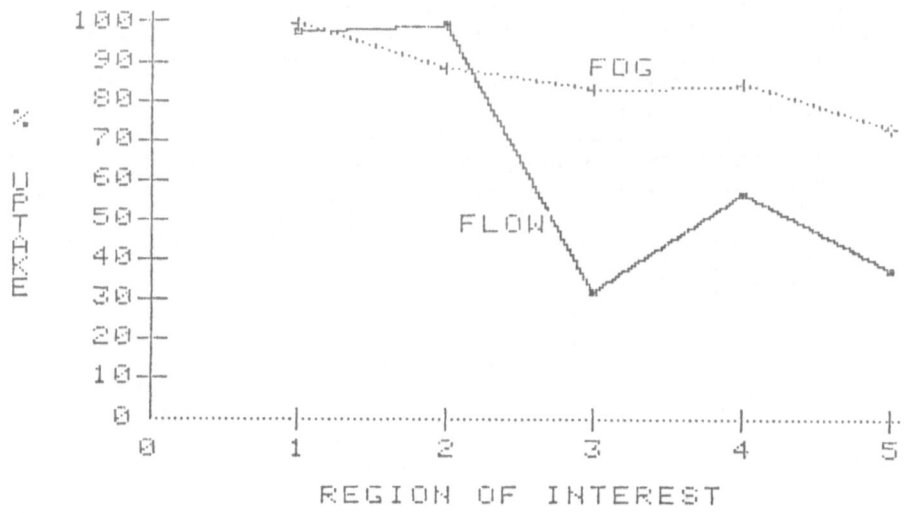

Fig. 6   Normalized uptake of potassium-38 and 18F-deoxy-glucose in same patients as Fig. 5. The uptake of the glucose analogue is disproportionately high relative to flow in areas 3, 4, and 5 (anterior wall, anterior and posterior parts of the septum). This pattern suggests the presence of myocardial viability in the area of infarction and was confirmed by a post coronary artery bypass follow-up study.

ACKNOWLEDGEMENTS
    We thank everyone involved in the long process of tracers supply, from the acceleration of particles to the final radiochemistry production; we express also our gratitude to Dr. J.P. Chapelle who provided the results of enzyme analysis, Mr. R. Redote for technical assistance, Mr. A. Marchal for illustrations, Mr. C. Degueldre and Mr. P. Merlo for data computing.

REFERENCES

De Landsheere, C., Raets, D., Pierard, L. et al. 1985a. Residual
    metabolic abnormalities and regional viability after a myocardial
    infarction: a study using positron tomography, 18F-deoxyglucose
    and flow indicators. J. Am. Coll. Cardiol., 5, 451.
De Landsheere, C., Raets, D., Pierard, L. et al. 1985b. Fibrinolysis
    and viable myocardium after an acute infarction: a study of
    regional perfusion and glucose utilization with positron emission
    tomography. Circulation, 72, III 393.
Lerch, R.A., Ambos, H.D., Bergmann, S.R. et al. 1981. Localization of
    viable ischemic myocardium by positron emission tomography with
    11C-palmitate. Circulation, 64, 689-699.
Marshall, R.C., Tillisch, J.H., Phelps, M.E. et al. 1983.
    Identification and differentiation of resting myocardial ischemia
    and infarction in man with positron computed tomography, 18F-
    labeled deoxyglucose and 13N-ammonia. Circulation, 67, 766-778.
Moore, K.H., Radloff, J.F., Hull, F.E. et al. 1980. Incomplete fatty
    acid oxidation by ischemic heart: beta-hydroxy fatty acid
    production. Am. J. Physiol., 239, H257-265.
Opie, L.H. 1976. Effects of regional ischemia on metabolism of glucose
    and fatty acids. Relative rates of aerobic and anaerobic energy
    production during myocardial infarction and comparison with
    effects of anoxia. Circ. Res., 38 (Suppl. 1), 53-73.
Rigo, P., De Landsheere, C., Raets, D. et al. 1985. Demonstration by
    positron tomography and 18F-deoxyglucose of regional myocardial
    viability after myocardial infarction: influence of fibrinolysis
    and revascularization. J. Nucl. Med., 26, P87.
Sobel, B.E., Geltman, E.M., Tiefenbrunn, A.J. et al. 1984. Improvement
    of regional myocardial metabolism after coronary thrombolysis
    induced with tissue-type plasminogen activator or streptokinase.
    Circulation, 69, 983-990.
Vary, T.C., Reibel, D.K., Neely, J.R. 1981. Control of energy
    metabolism of heart muscle. Ann. Rev. Physiol., 43, 419-430.

PET IN THE EVALUATION OF MYOCARDIAL INFARCTION
- OBSERVATIONS IN ACUTE AND CHRONIC STAGE -

H. Sochor, M. Schwaiger, R. Brunken

Dept. of Cardiology, University of Vienna, Vienna, Austria
Div. of Nuclear Medicine and Biophysics, Dept. of Radiological Sciences
UCLA School of Medicine, University of California, Los Angeles, USA,
Laboratory of Nuclear Medicine, Lab. of Biomedical and Environmental
Sciences*, University of California, Los Angeles, USA

Coronary occlusion causes a sudden cessation of blood flow in the
areas distal to the occlusion site starting a dynamic process of bio-
electrical, biochemical, (ultra)structural and contractile changes.
During this evolutionary process, progressing in a "wave-front"-like
manner (Reimer et al., 1977) from endo- to epicardium initially
reversible phases of ischemic injury lead to the final stage of
completed infarction so that cellular viability is irreversibly lost.

However, a number of variables, as relation of oxygen demand and
supply, occlusion duration and location, amount of residual or
collateral flow, influence the severity of an ischemic injury.
Additional factors, as vascular tone, wall tension and the humoral
situation finally make the extent of actual tissue necrosis
unpredictable. This wide variety has been shown by several studies (Lee
et al., 1981) and thus, necrotic tissue and viable cells may persist at
least for some usually unknown amount of time.

Clinically, size and location of irreversibly lost myocardium and
the amount of ischemic tissue within the peri-infarction zone or in
remote myocardium are known to be important determinants for prognosis

*Operated for the US Department of Energy by the University of
California under contract no. DE-AC03-76-SF00012. This work was
supported in part by the Director of the Office of Energy Research,
Office of Health and Environmental Research, by NIH grant nos. HL 29845
and HL 33177, and by an Investigatorship Group Award by the Greater Los
Angeles Affiliate of the American Heart Association.

(Sniderman et al., 1983; Santiago et al., 1983). The advent of aggressive therapy, as PTCA or early aorto-coronary bypass grafting, has reinforced the search for methods to assess the ratio of irreversible and reversible injury. Despite an impressive armamentarium of diagnostic methods in modern cardiology, traditional indices, as ECG, assessment of regional function by echocardiography, and even coronary angiography have conceptual limitations and usually only outline some aspects of the complex pathophysiology of myocardial infarction.

More recently, metabolic imaging by positron emissi   tomography has offered the possibility to study non-invasively myocaı ᵤ.al necrosis but also viable myocardium recovering from an ischemic event (Schelbert et al., 1983; Marshall et al., 1983; Schwaiger et al., 1985; Bergmann et al., 1982). A series of animal and clinical studies have indicated the ability of PET to characterize reversible tissue injury by combined studies of blood flow and metabolism (Schwaiger et al., 1984).

METHODS AND RESULTS

In a series of studies the ability of PET to characterize infarcted and reperfused myocardium has been investigated by metabolic imaging with F18-deoxyglucose (FDG). Regional myocardial blood flow is defined by N13-ammonia and function by echocardiography. Based on previous clinical and experimental studies reversible tissue injury character-istically displays enhanced glucose utilization in excess of blood flow ("mismatch" pattern), whereas irreversible necrosis ("match") is showing a concordant decrease of blood flow and metabolism.

Acute observations

To test the hypothesis that early metabolic findings would correlate with the outcome of regional function, 13 patients with electrocardiographic or enzymatically proven infarct (10 anterior, 2 inferior localizations) were submitted within 72 hours of acute onset of symptoms (Schwaiger et al., 1986) to a N13-ammonia study and a subsequent F18-deoxyglucose study in 4-5 contiguous cross-sectional planes. Analysis by a circumferential profile technique (Marshall et al., 1983) defined infarction by PET criteria as concordant reduction of N13 and F18 uptake of 2 or more standard deviations below a pooled normal data base for at least 2 sectors, whereas viable but compromised myocardium was defined by a F18/N13 uptake difference greater than two standard deviations above normal. These tracer studies of glucose metabolism and blood flow were compared to 2D echocardiography at the day of the tomograms and 6 weeks later. The majority (9/13) of patients revealed some segments with "residual viability". 50 % of the segments with reduced flow showed a "matched" decrease of flow and glucose utilization whereas the remaining 50 % revealed the "ischemia pattern", suggesting potential recovery. While echo wall-motion scores improved in the majority of "PET viable" segments, follow-up evaluation of segmental function revealed no change in mean wall-motion score with "PET infarction".

The results of these observations indicate that metabolic imaging with PET can identify viable but compromised myocardium in patients with acute myocardial infarction. However, the data also illucidated the possible clinical consequences. Would an agressive treatment strategy in those patients with residual viability who finally did not improve functionally have changed the "natural" course of events? Is collateral flow or early recanalization a major cause for this pattern? Initial early angiographic data in a subset of these patients show a higher degree of patent infarct related vessels or significant collaterals in the "mismatch", i.e., "viability" group. Conversely, the majority of "PET-infarct" segments was associated with occluded vessels.

Chronic observations

The same approach was used in a different study in 20 patients with chronic electrocardiographic Q-wave regions. Surprisingly only on third (32 %) exhibited infarction by PET criteria, whereas 20 % revealed signs of ischemia or were even normal (Brunken et al., 1986). Neither ST-T changes in the surface ECG nor the degree of wall-motion abnormality could reliably distinguish between patients exhibiting the "ischemia" pattern from those with "tomographic infarct". Even when an analysis reassignment was made for Q-wave analysis to avoid a bias in favour of a tomographic technique (by assigning erroneously electrocardiographic Q-waves to normal PET regions), residual glucose metabolism was identified in 54 % of the regions. Wall-motion scores for ischemic regions were not significantly different from those in infarcted regions in both the Q-wave and non Q-wave regions. We concluded from these data, that commonly

used clinical tests in a routine assessment of "completed" infarction
may include a variety of cell populations with different viability
status.

DISCUSSION

Positron emission tomography may add a new dimension to the
assessment of myocardial tissue injury following an ischemic event.
These "metabolic fingerprints" (Schelbert, 1986) are apparently more
sensitive for detection of viable tissue than conventional methods.
Importantly this pattern has been shown to be associated in quite high
proportions with subsequent functional recovery also in patients with
decreased left ventricular function scheduled for bypass surgery
(Tillisch et al., 1986). However, previous generations of PET tomographs
with limited spatial and temporal resolution precluded the development
of quantitative criteria for a metabolic threshold beyond which
functional improvement is unlikely to occur.

Also, further experimental evidence (Sochor et al., 1985) suggest
the coexistence of amounts of viable cells even within reperfused
segments with flows as low as 30 % of control. However, the outcome of
individual segments is variable and difficult to predict. Nevertheless,
these observations are consistent with previous studies showing a
"stunning" effect of ischemia (Braunwald and Kloner, 1982) with a
decrease of perfusion, temporary loss of function but potential slow
recovery since accelerated glycolytic flux in ischemic tissue is present
leading to impaired fatty acid oxidation (and thus contraction) whereas
aerobic or anaerobic glycolysis may preserve membrane integrity
(Liedtke, 1981).

Similar data were reported in experimental studies (Schwaiger et
al., 1984) of coronary reperfusion in chronically instrumented dogs and
in a 3 hour occlusion/reperfusion model by studying blood flow with N13-
ammonia, fatty acid metabolism with C11-palmitate and glucose
utilization again with F18-FDG. Absence of blood flow and C11-palmitate
uptake at 24 hours correlated with extensive necrosis while uptake of
fatty acids with delayed C11 clearance but increased FDG accumulation
identified reversibly injured tissue which then subsequently would
recover also functionally.

CONCLUSION

The impact of these studies is quite obvious: an approach using PET and its unique capability of exceeding the conventional anatomical and morphological connotations, seems to be feasible by applying several tracers of blood flow and metabolism early and late after infarction which might be predictive of later outcome of a given segment. Therefore, this new technology may offer a powerful tool for patient management and stratification and to assess the risk-benefit ratio of interventions in the time course of an ischemic myocardial event.

REFERENCES

Bergmann, S.R., Lerch, R.A., Fox, K.A. et al. 1982. Temporal dependence of beneficial effects of coronary thrombolysis characterized by positron tomography. Am. J. Med., 73, 573-581.

Braunwald, E., Kloner, R.A. 1982. The stunned myocardium: prolonged, post-ischemic ventricular dysfunction. Circulation, 66, 1146-1149.

Brunken, R., Tillisch, J., Schwaiger, M. et al. 1986. Regional perfusion, glucose metabolism, and wall motion in patients with chronic electrocardiographic Q-wave infarctions: evidence for persistence of viable tissue in some infarct regions by positron emission tomography. Circulation, 73, 951-963.

Lee, J.T., Toleker, R.E., Reimer, K.A. 1981. Myocardial infarct size and location in relation to the coronary vascular bed at risk in man. Circulation, 64, 526-534.

Liedtke, A.J.. 1981. Alterations of carbohydrate and lipid metabolism in the acutely ischemic heart. Prog. Cardiovasc. Dis., 23, 321-336.

Marshall, R.C., Tillisch, J.H., Phelps, M.E. et al. 1983. Identification and differentiation of resting myocardial ischemia and infarction in man with positron computed tomography, F18 labeled fluorodeoxyglucose and N13-ammonia. Circulation, 67, 766-777.

Reimer, K.A., Lowe, J.E., Rasmussen, M.M. et al. 1977. The wavefront phenomenon of ischemic cell death. I. Myocardial infarct size vs duration of coronary occlusion in dogs. Circulation, 56, 786-794.

Santiago, C., Castaner, A., Gines, S. et al. 1983. Prevalence and prognosis after a first non-transmural myocardial infarction. Am. J. Cardiol., 51, 1584.

Schelbert, H.R. 1986. Evaluation of "metabolic fingerprints" of myocardial ischemia. Can. J. Cardiol., 7, 121A-130A.

Schelbert, H.R., Phelps, M.E., Shine, K.I. 1983. Imaging metabolism and biochemistry - a new look at the heart. Am. Heart, 105, 522-526.

Schwaiger, M., Brunken, R., Grover-McKay, M. et al. 1986. Regional myocardial metabolism in patients with acute myocardial infarction assessed by positron emission tomography. J. Am. Coll. Cardiol., 8, 800-808.

Schwaiger, M., Hansen, H.W., Sochor, H. et al. 1984. Delayed recovery of regional glucose metabolism in reperfused canine myocardium by positron-CT. J. Am. Coll. Cardiol., 3, 552.

Schwaiger, M., Schelbert, H.R., Ellison, D. et al. 1985. Sustained regional abnormalities in cardiac metabolism after transient ischemia in the chronic dog model. J. Am. Coll. Cardiol., 6, 336-347.

Sniderman, A.D., Beaudry, J.P., Rahal, D.P. 1983. Early recognition of the patient at late high risk: incomplete infarction and vulnerable myocardium. Am. J. Cardiol., 52, 669-673.

Sochor, H., Schwaiger, M., Schelbert, H.R. et al. 1985. Assessment of tissue viability in reperfused canine myocardium by a multiple radiotracer technique. J. Am. Coll. Cardiol., 5, 451.

Tillisch, J., Brunken, R., Marshall, R. et al. 1986. Prediction of the reversibility of cardiac wall motion abnormalities using positron tomography, 18fluorodeoxyglucose and 13N-ammonia. N. Engl. J. Med., 314, 884-888.

APPLICATION OF PET TO THE STUDY OF HEART DISEASE

B. Lösse

Dept. of Cardiology, Pneumology and Angiology,
University of Düsseldorf, FRG

The purpose of this summary should not be a simple review of the heart session's papers in detail; rather I like to point out some questions derived from the vivacious discussions of the papers with regard to the future application of PET.

In the various papers a lot of information has been presented dealing predominantly with PET measurements in coronary artery disease. Different tracers for the assessment of regional myocardial flow and regional myocardial metabolism have been used in patients with stable and unstable angina pectoris, with and without myocardial infarction before and after interventional procedures like percutaneous trans-luminal coronary angioplasty (PTCA) and thrombolysis in acute myocardial infarction. The results indicate that such measurements may be more sensitive and more accurate than currently available methods in a number of pathophysiologically and clinically important questions, i.e., the detection of ischemia, the differentiation of reversibly from irre-versibly damaged myocardium after myocardial infarction, the natural course of restoration of myocardial function after myocardial infarction and interventional procedures.

Very exciting preliminary data have been presented on receptor studies relating to catecholamine and acetylcholin receptors, and the suggestion has been proposed that even studies of the membrane potential may be possible with PET.

From the data presented several questions may be raised:

1) Should PET be used only as a research tool to clarify patho-physiological mechanisms or should it also be applied for diagnostic use and compared in its diagnostic accuracy with currently available methods?

2) What diseases should be investigated?

3) What tracers should be used?

Previous work in coronary artery disease suggest convincingly that the application of PET as a pure research tool should be extended in favour of a broader clinical application. This pertains particularly to such questions of diagnostic and therapeutic relevance, in which the information gained by PET measurements appears to surpass that of the traditional methods, i.e., with regard to the detection of ischemia and irreversibly damaged tissue. Properly designed comparative studies should be done to correlate the results of PET measurements with those of conventional methods to establish the disease conditions in which PET studies will be helpful and in which they will not contribute further benefit. This has to go along with further research work relating to comparisons of different tracers in various pathophysiological subsets of the disease to define better the proper usefulness of each tracer.

Probably due to the restricted availability of the method previous work has been confined with few exceptions on coronary artery disease. There are however a lot of other disease processes, the pathophysiology of which is difficult or not at all to assess with traditional methods, i.e., cardiomyopathies, angina pectoris despite normal coronary arteries, or rhythm disorders. Assessibility of metabolic impairments, myocardial receptor binding and membrane potential changes as indicated by the presented work justify further intense research by PET with regard to the clarification of as yet poorly understood pathophysiological processes.

It is clear that such extensive work requires an extension of personal and equipment ressources.

SUMMARY of Discussion on Heart

L.E. Feinendegen, Institut für Medizin der Kernforschungsanlage Jülich GmbH, Jülich, FRG

The session discussed angina pectoris and myocardial infarction. In the first address regarding coronary artery disease, Dr. Maseri, London, summarized the expectations a cardiologist places on nuclear medical methods, especially on PET. From a clinical point of view information is needed on blood flow that should be presented as a three-dimensional image, for the purpose of delineating ischemic zones. Moreover, for classifying disease, monitoring progress and studying effects of therapy it is of special interest, and properly answerable by PET to investigate myocardial metabolism in its various aspects. Specifically there appears to be a need to relate uptake and consumption of glucose to that of free fatty acids. Also more work is asked for with regard to investigating neuronal activity and the binding of specific ligands to their proper receptors within the myocardium.

In order to pursue such suggested studies, they should be correlated with data obtained with other detection systems and from histolocigal specimen, and the suggestion was made to collaborate with cardiac surgery, especially regarding heart transplantation.

In discussing own data, Dr. Maseri demonstrated the differential diagnosis between unstable angina and stable angina by quantitatively measuring the uptake of 18-F-deoxyglucose. In unstable angina the uptake is higher compared to the uptake seen in stable angina; this differentiation may be of clinically valuable diagnostic significance and may perhaps dispend with invasive methods here.

Dr. Tillmanns, Heidelberg, reiterated the need for studies of myocardial viability in ischemic myocardial regions. In testing for the various approaches and possibilities, regional blood flow and metabolism need to be compared. Thus, for regional blood flow there is available 82-Rb, 15-O labelled water and 13-N labelled ammonia. For metabolic studies he cited the use of 18-F labelled deoxyglucose, 11-C labelled palmitic acid and 13-N labelled glutamate. In previous work, the Los Angeles group with Dr. Schelbert had shown the peculiar mismatch between flow and metabolism by using labelled ammonia and labelled deoxyglucose, in diagnosing ischemic regions distinct from scarred tissue. - The speaker, in testing labelled glutamate, takes advantage of glutamate being the donor of the ammonia group to pyruvate. The depression of oxidative metabolism leads to a relative decrease in transamination with the consequent retention of ammonia on glutamate. Thus, tracer accumulation following intravenous injection of 13-N labelled glutamate, signals the depression of oxidative metabolism. The data for ischemic regions were similar to those obtained by labelled deoxyglucose when uptake was plotted against local perfusion. The technique was demonstrated to be well applicable to checking the therapeutic efficacy of percutaneous transluminal coronary angioplasty (PTCA). It could be observed that there was delayed recovery of tissue following a reconstitution of flow. The latter alone can be well studied by the classical technique using 201-Tl. It was emphasized that following ischemia there is a change of capillary permeability with platelet accumulation and increase in oxygen radical concentration; then therapy should involve application of a xanthine oxidase inhibitor, free radical scavengers, platelet protectors in addition to classical treatment.

Dr. Syrota, Paris, emphasized the particular advantages of PET for mapping receptors for example for acethylcholine, benzodiazepine, beta-adrenergic substances, alpha-adrenergic substances, and serotonin. - In conducting such studies he emphasized the need of understanding the problem of drug displacement, regional distribution, subcellular distribution, stereospecificity of the compound, saturability of the receptors, reversibility of the binding, and the degree of affinity.

The acethylcholine antagonist QNB was labelled in Paris with 11-C and studied in detail. Thus, it could be shown that already 3 min after intravenous injection the labelled QNB was found to be bound in the left ventricular myocardium and accurate measurements of the saturability could be made. Following injection of 200-300 nMol/m² the receptors were seen to become saturated. The bound QNB could be displaced by atropin in the myocardium but not in the liver. Displacement depended on the amount of atropin injected (0.25-0.5 mg). There was also a relationship between the degree of binding and the heart rate, and with increasing heart rate the binding of the compound decreased, probably by a withdrawal of the vagal tonus so that there was a difference in affinity between agonist and antagonist, i.e. vagal versus sympathic stimuli. Indeed, QNB could be displaced by dexetimide.

Besides propanolol, practolol, and pindolol a new cell surface seeker, namely CGB-12-177, was tested. It was found that this compound has the advantage of only binding to the cell surface and therefore promises to be an ideal ligand. It is rather hydrophilic and it measures in vivo beta-1 plus beta-2 receptors. It is not yet clear, whether pathological signals may be obtained from such beta adrenergic receptors. So far only two human studies have been performed.

Dr. Camici, Pisa, addressed himself to the question why PET studies of the heart demand particular attention when compared to PET studies of the brain; thus, partial volume effects and motion effects must be corrected for, and radioactive tracer concentration must be graded between tissue and cardial blood pool. What has been learned was made clear by regarding the success of applying PET to studies of flow, for example with 82-Rb and 13-N labelled ammonia and of metabolism for example with 18-F labelled deoxyglucose. Reiterating Dr. Maseri's statement, he showed that in unstable angina there is no change in local perfusion, but a highly significant increase of uptake of labelled deoxyglucose in many patients. The respective images lucidly demonstrated this particular reaction. Dr. Camici pointed to future needs: quantification, multi parametric approach for understanding physiology, and to correlate PET with other techniques.

Regarding myocardial infarction. Dr. Parodi, Pisa, first drew comparisons between ECG findings and PET studies. Indeed, PET assesses viability in infarcted regions and also can predict the reversibility of local myocardial insufficiency after coronary bypass surgery.

It is generally difficult to identify non-Q wave subendocardial infarction, on the basis of the ECG alone. Better information is needed. Indeed, the prognosis is quite difficult without additional data, and these can be supplied by PET. Dr. Parodi suggested the following sequence of investigation: ECG, 201-Tl perfusion scintigraphy, PET studies with labelled ammonia or with labelled 68-Ga microspheres. Of particular importance is an early assessment of viability and coronary reserve and its temporal sequence of changes. Quantification and three dimensional imaging is of great help just there.

Following this presentation, a larger discussion evolved around using 82-Rb as a flow marker. It became clear, that using this tracer quantification is difficult because of lack of proper models; also fast scanning is required. In this context it was stated that perhaps changes in flow resulting in ischemia, may be detected by measuring membrane potential by PET, as suggested by Dr. Syrota in 1985.

Dr. De Landsheere, Liège, continued the discussion by specifically reporting on measuring myocardial viability in groups of patients with acute myocardial infarction treated in 3 ways: 1. no streptokinase treatment, 2. streptokinase treatment, 3. streptokinase treatment plus percutaneous transluminal coronary angioplasty (PTCA). Measurements were made 10 days after the infarction and checked for local myocardial perfusion and uptake of 18-F-deoxyglucose. The ratio between local uptake of labelled deoxyglucose to local flow, when above 1.5, was considered to be abnormal. It appeared clinically that the therapeutic effect was greatest in the patient group 3 and lowest in patient group 1. Despite these findings, all patients were reported to still have a diminished flow as measured by PET, and thus the metabolism/flow ratio appeared to remain pathological. The speaker pointed out that the study will continue to collect enough information for a reasonably good statistical analysis.

In the discussion it appeared again that only PET may presently access myocardial viability. An important question remains why in subendocardial infarction some patients develop transmural infarction soon and others later; it would be of great help to find some prognostic clue, and PET here promises to be important.

Dr. Sochor, Vienna, reiterated the main questions that should be addressed to PET: how can one specify diagnosis, how can one derive at a reliable prognosis, how can one efficiently evaluate therapy. Important in this context are studies regarding myocardial viability, the mass of ischemic involvement within the myocardium, the cause of the disease, particularly with the view of identifying those patients that should receive aggressive therapy. Again, the metabolism/flow ratio appears of great clinical value since it obviously identifies ischemia and infarction. An elevated ratio indicative of a mismatch between the two parameters may be also seen soon in patients with infarction when there is preserved viable tissue within the infarcted region. This can pose diagnostic problems. In general, an increased uptake of labelled deoxyglucose, i.e. ischemia, correlated well with wall motion abnormalities and it was rare when there was normal wall motion. Of course, wall motion alone does not give the full diagnostic answer and it should be related to studying the metabolism/flow ratio. The speaker also tried to relate uptake and turnover of 11-C labelled palmitic acid to the uptake of 18-F labelled deoxyglucose. Indeed, as shown previously, an increased uptake of labelled deoxyglucose correlated with altered kinetics of labelled palmitic acid showing a depressed uptake and a prolonged turnover time.

In the final discussion of this paper the need for an optimal resolution of PET images was emphasized in order to pick up islands of diseased muscle and to assess thickness of the myocardial wall; it is important always to link function to the proper structure. Thus, pitfalls regarding PET were related to a relatively low uptake of palmitic acid implying a relatively unfavourable signal to noise ratio, whereas uptake of labelled deoxyglucose permits relatively good statistics. Simplification of diagnostic procedures is important for clinical practice.

In his final summarizing responding remarks Dr. Lösse, Düsseldorf, posed questions from the clinician as listed before, but stressed particularly the need for recognizing the early phase of the disease, for specifying the recovery phase and for following up the chronic phase. For each of these disease phases the clinical questions are different. For the acute phase of the disease, the application of PET is restricted for ethical and practical reasons, since patients would need to be transported to the equipment. As a help in identifying risks following acute infarction, the correlation between left ventricular ejection fraction, myocardial ischemia, and the number of extrasystoles per hour, should be noted. Thus, the risk of fatality is less than 5 % when the ejection fraction is above 50 %, if there is no clear sign of ischemia and when ventricular ectopic beats are lower than 10 per hour. The risk rises up to 20 % if the left ventricular ejection fraction falls to 35-50 %, when ischemic signs are present and when the ventricular ectopic beats rise to 10-30 per hour. Risks appear greater than 20 % if the left ventricular ejection fraction is lower than 35 %, when the regional ischemia is extensive and when ventricular ectopic beats number more than 30 per hour.

In general, myocardial scintigraphy in case of inferior, anterior, and posterior wall infarction is more sensitive than the electro-cardiogram, whereas the latter appears to be more sensitive in case of small apical infarctions. Since exercise tests are generally important, PET has its limitations since it cannot be done during exercise.

PET may help in unravelling the mechanisms of infarction in patients with normal coronary arteries and in determining the patho-genesis of complex arrhythmias.

In summary, the session in general brought out the great progress that has been made in applying PET to comparing metabolism with flow and to differentiating unstable from stable angina. Many mechanisms may be involved in causing this particular phenomenon, such as cross membrane transport, differences in work load, and local hypoxia. Future work will surely add more information on left ventricular receptor typing and distribution, to amino acid utilization, and to lipid synthesis and turnover in various forms of myocardial disease, where the group of cardiomyopathies is still a nearly unknown territory. It is foreseen that a large number of small molecular metabolic substrates will be labelled with positron emitting radionuclides and become available for analysing myocardial metabolism so that the correlation between local blood flow, tissue transport, local metabolism, and humoral and nervous control in vivo may be better understood in the various forms and stages of myocardial disease.

LUNGS

CORRELATION OF STRUCTURE AND FUNCTION IN PULMONARY DISEASE

J.M.B. Hughes, C.G. Rhodes, L.H. Brudin, P.D. Buckingham, T. Jones

Dept. of Medicine, Royal Postgraduate Medical School,
and MRC Cyclotron Unit, Hammersmith Hospital, London, U.K.

INTRODUCTION

From the point of view of positron emission tomography, the lung is not the easiest of organs to study. First, like the heart, it is a moving structure and data collection takes much longer (2-8 min) than the breath-holding time (10-30 sec). This means some degradation of the spatial resolution particularly near the edges of the lung. Secondly, the lung has a density about one-third of that of other tissues; the partial volume effect in passing from a low lung density to the high density of the chest wall, mediastinum and myocardium is another reason for excluding the periphery of the lung from data analysis. Similarly, small regions of abnormally low density (emphysematous bullae) or high density (fibrosis) surrounded by normal lung, are difficult to resolve accurately. The low density of normal lung means that positrons travel a distance > 1.2 mm before annihilating with a tissue electron; thus, there is a biological limit to the spatial resolution which can be achieved in the lung. Although the ECAT II scanner used by us has a spatial resolution (FWHM) of 1.7 cm in all directions, the smallest regions which can be assessed accurately are about 8-10 cm^3. Finally, the lung is a very vascular organ, the ratio of blood to tissue weight being 1.6, and pulmonary tissue itself contributes only 10 % to the lung volume.

There are several reasons why PET studies of the lung are of intrinsic interest. Although the lung from lobe to lobe is structurally homogeneous (unlike the brain) its function, in terms of blood flow (Q) and ventilation (V), alters systematically from region to region under the influence of gravity, i.e., from ventral to dorsal in the supine posture (all our PET studies are made in this position). Matching of V and Q, region by region, is required for efficient pulmonary gas exchange. The metabolic functions of the lung, particularly the endothelial cell, have been the subject of intense research interest in recent years (Ryan et al., 1985). The lung carries the whole cardiac output and has the largest vascular surface area of any organ. The ability of the pulmonary endothelium to extract amines such as serotonin and catecholamine is well known. The surface of the endothelial cell presents to the flowing blood a variety of receptors which process many substances (bicarbonate, angiotensin I, bradykinin, ATP, ADP). In addition, endothelial cells take up arachidonic acid and synthesize prostacyclin (PGI_2) in the endoplasmic reticulum. Subsequent release of PGI_2 is stimulated by bradykinin whose inactivation is itself controlled by the endothelial cell.

Measurement of the density and distribution of pulmonary adrenergic, muscarinic and histamine receptors, which are of great relevance to asthma and other chronic pulmonary conditions, has not been achieved and remains a challenge for the PET-educated pulmonary investigator!

Measurements of regional lung structure

The first step towards quantification of regional pulmonary function is the definition of the structural compartments of the lung. Rhodes et al. (1981) showed that regional lung density (D_L), as $g.cm^{-3}$ thorax, could be measured with PET using the transmission scan (obtained with a ring source of $^{68}Ge/^{68}Ga$) which is required for attenuation correction. After a measurement of vascular volume (V_B), as $ml.cm^{-3}$, using inhaled ^{11}CO to form ^{11}C-carboxyhemoglobin, they showed that extravascular (tissue) density (D_{EV}) could be derived as $D_L - V_B \times 1.06$ where 1.06 is the density of whole blood. Table 1 shows mean values for these three compartments in normal supine subjects, smokers, patients with chronic airflow obstruction and interstitial lung disease. In normal subjects there is a clear gradient of density in the gravity axis with a ventral/dorsal ratio 0.53 for D_L, 0.36 for V_B and 0.75 for D_{EV}, but the influence of gravity has been ignored in Table 1 which presents average values for a single transaxial section. An important influence on any value of lung density is the state of lung inflation. In order to distinguish a low value of D_{EV} caused by lung destruction (e.g., emphysema) from that associated with bronchial obstruction and air trapping (e.g., asthma), Brudin (personal communication) has calculated an expansion index, based on body height and the number of pixels in the mid-thoracic cross section, from which a value of tissue density (D_{EV} norm) can be derived, appropriate for any level of expansion.

TABLE 1 Lung density and its components (tissue (extravascular) density and vascular volume), expansion ratio (actual/predicted area of transaxial section) and tissue density corrected to a normal level of end-expiratory inflation (D_{EV} norm) for normal subjects, asymptomatic smokers, patients with different clinical patterns of airflow obstruction and interstitial lung disease. Mean values for R. lung (1.7 cm transaxial section) at mid-thoracic level.

	n	Lung density g.cm^{-3}	Extravasc. density (D_{EV}) g.cm^{-3}	Vascular volume ml.cm^{-3}	Expansion ratio	D_{EV} (norm.) g.cm^{-3}
Normal	15	0.30	0.13	0.16	1.0	0.13
Smokers	15	0.29	0.14	0.16	1.1	0.15
Asthma	10	0.27	0.15	0.12	1.4	0.19
Chronic bronchitis	4	0.24	0.12	0.11	1.9	0.18
Emphysema	4	0.16	0.07	0.08	1.8	0.11
Sarcoidosis	7	0.50	0.34	0.16	-	-
Fibrosing alveolitis	9	0.44	0.29	0.15	-	-

Table 1 shows that mean D_L in patients with asthma and chronic bronchitis is slightly reduced compared to normals but that tissue density, normalized for the high expansion ratio, is significantly increased. This suggests the presence of inflammatory tissue in the lung periphery. D_{EV} is low in emphysema, as expected, but the exceedingly low values of D_L and V_B make the derivation of D_{EV} norm a little suspect. High values of tissue density, with normal vascular volume, were found in interstitial lung disease.

The vascular compartment has been subdivided by making sequential measurements of red cell density (using ^{11}CO-Hb) and plasma density (i.v. ^{11}C-methylalbumin). Brudin et al. (1986) computed regional lung hematocrit (as a fraction of venous blood Hct) from their measurements. In 5 normal subjects the average value of 0.9 was found which suggests that the Hct in pulmonary capillary vessels (assuming Hct in larger vessels equals venous blood Hct) is about 0.67 of venous Hct, or about 0.3 in absolute terms.

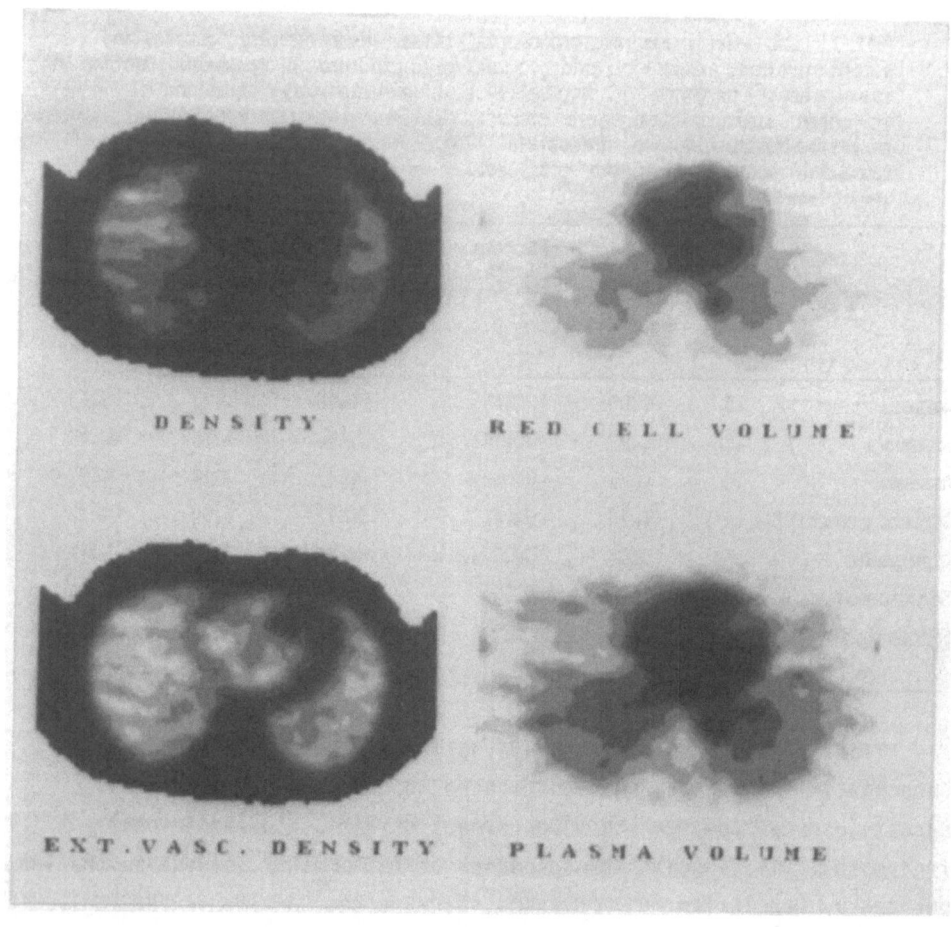

Fig. 1 Transaxial plane at midheart level in normal subject (1.7 cm slice thickness) supine. Density is obtained from a transmission scan, red cell volume from emission scan after 11CO inhalation, plasma volume after 11C-methylalbumin. Extravascular density is obtained by subtraction of red cell volume scan (after Hct correction) from density scan. Note vertical gradients from ventral to dorsal for density and blood volumes. Heart chambers are prominent except in extravascular density scan where only muscle of left ventricular free wall appears (from Hughes et al., 1985, with permission).

The last compartment to be considered is the regional pulmonary gas volume, usually called alveolar volume (V_A). It is derived in $ml.cm^{-3}$ as $1 - D_L/1.04$ where 1.04 is the physical density of lung tissue plus blood. In normal lungs the ratio V_A/D_{EV} ($ml.g^{-1}$) reflects the gas/tissue volume ratio of the gas exchanging units, or more collo- quially "alveolar size". With the quantification afforded by the positron camera, regional expansion of the lung (V_A) can be analyzed for the first time in terms of the number of gas exchanging units (D_{EV}) and their individual size (V_A/D_{EV}).

Application of structural indices to functional measurements

Analysis of structure, apart from its intrinsic physiological interest and importance, is necessary in the quantification of functional parameters. A good example is the study of Wollmer et al. (1982) in which i.v. ^{11}C-erythromycin was given to patients with unilateral pneumonia. To calculate the concentration of [11]C- erythromycin in lung tissue, the intravascular component within each pixel must be subtracted by a) measuring ^{11}C-erythromycin levels ($\mu Ci.ml^{-1}$) from a peripheral blood sample in a well counter and b) measuring, in a subsequent vascular volume scan with [11]CO-Hb, the ratio of lung pixel counts to peripheral blood counts for [11]CO-Hb. After making this correction, Wollmer et al. (1982) found that the thoracic concentration of ^{11}C-erythromycin was higher in the pneumonic lung (Table 2). Nevertheless this lung was consolidated with a high tissue density (D_{EV}) and per gram of tissue, the ^{11}C-erythromycin concentrations were approximately equal. In addition, since the total amount of erythromycin given was known, it was possible to predict that the concentrations of erythromycin in lung tissue would be bactericidal within 10 min following injection when administered in the usual therapeutic doses.

Structure-function correlations
1. Pulmonary gas exchange

Regional ventilation (V_A) has been measured during continuous inhalation of [19]Ne ($t_{1/2}$ = 17 sec) (the theory and practice is similar to that used for Krypton[81m], $t_{1/2}$ = 13 sec). Regional ventilation-perfusion (V_A/Q) ratio has been assessed during continuous i.v.infusion of a ^{13}N solution; regional Q was derived

TABLE 2 Erythromycin concentrations in pneumonic and unaffected lung in 5 patients following i.v.injection of 250 mg erythromycin lactobionate plus 20 mg (2-4 mCi) of 11C-erythromycin. Note concentrations in pneumonic lung are high (Ryan et al., 1985) but appropriate (Brudin et al., 1986)) for the increased tissue density (Rhodes et al., 1981). From Wollmer et al., 1982.

	Pneumonic lung	Unaffected lung
1. Extravascular erythromycin conc. (μg per cm³ thoracic volume)	2.24	0.82
2. Extravascular density (g per cm³ thoracic volume)	0.43	0.14
3. Extravascular erythromycin conc. (μg per g lung tissue)	5.5	6.6

from measurements of V_A/Q and V_A. Further details can be found in a recent review (Hughes et al., 1985). Because the input concentration of ^{13}N (mixed venous) can be measured if the transaxial slice includes the right ventricle, the regional V_A/Q ratio can be calculated in absolute rather than arbitrary units. In addition, regional V_A and Q as ($ml.min^{-1}.cm^{-3}$ thorax) can be re-expressed as $ml.min^{-1}$ per unit alveolar gas volume (e.g., V_A/V_A: $ml.min^{-1}.ml^{-1}$) or as $ml.min^{-1}$ per unit weight of tissue, or "per alveolus" (using D_{EV}). The expression "per cm³ thorax", implying regional flow, and "per g tissue" for V and Q can only be derived with tomographic techniques and can only be assessed quantitatively with PET.

Examples of measurements of V_A and Q per g lung tissue in Table 3 show surprisingly low values in asthmatic subjects, possibly related to their increase in D_{EV} (Table 1). Conversely, the apparently normal value for V_A in emphysema is related to the low D_{EV} which is associated with parenchymal destruction. As regards gas exchange, the dispersion (SD) of V_A/Q ratios is more important than the mean. Note that although the mean V_A/Q in emphysematous subjects (1.3) appears favourable (the greater the V_A/Q, the higher the oxygen tension), the large SD implies severe inefficiency of oxygen exchange.

TABLE 3. Alveolar ventilation (V_A) and perfusion (Q) (ml.min^{-1} g^{-1} extravascular lung tissue), ventilation-perfusion ratio (V_A/Q) and the standard deviation (SD) around the mean V_A/Q for normal subjects, asymptomatic smokers and patients with different clinical patterns of airflow obstruction. Mean values for R. lung (1.7 cm transaxial section) at mid-thoracic level.

	n	V_A ml.min^{-1}g^{-1}	Q ml.min^{-1}g^{-1}	V_A/Q	SD (V_A/Q)
Normal	15	14.1	17.6	0.8	0.15
Smokers	15	10.5	16.7	0.66	0.13
Asthma	10	4.75	7.19	0.69	0.21
Chronic bronchitis	4	9.0	14.6	0.65	0.22
Emphysema	4	12.5	10.3	1.3	0.47

2. Regional metabolic rate for glucose

Somewhat to our surprise, in view of the high blood to tissue ratio in normal lungs (1.6:1, see Table 1) and the small fraction of tissue, the metabolic rate for glucose can be measured in the lung using ^{18}FDG. As with the ^{11}C-erythromycin studies, the extravascular ^{18}F concentration per pixel is computed after subtraction of the vascular ^{18}F and divided by extravascular density. Serial scans are obtained for 60 min following the initial i.v.injection. From the slope of the increase in the tissue to plasma ^{18}F ratio plotted against the cumulative input (area under the plasma curve) to plasma ratio the regional metabolic rate (MRg) is derived. Rhodes (personal communication) has compared MRg (nmol.g^{-1}. hr^{-1}) in the lung with MRg in the chest wall and myocardium in normal subjects in both fasting and fed conditions. The increase in MRg after feeding is x 2.7 (lung), x 5.9 (chest wall) and x 15.3 (myocardium).

Clinical application in the lung has concentrated so far on inflammatory and neoplastic conditions because the energy metabolized in these cells is derived almost entirely from glycolysis. Values for fasting normal subjects and patients with chronic interstitial inflammatory disease are summarized in Table 4. Those regions with the highest glucose utilization tended in sarcoidosis to have the highest values for tissue density (D_{EV} of max MRg). This was not the case in fibrosing alveolitis, when the areas of highest tissue density may reflect fibrosis in addition to inflammation.

TABLE 4 Regional metabolic rate for glucose (MRg), measured with c. 4 mCi i.v. 18F-deoxyglucose (18FDG) in normal fasting subjects and in patients with sarcoidosis and interstitial lung disease, with measuements of tissue (extravascular) density in single transaxial slice (1.7 cm thick) at mid-thoracic level. Average values and range ( ) for each group for whole slice (mean) and maximal regional value (max) within the slice.

	n	MRg(mean)	MRg(max)	D_{EV}(mean)	D_{EV}(of max MRg)
		$\mu mol \ g^{-1} \ hr^{-1}$		$g \ cm^{-3}$	
Normal	9	1.21	1.73	0.15	0.15
		(0.62-1.91)	(1.0-2.37)	(0.12-0.18)	(0.11-0.22)
Sarcoidosis	7	3.24	5.3	0.34	0.46
		(2.0-4.85)	(2.4-9.5)	(0.29-0.43)	(0.28-0.65)
Fibrosing alveolitis	9	2.17	3.5	0.29	0.25
		(1.14-3.75)	(2.0-7.1)	(0.22-0.41)	(0.12-0.33)

CONCLUSION

It would be rather premature to reach conclusions about the clinical efficacy of lung PET studies on the basis of the data which we have just summarized. In spite of the difficulties to be overcome, we believe that unique physiological and pathophysiological information will emerge from the application of PET to the lung.

REFERENCES

Brudin, L.H., Valind, S.O., Rhodes, C.G. et al. 1986. Regional lung hematocrit in humans using positron emission tomography. J. Appl. Physiol., 60, 1155-1163.
Hughes, J.M.B., Brudin, L.H., Valind, S.O. et al. 1985. Positron emission tomography in the lung. J. Thoracic Imag., 1, 79-88.

Rhodes, C.G., Wollmer, P., Fazio, F. et al. 1981. Quantitative measurement of regional extravascular lung density using positron emission and transmission tomography. J. Comput. Assist. Tomogr., 5, 783-791.

Ryan, U.S., Ryan, J.N., Crutchley, D.J. 1985. The pulmonary endothelial surface. Fed. Proc., 4, 2603-2609.

Wollmer, P., Rhodes, C.G., Pike, V.W. et al. 1982. Measurement of pulmonary erythromycin concentration in patients with lobar pneumonia by means of positron tomography. Lancet, II, 1361-1364.

LUNG EDEMA: CLINICAL EFFICACY OF POSITRON EMISSION TOMOGRAPHY

O. Schober, G.-J. Meyer
Med. Hochschule, Nuklearmedizin,
Hannover, FRG

INTRODUCTION
Physiology.

The prime function of the lung is to exchange gas between the inspired air and the venous blood. Therefore, 60-75 % of the lung volume is taken up by gas and blood. Blood free lung tissue consists to approximately 80 % of water, of which 30-50 % is in the interstitial space and lymphatics while the remainder is intracellular. In addition the lung plays a major role in the regulation of a number of circulating mediators (Staub, 1974, 1978; Fishman and Renkin, 1979; Valind et al., 1985; Coates, 1986; Rahinian et al., 1986).

Pathophysiology.

As early as 1819 Laennec defined a pathological state in which there is abnormal extravascular storage in the lungs, the "pulmonary edema" as an infiltration of serum into the pulmonary tissue to such a degree that it significantly diminishes its permeability to air (Laennec, 1891; Guyton and Lindsey, 1959; Visscher et al., 1956; Staub, 1974). This already formulates the clinical problem. Staub (1974, 1978) and Snashall and Hughes (1981) describe and review several specific forms of pulmonary edema from the point of clinical physiology, with concepts including changes in the rate of fluid and protein flow through the lung's interstitium as well as changes in fluid and protein content. A clinical important finding is that an increase in interstitial water is the primary abnormality in pulmonary edema, while an increase in cellular water is an important feature of deranged cell metabolism. Most of the information has been obtained from experimental animal models, partly with direct destructive qualitative and quantitative methods (gross and microscopic appearence, lymph flow and composition, lung weight or weight change, lung water; Staub, 1974, 1978).

The basis for the understanding of fluid and protein exchange across a membrane under steady state conditions is described by Starling's general equation including the factors that control lung water balance. The net transvascular fluid flow is a function of the

filtration coefficient, the effective reflection coefficient of the
membrane, the hydrostatic pressures and the protein osmotic pressures on
each side of the membrane (Starling, 1896).

From a clinical point of view different pathophysiological mechanisms are discussed, which are causing pulmonary edema: raised left
arterial pressure, raised pulmonary arterial pressure, increased micro-
vascular permeability, lymphatic obstruction and other influences, e.g.,
lung inflation, body position, alveolar and airway epithelium, and
bronchial circulation. In clinical routine work the primary aetiology of
pulmonary edema is furthermore discussed in terms of cardiogenic or
noncardiogenic edema, and an important distinction must be made between
interstitial and alveolar edema.

Detection on lung fluid

Of the several noninvasive methods which are based on the measurement of changes in the physical properties of the lung related to extravascular water accumulation, clinical examination and the study of the
chest radiographic pattern are the only methods commonly used in routine
clinical work. Radiological criteria used are: hila, Kerley's lines,
micronuduli, widening of scissurae, peribronchial and perivascular
cuffs, extensive perihilar haze, subpleural effusion, and diffuse
increase of density (Stender and Schermuly, 1969; McCredie, 1967, 1974;
Pistolesi and Giuntini, 1978).

Up to now it is generally believed that the excess water in the interstitial spaces of the lung is not clinically apparent until the lung
interstitial fluid has increased fivefold to sixfold (Fishman and
Renkin, 1979). However, Coates et al. (1983) examined the effect of only
15 % increase in extracellular fluid volume with indirect qualitative
and quantitative tests, such as lung volume measurement, lung function
test (nitrogen washout), chest radiographs, and computerized tomography
scans of the thorax. The analysis of the sensitivity of these techniques
demonstrated that the tests of small airway function, residual volume
and nitrogen washout, are more sensitive than radiographic techniques to
a small increase (< 15 %) in lung water. These results are supported by
different studies on techniques (compton scatter densitometry, attenuation of gamma rays, transvascular protein flux, impedance) which have
not been widely applied in clinical practice, as well as the invasive

thermo-dye dilution technique (Staub, 1978; Snashall and Hughes, 1981; Lewis et al., 1982; Creutzig et al., 1984; Schober et al., 1985).

Positron emitters

Positron emission tomography provides means to map and measure quantitatively physiologic and pathophysiologic data, rates and functions with physiologic tracers. Studies can be conducted in both, animals and humans.

The measurement of pulmonary extravascular water with positron emitters is described since the early 70's (Jones et al., 1972; Cooper et al., 1982). The measurement of extravascular lung water has been approached by using the volume of dilution principle for two indicators, one intravascular (nondiffusible: $C^{15}O$ erythrocytes) and one extra-vascular (diffusible: $H_2^{15}O$). The disadvantages and constraints of all described invasive first-pass indicator dilution measurements are the limited exchangeability of the water space during the first pass and the lack of regional data. Further sources of error are inherent to most of the first-pass measurements: separation of recirculation, onset of the curve and recovery problems, validity of different methods for data analysis: height over area versus ratio of moments, patients with low cardiac output, sludge phenomenon, and the regional distribution in a multiphase system (Jones et al., 1972; Cooper et al., 1972; Staub, 1974; Hughes, 1979; Snashall and Hughes, 1981; Lewis et al., 1982; Helmeke et al., 1982).

To overcome these problems, Rhodes et al. (1981) proposed a technique for the measurement of regional values of extravascular lung density using PET and transmission tomography. Schober et al. (1983) and Meyer et al. (1984) developed steady state technique for the quantifi-cation of the extravascular lung water with a constant infusion of ^{15}O-labelled water.

POSITRON EMISSION TOMOGRAPHY
Extravascular lung density. Methods

Intravascular space. In order to determine extravascular density or lung water, the total density or water pool must be corrected for the intravascular space. Neglecting regional differences of the hematocrit in the lungs, in vivo labelling with ^{11}CO, i.e., the formation of carboxyhemoglobin, seems to be the most suitable method following an equilibration period. The tracer is chemically stable and the half-life of ^{11}C allows a smooth administration of approximately 5-10 mCi ^{11}CO via a disposable face mask.

For absolute quantification of regional blood volume (ml/cm³) the absolute intravascular count density is calculated from venous and arterial blood samples, taken during the blood pool measurement, and a camera calibration factor, obtained from phantom studies. With activities used in patient studies there is a linear relationship between the camera sensitivity (counts/voxel) in reconstructed slices, regions of the aortic arch, atrium or left ventricle to ensure full quantitative recovery, and the venous and arterial blood activity (μCi/cm³), measured in a calibrated well type NaI counter (Rhodes et al., 1981; Schober et al., 1983; Meyer et al., 1984).

Lung density and extravascular lung density distribution

The lung density is measured either with a ring source of positron emitting ^{68}Ga, or a conventional transmission CT scanner. The (linear) relationship between the distribution of attenuation, and known densities of various phantoms (g/cm³) has to be shown.

The extravascular lung density distribution (D_{EV}) is defined by the difference on a voxel by voxel basis

$$D_{EV}: = D_{(V + EV)} - D_V$$

where D_{EV}: extravascular lung density, $D_{(V + EV)}$: normalized lung density (vascular plus extravascular), and D_V: blood density, which is calibrated versus the fractional blood volume. This number can be converted to units of mass density after a linear relationship is shown to exist between blood densities (normals: 1.060 ± 0.04 g/cm³) and isotope concentrations in the blood pool scan (Rhodes et al., 1981; Schuster et al., 1986).

Total lung water and extravascular lung water

Constant infusion of ^{15}O-labelled water allows a direct quantification of the total water volume. The principal assumption is, that the tracer for water euqilibrates with the water tissue very rapidly in relation to the intravascular transit time through the lung microcirculation. Owing to short transit times in the pulmonary and

heart systems and the high permeability and short diffusion pathways in
the lung parenchyma, the unavoidable concentration gradients are quite
small.

The trapping of ^{15}O labelled water in a small buffer reservoir of
0.9 % saline fed by a peristaltic pump and its continuous withdrawal at
the same rate by a precision pump results in a constant flow of tracer,
approximately 6 ml/min and 3 mCi/min. After 10 min of intravenous
infusion a steady state is reached with a deviation less than ± 5 %
(Schober et al., 1983, 1985; Meyer et al., 1984, 1985).

Neglecting regional differences of the hematocrit of the lungs, the
regional extravascular lung water (rELW) is defined as the difference
between calibrated values of the reconstructed total lung water (TLW)
and the normalized reconstructed blood volume (BV).

$$ELW: = TLW - BV$$

The emission scans have to be corrected for attenuation in the
usual way by transmission scans.

VALIDATION
Extravascular lung water

The method was validated in an experimental noncardiac canine
pulmonary edema. The dogs were measured before and after induction of
lung edema by intravenous injection of oleic acid. The increase of
extravascular lung water was monitored by thermo-dye-method. The
correlation of extravascular lung water as measured by indicator
dilution and PET measurements is good (r=0.94). The PET values agree
also with the "gold standard", the gravimetric lung water determination. In this study the uncertainty in the absolute quantification is
estimated to be ± 20 %. In the experiments the mean extravascular lung
water was 0.13 ml/cm³ before and 0.25 ml/cm³ after induction of lung
edema (Schober et al., 1983; Meyer et al., 1984).

Extravascular lung density

In a recent study, regional lung density and lung water measurements were correlated in normal and edematous dogs. A comparison was
made between densities, measured by X-ray CT and PET, respectively. Mean
lung water was measured to be 0.25 ml/cm³ lung tissue, mean density to
be 0.32 g/cm³ with an antero-posterior, gravity-dependent gradient and a
high correlation between regional lung water (PET) and regional lung

density (CT) in both, normal and edematous dogs (r=0.89) (Schuster et al., 1986a).

CLINICAL MEASUREMENTS
Normal subjects

Pulmonary blood volume. In supine controls a progressive decrease from the basal (0.26 g/cm³) to apical regions (0.16 g/cm³) is observed. The variations of blood density rise from 0.08 g/cm³ anteriorly to 0.21 g/cm³ posteriorly lower (caudal) parts of the lung.

Extravascular lung water. The differences in the regional extra-vascular lung water are rather small, with a tendency to higher values at the base of the lung (0.13 g/cm³) compared with apical regions (0.11 g/cm³).

Lung density. In a supine control subject there is a progressive increase from front to back in lung density. This is explained due to differences in blood content between the anterior and posterior part of the lung. The regional differences in extravascular lung density (0.14 g/cm³) have been found to be rather small, rising from 0.12 g/cm³ anteriorly to 0.16 g/cm³ posteriorly (Rhodes et al., 1981; Wollmer et al., 1983, 1984; Schober et al., 1985).

Patients with cardiac lung disease

Blood volume. In the basal lung regions of patients with chronic heart failure (stage III, according to the New York Heart Association) the blood volume (0.18 g/cm³) was reduced by about 30 %. Instead of the normal baso-apical gradient of blood volume, these patients showed a rather flat regional distribution. The normal ventrodorsal gradient of the blood pool was also missing. Instead the blood volume shows a rather flat distribution and is reduced to about half of the normal value in the dorsal part of the lungs (Wollmer et al., 1983; Schober et al., 1985).

Extravascular lung water and density. In the same patients with chronic heart failure, the level of extravascular lung water in the basal parts of the lung was found to be markedly increased (0.20 g/cm³), whereas in the apical regions (0.14 g/cm³) only minor deviations from the levels observed in the controls were measured (Table 1). The in-crease of extravascular lung density is significant and greater in the posterior part (50 % : 0.28 g/cm³) than in the anterior part of the lungs (30 %: 0.19 g/cm³) (Wollmer et al., 1983; Schober et al., 1985).

Hemodynamic data. To investigate different mechanisms causing pulmonary edema patients with chronic heart failure and hemodynamic imbalance were studied with PET immediately after angiography. Table 1 lists the mean values of the cardiac index (CI), the pulmonary artery pressure (PA), the pulmonary capillary wedge pressure (PC), and the angiographically determined ejection fraction (EF) found in controls and patients with coronary artery disease and aortic/mitral valve disease. The relationship between these parameters, along with the classification according to the NYHA are shown in Table 2. The correlation with single hemodynamic data is rather poor, but significant (r>0.55, p<0.01). After normalizing the extravascular lung water with respect to the blood volume, a high correlation (r=0.87) between this ratio and the grade of the heart failure (NYHA) was found (Schober et al., 1985).

TABLE 1   Group 1: non-hemodynamic significant stenosis of coronary arteries; group 2: coronary heart disease (CHD: n=5); mitral/aortic valve disease (n=3); group 3: CHD: (n=1); mitral/aortic valve disease (n=5). Clinical, hemodynamic and PET data (regional extravascular lung water/blood volume) (mean ± one SD, range). Legend see Table 2.

	Group 1	Group 2	Group 3
Clinically	NYHA = 1	I<NYHA<III	III<NYHA
Age (y)	41-62	48-63	53-82
	5 m	2 f; 6 m	4 f; 2 m
CI (ml/min.m²)	2.7 ± 0.4	2.6 ± 0.4	1.8 ± 0.2
PC (mm Hg)	5 ± 2	12 ± 8	18 ± 10
PA (mm Hg)	12 ± 2	19 ± 11	33 ± 14
EF (%)	69 ± 9	52 ± 23	48 ± 7
rELW (g/cm³)	0.11 ± 0.02	0.14 ± 0.02	0.17 ± 0.02
	0.06 - 0.17	0.07 - 0.21	0.09 - 0.24
rBV (g/cm³)	0.21 ± 0.02	0.21 ± 0.03	0.17 ± 0.02
	0.12 - 0.27	0.17 - 0.26	0.14 - 0.21
rELW/rBV	0.52	0.67	1.00

TABLE 2   Correlation coefficient pearson "r": Mean extravascular
lung water versus different hemodynamic parameters. r > 0.55 indicates:
p < 0.01. ELW: Extravascular lung water, CI: Cardiac index, PA:
Pulmonary artery pressure, EF: Ejection fraction, PC: Pulmonary
capillary wedge pressure, NYHA: Severity of the disease, New York Heart
Association

	CI (1/min.m²)	PC (mm Hg)	PA (mm Hg)	EF (%)	NYHA (I-IV)
ELW (g/cm³)	0.45	0.47	0.57	0.60	0.69

Radiographic findings. Retrospective radiographic findings of
pulmonary edema generally appeared together with a global extravascular
lung water excess of more than 30 %, i.e., greater than 0.14 ml/cm³
(9/10 patients). In two patients with an ELW of 0.14 ml/cm³ the chest
radiograph appeared to be possibly positive, i.e., apparently abnormal
shadowing but insufficient to blurr or obscure vessel shadows, or
cardiac or diaphragmatic outlines. In controls and patients with an ELW
of less than 0.14 ml/cm³ (8/8 patients), there was no radiographic
detection of pulmonary edema. In summary, radiographic correlates of
excess water is detected, when the local water content in at least a
part of the lungs is approximately doubled (Schober et al., 1985).

Patients with interstitial diseases

In patients with interstitial disease of the lung extravascular
lung density was found to be increased and large variations were
observed. The blood volume was markedly reduced in patients with
pulmonary fibrosis. In patients with sarcoidosis, a reduction in
extravascular lung density occurred after treatment with oral
prednisone. The abnormalities correlated with those shown by tests of
the overall pulmonary function, as tests for vital capacity, total lung
capacity, and transfer factor for carbon monoxide. There was no common
pattern of regional abnormalities in the investigated groups (Wollmer et
al., 1984).

DISCUSSION

There is little information on regional variations in lung water, in normals and patients, measured with non-invasive methods. Chest X-ray is routinely used, and in some clinical problems absolute measurements of density, in terms of secondary units, e.g., Hounsfield unities, and/or proton densities and relaxation times are given. Nevertheless, because of their qualitative nature, the results obtained with conventional methods need to be compared with quantitative measurements which are methodologically more demanding. From measurements with positron emission tomography, regional quantitative data of the extravascular lung density or water can be derived.

Phelps et al. (1985) specified four phases of an establishment of a clinically procedure in an espousal for positron emission tomography.

1. Basic research where the fundamental principles and precision of a technique are performed,
2. clinic research where the ability to separate normal from abnormal tissue is explored,
3. clinical trials where the sensitivity and specifity of a technique are determined,
4. clinical utility determinations where the impact of the procedure on mortality, morbidity, and medical economics are assessed.

The experiments and tests carried out so far demonstrate that we have to consider these stages carefully in order to determine whether these tests are clinically useful.

Extravascular lung density

Values for lung density by positron emission tomography are consistently higher than those values obtained for lung density by X-ray CT. These differences are probably due to beam-hardening effects with CT, and partial-volume averaging and scattered radiation effects with PET (Schuster et al., 1986). The same authors demonstrate in an animal study with normal and edematous dogs that PET lung density measurements are a satisfactory method for following acute changes in lung water or for normalizing other PET derived data.

PET data are given up to now in terms of volume instead of lung weight (Rhodes et al., 1981; Schober et al., 1983, 1985). Wollmer et al.

(1983) argued that the reduced lung inflation made only an unimportant contribution to their findings; on the other hand Meyer et al. (1984) found a significantly increased level for extravascular lung water in a dog due to constriction of its chest. Schuster and Marklin (1986) evaluated the changes of total and extravascular lung density before and after changes in either lung inflation or blood volume. Large changes in tidal volume, modest amounts of positive end-expiratory pressure, and significant decreases in blood volume produced only small effects on total lung density, while regional extravascular lung density remained unchanged.

Extravascular lung water

In order measure the exchangeable water content of lung tissue directly and not densities, which yield of course a measure of extravascular water, and to assess specific structural changes in the lung, a method for the constant infusion of ^{15}O-labelled water was developed (Schober et al., 1983; Meyer et al., 1984).

In this approach with short lived radioisotopes the quantitative analysis necessitates the evaluation of potential error sources, as the concentration gradients, caused by decay along the transit pathway, partition coefficients, and the extraction fraction. Furthermore, inherent partial volume effects, normalization and calibration factors, and absorption corrections play an important role in the estimation and quantification of regional extravascular lung water. However, when compared with clinical pathophysiological differences, the influence of these factors seems to be acceptable.

In absolute ELW measurements, the overall estimated error is in the range of $\pm$ 30 %. As to whether this is also true in later stages of edema when alveolar flooding occurs with changed transit times and diffusion pathways, has been discussed. In the range of normal transit times (8-15 sec) reduced extraction fractions or partition coefficients of 0.9 lead to an underestimation of the extravascular water volume by 15-20 %. In the case of prolonged transit times (20-30 sec) the effect increases, leading to errors of 30-40 % (Meyer et al., 1985).

As shown in the experiments with dogs the PET technique is more sensitive than any other nondestructive method for the detection of differences of the extravascular lung water, and is accurate enough to allow topographic mapping of the distribution of ELW in advanced pulmonary edema (Schober et al., 1983; Meyer et al., 1984).

Normal subjects, patients with cardiac and interstitial lung disease. As has been demonstrated by radiological and morphological studies, chronic heart failure is accompanied by regional structure changes in the lung parenchyma. The thickening of vessel walls and interstitial fibrosis have been described. These changes correspond to a lower regional blood volume in the basal parts of the lungs. The radiographic pattern of the cranialization of the blood volume may be due to distensibility of the pulmonary vessels or functional changes of the pulmonary vasculature. This seems to be reflected in a relatively enhanced regional blood volume compared to that in the basal parts. The highest values of extravascular lung water were noticed at the lung base (Wollmer et al., 1983, 1984; Schober et al., 1985).

Different measurements with different techniques assess different distribution volumes of biochemically different and physiologically distinguishable water compartments in the lung.

A detailed discussion of the various methods and their limitations is beyond the scope of this presentation. However, the PET results are in reasonable agreement with the published results obtained by the different qualitative and quantitative, nondestructive and invasive destructive techniques (Staub, 1974, 1978; Hughes, 1979; Snashall and Hughes, 1981).

The published qunatitative data and correlations to human hemodynamic data do not allow a detailed discussion of the factors which control the lung water balance in terms of concepts including changes in the rate of fluid and protein flow through the lung's interstitium as well as changes in fluid and protein content (Starling equation) (Hughes, 1979; Snashall and Hughes, 1981; Wollmer et al., 1983, 1984; Schober et al., 1985).

CONCLUSIONS

Physiology and pathophysiology. It has already been demonstrated that measurement of extravascular lung water with positron emission tomography can yield new insights in lung water balance.

Calibration of conventional imaging methods. Other imaging techniques, such as conventional X-ray, X-ray computed tomography (CT),

and magnetic resonance imaging (MRI) can be calibrated against quantitative, regional, and physiological measurements with positron emission
tomography.

Therapy control. The medical treatment of the patients and the
sensitivity of regional extravascular lung water to pharmacological
influences can be followed quantitatively by positron emission
tomography.

Future. More clinical trials are needed in order to determine the
clinical utility of the method, which implies a demonstration on an
impact on mortality, morbidity, and medical economics.

REFERENCES

Coates, G., Powles, A.C.P., Morrison, S.C. et al. 1983. The effects of
    intravenous infusion of saline on lung density, lung volumes,
    nitrogen washout, computed tomography scans, and chest radiography
    in humans. Am. Rev. Respir. Dis., 127, 91-96.
Coates, G. 1986. Quantitative studies of aerosol clearance in pulmonary
    disease. Sem. Nucl. Med., 16, in press.
Cooper, J.C., McCullogh, N.J., Lowenstein, E. 1982. Determination of
    pulmonary extravascular water using oxygen 15-labeled water. J.
    Appl. Physiol., 33, 842-845.
Creutzig, H., Sturm, J.A., Schober, O. et al. 1984. Nuklearmedizinische
    Diagnostik des "pulmonary capillary protein leakage". Nucl. Med.,
    23, 253-256.
Fishman, A.P., Renkin, E.E. 1979. Pulmonary Edema. Am. Physiol. Soc.,
    Bethesda.
Guyton, A.C., Lindsey, A.W. 1959. Effect of elevation of left arterial
    pressure and decreased plasma protein concentration on the
    development of pulmonary edema. Circ. Res., 7, 649-657.
Helmeke, H.J., Schober, O., Lehr, L. et al. 1982. Measurement of
    regional lung water with 150-labeled water and C150-labeled
    carboxyhemoglobin. In "Radioaktive Isotope in Klinik und
    Forschung". (Eds. R. Hoefer, H. Bergmann). (Egermann-Verlag). pp.
    635-642.
Hughes, J.M.B. 1979. Short-life radionuclides and regional lung
    function. Brit. J. Radiol., 52, 353-370.
Jones, T., Clark, J.C., Buckingham, P.D. et al. 1972. The use of oxygen-
    15 labelled water for the measurement of pulmonary extravascular
    water. Brit. J. Radiol., 45, 630.
Laennec, R.T.H. 1819. Traité de l'Ausculation médiate. Brosson and
    Chaude, Paris.
Lewis, F.R., Elings, V.B., Hill, S.L. et al. 1982. The measurement of
    extravascular lung water by thermal-green dye indicator dilution.
    Ann. N.Y. Acad. Sci., 80, 394-410.

McCredie, R.M. 1967. Measurement of pulmonary edema in valvular heart disease. Circulation, 36, 381-386.

McCredie, R.M. 1974. Measurement of lung water. In "Progress in Cardiology". (Eds. P.N. Yu, J.F. Odwin). (Lea and Febiger, Philadelphia). pp. 331-339.

Meyer, G.-J., Schober, O., Bossaller, C. et al. 1984. Quantification of regional extravascular lung water in dogs with positron emission tomography, using constant infusion of 150-labeled water. Eur. J. Nucl. Med., 9, 220-228.

Meyer, G.J., Schober, O., Hundeshagen, H. 1985. Gradient effects in extravascular water determination using 150-labelled water under steady state conditions: Theory and error sensitivity. Eur. J. Nucl. Med., 10, 77-80.

Phelps., M.E., Mazziotta, J.C., Schelbert, H.R. et al. 1985. Clinical PET: What are the issues? J. Nucl. Med., 26, 1353-1358.

Pistolesi, M., Giuntini, C. 1978. Assessment of extravascular lung water. Radiol. Clin. North Am., 16, 551-574.

Rahinian, J., Glass, E., Touya, J. et al. 1986. Metabolic lung function studies with radiotracers. Sem. Nucl. Med., 16, in press.

Rhodes, C.G., Wollmer, P., Fazio, F. et al. 1981. Quantitative measurement of regional extravascular lung density using positron emission and transmission tomography. J. Comput. Assist. Tomogr., 5, 783-791.

Schober, O., Meyer, G.-J., Bossaller, C. et al. 1983. Quantitative Messung des regionalen extravaskulären Lungenwassers bei Hunden mit der Positronen-Emissions-Tomographie. Fortschr. Röntgenstr., 139, 117-126.

Schober, O., Meyer, G.-J., Bossaller, C. et al. 1985. Quantitative determination of regional extravascular lung water and regional blood volume in congestive heart failure. Eur. J. Nucl. Med., 10, 17-24.

Schuster, D.P., Marklin, G.F., Mintun, M.A. et al. 1986. PET measurement of regional lung density: 1. J. Comput. Assist. Tomogr., 10, 723-729.

Schuster, D.P., Marklin, G.F. 1986. Effect of changes in inflation and blood volume on regional lung density - A PET study: 2. J. Comput. Assist. Tomogr., 10, 730-735.

Snashall, P.D., Hughes, J.M.B. 1981. Lung water balance. Rev. Physiol. Biochem. Pharmacol., 89, 5-62.

Starling, E.H. 1895-96. On the absorption of fluids from the connective tissue spaces. J. Physiol., 19, 312-326.

Staub, N.C. 1974. The pathophysiology of pulmonary edema. Physiol. Rev., 54, 674-811.

Staub, N.C. 1978. Lung Water and Solute Exchange. Marcel Dekker, New York, Basel.

Stender, H.S., Schermuly, W. 1969. Allgemeine Röntgensymptomatologie der Lungenerkrankungen. In "Encyclopedia of Medical Radiology". (Ed. L. Diethelm). (Springer, Berlin, Heidelberg, New York). pp. 226-339.

Valind, S.O., Wollmer, P.E., Rhodes, C.G. 1985. Application of positron emission tomography in the lung. In "Positron Emission Tomography". (Eds. M. Reivich, A. Alavi). (Allan R. Riss, New York). pp. 387-412.

Visscher, M.B., Haddy, F.J., Stephens, G. 1956. The physiology and pharmacology of lung edema. Pharamcol. Rev., 8, 389-434.

Wollmer, P., Rhodes, C.G., Allan, R.M. et al. 1983. Regional
    extravascular lung density and fractional pulmonary blood volume
    in patients with chronic pulmonary venous hypertension. Clin.
    Physiol., 3, 241-256.
Wollmer, P., Rhodes, C.G., Hughes, J.M.B. 1984. Regional extravascular
    density and fractional blood volume of the lung in interstitial
    disease. Thorax, 39, 286-293.

PHARMACOLOGICAL STUDIES OF THE LUNG WITH PET

A. Syrota
Service Hospitalier Frédéric Joliot
Département de Biologie du Commissariat à l'Energie Atomique
Orsay, France

Positron emission tomography (PET), known to be used for lung
ventilation and perfusion studies (West, 1967), can also be used in
pharmacology to obtain information that is otherwise not available. The
lung takes up biologically active substances which can be inactivated or
activated, and synthesises and releases others (Alabaster, 1977). Such
information in man has been obtained from samples of human lungs (Al-
Ubaidi and Bakhle, 1980), or from in vivo first-pass studies, invasive
(Jorfeldt et al., 1979; Gillis et al., 1979; Geddes and Blackburn, 1979)
or not (Syrota et al., 1981), as well as from in vivo kinetic studies
using external detection methods with scintillation cameras (Gallagher
et al., 1977; Winchell et al., 1980). PET provides now quantitative
regional data in the human lung.

Uptake of basic amines
        Two basic amines, imipramine, a tricyclic antidepressant, and
propranolol, a high affinity beta-adrenergic antagonist were labeled
with carbon-11 (Berger et al., 1979, 1982) and injected in nonsmoking
subjects, in smoking patients with pulmonary centrilobular emphysema and
in patients with pulmonary sarcoidosis (Pascal et al., 1981, 1982;
Syrota et al., 1982).
        In controls, the chest PET scans showed high pulmonary and low
cardiovascular concentrations. The tissue-to-blood concentration ratio
increased from the first to the 10th min.and then leveled off, remaining
between 80 and 150. Such a very high uptake is also found in in vitro
studies on perfused isolated rat or rabbit lungs (Eling et al., 1975;
Blanck and Gillis, 1979; Dollery and Junod, 1976; Anderson et al.,
1974).
        The lung activity versus time curves could be fitted with single
decreasing monoexponential curves with a correlation coefficient greater

than 0.85 (p<0.001). Each curve was characterized by the initial value (uptake extrapolated at time of injection: U_o) and by the efflux half-life (T). U_o was similar for all subjects (Mean: 22.9; Range: 8.5-38.6) and was expressed as 10^{-3}% of the injected dose/g of lung. T (in min) was significantly different (p<0.025) when subjects with sarcoidosis (M: 236; R: 53-486) were compared to control subjects (M: 45; R: 20-68). In the group of patients with sarcoidosis, no linear correlation was found between the values of T and either the values of serum angiotensin converting enzyme or the percentage of lymphocytes in the bronchoalveolar fluid.

No change of slope was observed on the efflux curves after loading with an excess of unlabeled molecule although blood pressure decreased by 20 % after chlorpromazine infusion and heart rate decreased by 20 % after propranolol infusion.

The uptake of ^{11}C imipramine and of ^{11}C propranolol was therefore mainly non-specific since 1. the lung concentration as a function of time did not change after loading with 10^{-6}M unlabeled molecules, and 2. the amine pulmonary concentration expressed as pmol/g of lung was linearly related to the amount of injected amines. The human lung took up about 20 % of the intravenously injected amines (the uptake extrapolated at t = 0 corresponded to 23 x 10^{-3}% of the injected dose per gram of lung and the entire lung weighed nearly 1000 g). This non-specific uptake may be related to the high lipid solubility of imipramine and propranolol (the oil-to-water partition coefficient is 100 for imipramine and 90 for propranolol, Eling et al., 1975; Anderson et al., 1974; Oldendorf, 1974).

For imipramine and propranolol, a higher uptake (nearly 100 %) was observed in first-pass studies in the isolated perfused rat lung (Syrota and Yudilevich, 1983), it was not inhibited by infusing unlabeled imipramine or chlorpromazine (10^{-4}M). A high chlorpromazine extraction (80 %) was also seen in in vivo human studies using the multiple indicator dilution technique (Syrota et al., 1981). This extraction was not modified by an infusion of 10^{-6}M chlorpromazine just before the test. A similar high extraction was also seen with imipramine and propranolol (unpublished observations). In subjects taking propranolol regularly, Geddes reported that the propranolol first-pass extraction is lower than that observed in controls (Geddes and Blackburn, 1979). This could suggest either the presence of specific fixation sites or a membrane modification by propranolol (Surewicz and Leyko, 1981).

From the results showing an extraction of 80 % during the first-pass and from our results showing an uptake (extrapolated at t = 0) of 20 %, we are led to suppose that the lung amine pool consists of two compartments : 3/4 of the total capacity could correspond to a pool of rapid efflux (half-life shorter than 1 min), non detectable with PET, and 1/4 to a slow effluxable pool (efflux half-life: 45 min), which can be observed with PET and which corresponds to a non-specific binding. These hypotheses are consistent with those suggested from studies in isolated rat and rabbit lung (Eling et al., 1975; Blanck and Gillis, 1979; Dollery and Junod, 1976; Anderson et al., 1974).

In 3 subjects, pulmonary blood pool volume was also measured by PET after injection of ^{11}C-autologous red cells. 99 % of the molecules of imipramine were found in the extravascular compartment. The technique used in the other studies provides information on the amount of amine present per gram of lung in both the extravascular and vascular compartments. When both compartments were considered together, the uptake per gram of lung was found to be similar in subjects with low lung density (emphysema), high density (sarcoidosis) and in control subjects.

Patients with sarcoidosis had a 5-fold slower efflux than control subjects. Such a modification could not be related only to a lower rate of efflux but is probably also due to a change in the non-specific binding characteristics of the amines and of their extrapulmonary metabolites. This could be related to a modification of the cell membrane composition which might be specific to sarcoidosis.

Serotonin receptors in the human lung

Serotonin receptors known to be present on the membrane of the pulmonary alveolar macrophages were identified after i.v.injection of ^{11}C-ketanserin, a potent antagonist of S2 receptors (Berridge et al., 1983). After injection at high specific activity ^{11}C-ketanserin was concentrated in the myocardium and the ^{11}C-ketanserin pulmonary concentration was very low. However, this pattern was observed only in nonsmokers. High concentrations of ^{11}C-ketanserin were found in the lungs of smokers compared to nonsmokers (Charbonneau et al., 1986). The lung/heart ratio of ^{11}C-ketanserin concentration was 0.64 ± 0.04 (n=7) in the nonsmokers group and 1.40 ± 0.35 (n=7) in the smokers group. The radioactive ligand concentration in the lungs of smokers was linearly correlated (r=0.901, n=7, p <0.001) to the amount of the tobacco smoke absorption (expressed as a multiple of 20 cigarettes a day smoked regularly for one year). The very high ^{11}C-ketanserin concentration in the lungs of smokers seems to reflect the increased cellularity induced by cigarette smoking. These results concord with the accumulation of alveolar macrophages previously described in vivo in bronchial lavage cell sediments. In similar circumstances studying brain and heart receptors, the ligand may become specifically bound to receptors in the lungs, since the injections are given i.v. Moreover, PET opens the way to noninvasive investigations of the effects of atmospheric pollution on human lungs.

In many aspects of physiology and biochemistry the behavior of a system in vivo is often dramatically different from that observed in vitro. The studies of in vivo systems are more complex because it is difficult to control the conditions of a particular experiment. Results obtained in in vivo studies of metabolic functions of the lung with PET suggest that the physiological data obtained in vitro on isolated perfused lungs are helpful for the understanding of results observed in clinical situations (Syrota and Yudilevich, 1981; Syrota et al., 1982; Syrota, 1985). An explanation of this approximation between in vitro and in vivo findings relies in the fact that radioligands are intravenously injected and that the lung is the organ where solute transfer from blood to tissue first occurs. The lungs thus acts both as a capacitor and as a site of enzymatic reactions.

REFERENCES

Alabaster, V.A. 1977. Inactivation of endogenous amines in the lungs. In "Metabolic Functions of the Lung". (Eds. Y.S. Bakhle, J.R. Vane). (M.Dekker, New York). pp. 3-31.

Al-Ubaidi, P., Bakhle, Y.S. 1980. Metabolism of vasoactive hormones in human isolated lung. Clin. Sci., 58, 45-51.

Anderson, M.W., Orton, T.C. et al. 1974. Accumulation of amines in the isolated perfused rabbit lung. J. Pharmacol. Exp. Ther., 189, 456-466.

Berger, G., Mazière, M., Knipper, R. et al. 1979. Automated synthesis of 11-C labeled radiopharmaceuticals: imipramine, chlorpromazine, nicotine and methionine. Int. J. Appl. Rad. Isot., 30, 393-399.

Berger, G., Mazière, M., Prenant, C. et al. 1982. Synthesis of 11C
    propranolol. J. Radioanal. Chem., 74, 301-306.
Berridge, M., Comar, D., Crouzel, M. et al. 1983. 11C-labeled
    ketanserin, a selective serotonin S2 antagonist. J. Label. Comp.
    Radiopharm., 20, 73-78.
Blanck, T.J.J., Gillis, C.N. 1979. Beta-adrenergic receptor ligand
    binding by rabbit lung. Biochem. Pharmacol., 28, 1903-1909.
Charbonneau, P., Syrota, A., Boullais, C. et al. 1986. Serotonin
    receptors and lung phagocyte recruitment induced by cigarette
    smoking detected in vivo by positron emission tomography. J. Nucl.
    Med., 27, 950.
Dollery, C.T., Junod, A.F. 1976. Concentration of + propranolol in
    isolated perfused lungs of rat. Br. J. Pharm., 57, 67-71.
Eling, T.E., Pickett, R.D., Orton, T.C. et al. 1975. A study of the
    dynamics of imipramine accumulation in the isolated perfused
    rabbit lung. Drug Metab. Dispos., 3, 389-399.
Gallagher, B.M., Christman, D., Fowler, J.S. et al. 1977. Radioisotope
    scintigraphy for the study of dynamics of amine regulation by the
    human lung. Chest, 71, 282-284.
Geddes, D.M., Blackburn, J.P. 1979. First pass uptake of 14C
    propranolol by the lung. Thorax, 34, 810-813.
Gillis, C.N., Cronau, L.H., Mandel, S. et al. 1979. Indicator dilution
    measurement of 5 hydroxytryptamine clearance by human lung. J.
    Appl. Physiol. Respirat. Env. Exerc. Physiol., 46, 1178-1183.
Jorfeldt et al. 1979. Lung uptake of lidocaine in healthy volunteers.
    Acta Anaesth. Scan., 23, 567-574.
Oldendorf, W.H. 1974. Lipid solubility and drug penetration of the
    blood-brain barrier. Proc. Soc. Exp. Biol. Med., 147, 813-816.
Pascal, O., Syrota, A., Berger, G. et al. 1981. Lung uptake of 11C-
    propranolol in patients with sarcoidosis evaluated by positron
    emission tomography. In "Sarcoidosis and Other Granulomatous
    Disorders". (Eds. J. Marsac, J. Chretien). (Pergamon Press,
    Paris). pp. 404-408.
Pascal, O., Syrota, A., Berger, G. 1982. In vivo uptake of 11C-labeled
    amines by human lung. In "Nuclear Medicine and Biology". (Ed. C.
    Raynaud). (Pergamon Press). pp. 2558-2561.
Surewicz, W.K., Leyko, E. 1981. Interaction of propranolol with model
    phospholipid membranes. Biochem. Biophys. Acta, 643, 387-397.
Syrota, A. 1985. Solute transport and ligand-receptor interactions
    studied in man by positron emission tomography. In "Carrier-
    Mediated Transport of Solutes from Blood to Tissue". (Eds. D.L.
    Yudilevich, G.E. Mann). (Longman, New York). pp. 155-176.
Syrota, A., Girault, M., Pocidalo, J.J. et al. 1982. Endothelial uptake
    of amino acids, sugars, lipids and prostaglandins in rat lung. Am.
    J. Physiol., 243,
Syrota, A., Pascal, O., Crouzel, M. et al. 1981. Pulmonary extraction of
    11C-chlorpromazine, measured by residue detection in man. J. Nucl.
    Med., 22, 145-148.
Syrota, A., Pascal, O., Yudilevich, D.L. 1982. Evaluation of
    endothelial cell function in vivo with positron emission
    tomography. Microcirc. Clin. Exp., 1, 244.
Syrota, A., Yudilevich, D.L. 1983. In vivo characterization of the
    site of amine uptake in the rat lung. J. Physiol. (London), 342,
    30-31P.

Syrota, A., Yudilevich, D.L. 1983. In vivo characterization of the
site of amine uptake in the rat lung. J. Physiol. (London), <u>342</u>,
30-31P.
West, J.B. 1967. The use of radioactive material in the study of lung
function. UK. A.E.A. Medical Monograph 1. Amersham, England.
Winchell, H.S., Baldwin, R.M., Lin, T.H. 1980. Development of I-123-
labeled amines for brain studies. J. Nucl. Med., <u>21</u>, 940-946.

Respondent to Lungs:

POSITRON EMISSION TOMOGRAPHY OF THE LUNGS

G.J. Huchon

Université René Descartes, Unité INSERM U 214, Hopital Laënnec
Paris, France

The lung is an organ in motion during respiration. The respiratory
system is made of blood and cells, like other organs, but with the
particularity that there is as much blood as lung cells inside the
chest. In addition, the lung contains a huge amount of gas. Therefore, the blood-free pulmonary cell content per unit chest volume is
quite low: about 10% lung cells as compared to 10% blood and 80% gas.
There is considerable heterogeneity within the lungs, and airways
receiving their blood supply from the bronchial circulation are opposed
to the alveoli which receive their blood from the pulmonary system. Both
conducting airways and alveoli are located close to inspired air.

PULMONARY FUNCTIONS

The functions of the lungs that might be explored by positron emission tomography (PET), as well as by other techniques, are gas exchange,
pulmonary defense mechanisms, and metabolic functions. Gas exchange is
the main purpose of the lungs, and this function has been studied extensively; no major progress is likely to be made in that field in the
future. Two or three decades ago, some experts began to study non-respi-
ratory functions of the lungs, i.e., defense mechanisms and metabolic
functions, both in normal and abnormal lungs. Furthermore, extensive
studies on the pathophysiology of pulmonary diseases were performed.

CONTRIBUTION OF PET

Only a few teams used PET to study both normal and abnormal lungs.
That contribution was recently reviewed, demonstrating that PET provides
regional information on the lungs (Hughes et al., 1985, 1986): regional
blood volume, its components (red cell volume, plasma volume) and
hematocrit (Brudin et al., 1986), regional lung density and extravascular lung water (Meyer et al., 1984; Rhodes et al., 1981), regional
ventilation (Brudin et al., 1985b; Clark et al., 1983), regional venti-

lation/perfusion ratios $-V_A/Q-$ (Brudin et al., 1985b; Lavender et al., 1984; Rhodes et al., 1983), regional pulmonary blood flow (Mintun et al., 1984), regional rate of glucose consumption (Rhodes et al., 1984), and pulmonary extraction of chlorpromazine and amines (Pascal et al., 1982; Syrota et al., 1981) have been determined in the normal lung. In smokers, regional extravascular density was increased by 10 - 20%, ventilation and V_A/Q were normal (Brudin et al., 1985b), and the increase in serotonin receptors was related to tobacco consumption (Charbonneau et al., 1986); regional ventilation and V_A/Q were much more variable in asthmatics than in normal subjects, and the overall ventilation and perfusion per unit volume were low (Valind et al., 1984a); in chronic obstructive lung disease, extravascular density was either decreased - with high regional ventilation and normal or low V_A/Q - or normal, or increased with rather low V_A/Q (Brudin et al., 1985a); fractional blood volume was reduced and extravascular density was increased in vascular pulmonary diseases (Wollmer et al., 1983); in hemodynamic pulmonary edema, extravascular lung density was markedly increased in the basal parts of the lungs, whereas only minor deviations from normal values were observed in apical regions (Schober and Meyer, 1986); in fibrosing pneumonitis and sarcoidosis, extravascular density was increased and blood volume was decreased (Wollmer et al., 1984); in sarcoidosis, the pulmonary metabolic rate for glucose and the lung uptake of imipramine and propranolol were increased (Pascal et al., 1981; Valind et al., 1984b); in squamous cell carcinoma, the rate of glycolysis was increased by a factor of 9.1 (Nolop et al., 1985); in pneumonia, erythromycin in pneumonic foci was at the same concentration per unit volume of tissue as in normal tissue - clearly above the minimum inhibitory concentration for sensitive micro-organisms (Wollmer et al., 1982).

ORIGINALITY OF PET STUDIES

Did PET so far provide new knowledge on normal and abnormal lungs? The answer is probably no. Rather, PET confirmed previous works in a fancy manner, with a few exceptions, e.g., the pulmonary erythomycin pharmacokinetic study in pneumonia and the serotonin uptake in smoker lungs. Why did PET not contribute more to the knowledge of the physiology and pathophysiology of the lungs as it did for some other organs? There are several possible explanations: the first one is that a lot has al-

ready been done; the second one is that pneumologists did not ask
pertinent questions; the third one is that PET was not able to answer new
questions. In fact, it probably is a combination of all: first, lung
experts confirmed previous studies performed with older technologies and
only then started to ask new questions. This is were we stand, but we do
not know if PET can answer these questions, considering the low lung cell
contents per unit chest volume.

WHAT CAN BE DONE?

There still are plenty of studies to be performed in asthma, interstitial lung diseases and pulmonary edema. This is not a limited listing,
but those are lung diseases without any good animal model; therefore,
human studies are of particular importance. Similarly, some pharmacological studies on receptors, mediators, and the pharmacokinetics of
drugs within the lungs are needed. Asthma is one of the best examples of
the potential contribution of PET to lung diseases: we really know very
little about the location, density, distribution, functional effects of
stimulation and drug interactions on, receptors in that disease. Similar
statements can be made on other diseases, such as interstitial lung
diseases and permeability pulmonary edema. But is PET able to answer
those questions, considering the large pulmonary gas contents? These
problems illustrate that PET per se cannot provide the explanation for
a disease. But if PET is applied for that purpose, together with other
techniques, it may significantly contribute to the knowledge on lung
diseases, particularly those lacking an appropriate animal model.

REFERENCES

Brudin, L.H., Rhodes, C.G., Valind, S.O., et al. 1985a. Topographic relationships between ventilation, ventilation to perfusion ratio and
extravascular density in patients with emphysema and chronic
bronchitis using positron emission tomography (PET). Am. Rev. Resp.
Dis., 131, A67.

Brudin, L.H., Rhodes, C.G., Valind, S.O., et al. 1985b. Topographic relationships between ventilation, ventilation to perfusion ratio,
alveolar volume and extravascular density in man using positron
emission tomography (PET). Am. Rev. Resp. Dis., 131, A313.

Brudin, L.H., Valind, S.O., Rhodes, C.G., et al. 1986. Regional lung
hematocrit in humans using positron emission tomography. J. Appl.
Physiol., 60, 1155-1163.

Charbonneau, P., Syrota, A., Boullais, C., et al. 1986. Serotonin receptors and lung phagocyte recruitement induced by cigarette
smoking detected in vivo by positron emission tomography (PET).
J. Nucl. Med., 27, A300.

Clark, J.C., Hughes, J.M.B., Rhodes, C.G., et al. 1983. Quantitative measurements of topographic distribution of alveolar ventilation in normal subject using positron emission tomography. J. Physiol., 345, 82.

Hughes, J.M.B., Brudin, L.H., Valind, S.O., et al. 1985. Positron emission tomography in the lung. J. Thorac. Imag., 1, 78-88.

Hughes, J.M.B., Rhodes, C.G., Brudin, L.H., et al. 1987. Contribution of the positron camera to studies of regional lung structure and function. In "Clinical Efficacy of PET" (Eds. W.-D. Heiss, G. Pawlik, K. Herholz, K. Wienhard). (Martinus Nijhoff Publ., Dordrecht). 1987 in press.

Lavender, J.P., Al-Nahhas, A.M. and Myers, M.J. 1984. Ventilation perfusion ratios of the normal supine lung using emission tomography. Br. J. Radiol., 57, 141-146.

Meyer, G.J., Schober, O., Rossaller, C., et al. 1984. Quantification of regional extravascular lung water in dogs with positron emission tomography using constant infusion of 15-O-labelled water. Eur. J. Nucl. Med., 9, 220-228.

Mintun, M.M., Ter-Pogossian, M.M. and Schuster, D.P. 1984. Measurement of pulmonary blood flow with positron emission tomography. Am. Rev. Resp. Dis., 129, A329.

Nolop, K.B., Brudin, L., Rhodes, C.G., et al. 1985. Glucose utilisation by pulmonary squamous cell carcinomas in man. Clin. Sci., 69.

Pascal, O., Syrota, A., Berger, G., et al. 1981. Lung uptake of 11-C-imipramine and 11-C-propanolol in patients with sarcoidosis evaluated by positron emission tomography. In "Sarcoidosis and other Granulomatous Disorders". (Eds. J. Chrétien, J. Marsac, J.C. Saltiel). (Pergamon Press, Paris). pp. 404-408.

Pascal, O., Syrota, A., Berger, G., et al. 1982. In vivo uptake of 11-C-labelled amines by human lung. Nucl. Med. and Biol., 3, 2558-2561.

Rhodes, C.G., Valind, S.O., Barnes, P.J., et al. 1983. Regional mismatching between alveolar ventilation and perfusion in normal subjects using positron emission tomography. J. Physiol., 345, 82.

Rhodes, C.G., Valind, S.O., Suzuki, T., et al. 1984. Regional measurement of pulmonary glucose utilization rate and distribution volume in man. Am. Rev. Resp. Dis., 129, A309.

Rhodes, C.G., Wollmer, P., Fazio, F., et al. 1981. Quantitative measurement of regional extravascular lung density using positron emission and transmission tomography. J. Comput. Assist. Tomogr., 5, 783-791.

Schober, O. and Meyer, G.J. 1987. Lung oedema. In "Clinical Efficacy of PET" (Eds. W.-D. Heiss, G. Pawlik, K. Herholz, K. Wienhard). (Martinus Nijhoff Publ., Dordrecht). 1987 in press.

Syrota, A., Pascal, O., Crouzel, M., et al. 1981. Pulmonary extraction of C-11 chlorpromazine, measured by residue detection in man. J. Nucl. Med., 22, 145-148.

Valind, S.O., Rhodes, C.G., Barnes, P.J., et al. 1984a. Effects of inhaled salbutamol on the regional distribution of alveolar ventilation in asthma, studied with positron emission tomography. Thorax., 39, 222.

Valind, S.O., Rhodes, C.G., Pantin, C., et al. 1984b. Measurements of pulmonary glucose metabolism in patients with cryptogenic fibrosing alveolitis and pulmonary sacroiditis. Am. Rev. Resp. Dis., 129, A53.

Wollmer, P., Rhodes, C.G., Allen, R.M., et al. 1983. Regional extravascular lung density and fractional pulmonary blood volume in
patients with chronic pulmonary venous hypertension. Clin. Phys.,
3, 214-256.
Wollmer, P., Rhodes, C.G. and Hughes, J.M.B. 1984. Regional extravascular density and fractional blood volume of the lung in interstitial disease. Thorax., 39, 286-293.
Wollmer, P., Rhodes, C.G., Pike, V.W., et al. 1982. Measurement of
pulmonary erythromycin concentration in patients with lobar
pneumonia by means of positron tomography. Lancet, 2, 1361-1364.

SUMMARY of Discussion on Lungs

J.M.B. Hughes, RPMS, Dept. of Medicine, London, United Kingdom

The chairman (Dr. Hughes, London) welcomed the invitation to lungs and heart to join the brain at this PET congress, but wondered why liver and kidney were not at the party. He stressed the difficulties in working with the lung. It was a moving organ, two-thirds of which was gas. Only 10 % of the lung volume was composed of non-vascular tissue. As is well known, regional structure and function in the lung is distorted by gravity. Nevertheless, the lung carries the whole cardiac output and has a larger vascular surface area than any other organ for the uptake of lipophilic substrates from blood. The pulmonary endothelial cell has been the subject of intense study in the last decade and its cell surface is studded with receptors for bicarbonate (carbonic anhydrase), angiotensin I, bradykinin, ADP, ATP, CIq and it has procoagulant, immunologic and phagocytic properties.

Dr. Hughes discribed studies of "correlation of lung structure and function in pulmonary disease" carried out at the M.R.C. Cyclotron Unit at Hammersmith Hospital. For studies of lung structure it was necessary to define three compartments - gas volume, blood volume and tissue (extravascular) volume. This was achieved by two scanning procedures: 1. a transmission scan (also used for attenuation corrections) from which the topography of density (D-L) was determined and 2. a vascular volume (Vb) scan (following the inhalation of 11-CO gas to give 11-CO-Hb). Tissue density (g.cm³) was derived by subtraction regionally of Vb from D-L and gas volume as 1-D-L (Rhodes et al., 1981). These structural parameters were crucial in the analysis of regional function. For example, by knowing the relationship between 11-C-Hb concentration (mCi.cm³) in a peripheral venous blood sample and in any region of the lung being scanned, the pulmonary vascular contribution to the intrathoracic concentration of any radiolabel could be computed once its concentration in a peripheral blood sample was known. By "vascular subtraction" the pulmonary tissue concentration of tracers could be derived. If the regional tissue concentration (mCi.cm³) was subsequently divided by the regional tissue density (g.cm³) absolute radiotracer concentrations per g. of lung tissue could be obtained. As an example of this approach, Dr. Hughes cited the study of Wollmer at al. (1982) in which 11-C-erythromycin was given to patients with unilateral pneumonia. After subtraction of intravascular 11-C-erythromycin, the concentration (mCi.cm³) was much greater on the pneumonic side but, per g. lung tissue (consolidated lung being much denser), the concentrations were approximately equal to that in normal lung. It was also possible to calculate that at normal i.v. concentrations, a bactericidal level of the antibiotic would have been reached in the pneumonic lung.

The Hammersmith group have also studied the relationship between local tissue volume and gas volume and functional parameters such as ventilation and perfusion. 18-FDG has been used to define areas of pulmonary inflammation (in sarcoidosis and cryptogenic fibrosing alveolitis); lung tumours of various cell types have also been studied.

Dr. Schober, Hannover, described the contribution of PET to the study of extravascular water accumulation. He reviewed previous studies using H-2-15-O and C-15-O-red cells and single pass indicator-dilution techniques. The amount of regional information which can be obtained in this way is rather limited. The Hannover approach was to measure the steady state distribution of H-2-15-O during constant i.v. infusion.

After subtraction of blood volume (11-CO-erythrocytes) extravascular
water volume (EVLW) is obtained. Validation of lung water measurements
was carried out in dogs using the cold-dye injection method (giving
total lung water) and X-ray CT (for regional total water). In chronic
heart failure, EVLW increased much more in dependent (i.e. dorsal, all
patients being supine) than non-dependent regions. There were opposing
effects on the distribution of blood volume (BV) and the ratio EVLW/BV
correlated highly with the NYHA grading of heart failure. Local water
content must double in some part of the lungs before oedema is diagnosed
radiographically but one must remember that the normal value for EVLW is
very low < 0.12 g.cm³. Future work probably lies in correlating a rise
in EVLW with other parameters of local function, i.e. protein
permeability (11-C-methyl albumin), V-A/Q ratios (13-N), endothelial
cell function (11-C-labelled amines) and inflammatory cell infiltration
(18-FDG).

Dr. Syrota, Orsay, described lung PET work carried out at Orsay.
Interest has centered on the pulmonary uptake of 11-C-labelled amines.
For example, the extraction of 11-C-propranolol by normal lungs was
almost complete (98 %) in a single pass following i.v. injection. For
11-C-imipramine the pulmonary tissue/blood concentration ratio was 150.
The uptake of this amine was saturable implying a receptor-mediated
process. Following extraction by the lung, the subsequent clearance was
found to be prolonged in sarcoidosis where there is granulomatous
chronic inflammation.

Ketanserin is a lipophilic antagonist of 5-HT receptor
(predominantly the S-2 receptor). 11-C-ketanserin given i.v. is.
concentrated in the myocardium more than in the lung with a ratio of
0.64 but in smokers the lung/heart ratio is reversed (1.4). Dr. Syrota,
Orsay, speculated that the excess macrophages which are found in
smokers' lungs might have been responsible. The release of amines such
as 123-I-HIPDM is prolonged in smokers compared to non-smokers. Clearly,
these intriguing findings need further investigation and follow-up.

Dr. Huchon, Paris, in his capacity as respondent, felt that studies
of traditional parameters (tissue volumes, densities, V-a/Q, etc.) were
unlikely to break new ground. He was intrigued by the application of PET
to lung pharmacokinetics (e.g. 11-C-erythromycin) and metabolism (18-FDG
in inflammatory and neoplastic conditions). He felt that efforts should
be made to define the distribution, density and functional state of
receptors and mediators in immunological and allergic lung diseases,
especially asthma.

In Dr. Syrota's, Orsay, studies of muscarinic (11-C-MQNB) and
adrenergic (11-C-CGP 12177) receptors in the myocardium, no significant
signal coming from the lung had been noted. Nevertheless, as chairman of
the lung session, I believe that the distribution and density of beta-
adrenergic (and other) receptors will be mapped out in man in vivo using
positron emission tomography over the next five years.

REFERENCES

Rhodes, C.G., Wollmer, P., Fazio, F. et al. 1981. Quantitative
    measurement of regional extravascular lung density using positron
    emission and transmission tomography. J. Comput. Assist. Tomogr.,
    5, 783-91.
Wollmer, P., Rhodes, C.G., Pike, V.W. et al. 1982. Measurement of
    pulmonary erythromycin concentration in patients with lobar
    pneumonia by means of positron tomography. Lancet, II, 1361-64.

SOFT TISSUE TUMORS

CIRCULATORY AND METABOLIC STUDIES IN EXTRACRANIAL MALIGNANT TUMORS

K. Schelstraete

University Hospital, Dept. of Radiotherapy and Nuclear Medicine,
Ghent, Belgium

In a way a malignant tumor may be considered as an autonomous
entity having its own circulatory and metabolic characteristics. Yet,
very little is known about the pathophysiological behavior of a
particular cancer in the individual patient. Most of the knowledge on
the functional properties of tumors is based on animal studies and on in
vitro experiments, and not necessarily transferable to an individual
human cancer.

Both radiotherapy and chemotherapy have been used for decades on a
more or less empirical basis. Knowledge of some of the functional parameters of human cancers may possibly indicate their degree of
malignancy, allow a more rational approach of their treatment modalities
and provide means to monitor their response to various therapeutic
manipulations.

Since positron emission tomography (PET) has the capacity to
provide information on local or regional physiological processes in the
living subject it is obvious that this technique should also be applied
to the field of human cancer (Beaney, 1984). Among the functional
aspects of tumors which have been addressed by PET we note:
- blood flow and oxygen consumption (Beaney et al., 1984; Brownell et
  al., 1983),
- amino acid uptake (Kubota et al., 1984, 1985; Reiman et al., 1982;
  Sordillo et al., 1982),
- glucose metabolism (Ahonen et al., 1985; Fukuda et al., 1982, 1984,
  Paul et al., 1986; Som et al., 1980; Yonekura et al., 1982),
- uptake of labeled chemotherapeutic agents (Lieberman et al., 1979).

Further potential applications are the exploration of cell kinetics
using DNA-precursors such as ^{11}C-thymidine (Shields et al., 1984) and
the search for hormone receptors (Kiesewetter et al., 1984; Terpstra et
al., 1985).

Perfusion and oxygen consumption are among the most important
physiological parameters of a neoplasm, since the effectiveness of low

LET ionizing radiation is highly dependent on the available oxygen. Furthermore, regional blood flow also governs the supply of chemo-therapeutic agents to various parts of the tumor.

The subject of regional perfusion and oxygen consumption as studied by means of the steady state inhalation technique using $C^{15}O_2$ and $^{15}O_2$, will be discussed in depth by Beaney in the next presentation. We would like to concentrate on our personal experience of PET techniques as applied to the problem of tumor perfusion and metabolism.

I. Studies with ^{13}N-ammonia

In both the myocardium and the brain ammonia labeled with ^{13}N has been shown to be removed from the blood by first pass extraction and to be metabolically trapped within the tissues, by incorporation into the cellular pool of amino acids, the distribution of $^{13}NH_3$ being proportional to the regional capillary blood flow (Phelps et al., 1976; Schelbert et al., 1979). These observations have prompted us to investigate if $^{13}NH_3$ could also be used for physiological imaging of human cancers.

Time activity curves over neoplastic lesions after i.v.injection of NH_3 (Schelstraete et al., 1985) are of the same patterns as the curves which have been obtained in the brain (Phelps et al., 1976), the myocardium (Schelbert et al., 1979), and other organs, such as the liver and the skeletal muscles (Lockwood et al., 1979). Maximum activity over the tumor is attained 1 to 3 min after injection. In some cases this peak is followed by a slow decrease of the activity, half-times of the clearance phase ranging from 28 to 112 min (Fig. 1a). In other lesions, after the initial rapid rise of activity, a plateau formation or a continuous slight increase of the tracer concentration is observed (Fig. 1b). Of course, no disappearance rate of the tracer can be calculated in these cases during observation time of 30 min.

These differences observed in the washout rate of the tracer or its metabolites might be related to the turnover rate of the intracellular pool in which the $^{13}NH_3$ was incorporated; for those cases in which a continuing slight rise of the curve was seen, the small increase in activity might have been caused by uptake of recirculating labeled metabolites released from other sites in the body.

In our small group of 12 patients no correlation has been established between the height and the shape of the NH_3 curve and a particular tumor type except for a curve with a distinct vascular peak in a highly vascularized metastasis of a hypernephroma (Schelstraete et al., 1985).

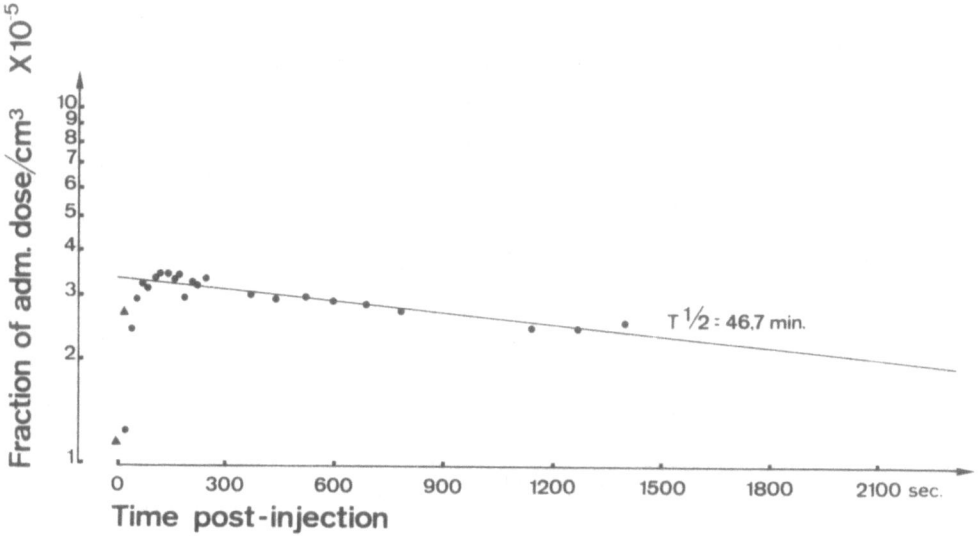

Fig. 1a: Time activity curve over a neck node metastasis of a squamous cell carcinoma after i.v.injection of 13NH3. Maximum activity is reached after 2 min; afterwards the tracer is cleared with a half-time of 46.7 min.

Tumor examination with $^{13}NH_3$ is a relatively simple procedure: imaging can be started 2 min after a single i.v.injection of the tracer; tracer concentration can be assumed to be relatively stable during the time of imaging.

In a case of huge fibrosarcoma involving the inner 2/3 of the left thigh a comparative study has been made with $^{13}NH_3$ i.v. and the

348

steady state inhalation technique using $C^{15}O_2$ and $^{15}O_2$. A very
good correlation was observed between the activity distribution as found
with $^{13}NH_3$ and with $C^{15}O_2$ and $^{15}O_2$ (Fig. 2), which seems to
indicate that ^{13}N-ammonia uptake is indeed related to both regional
blood flow and the general metabolic activity of the substrate.

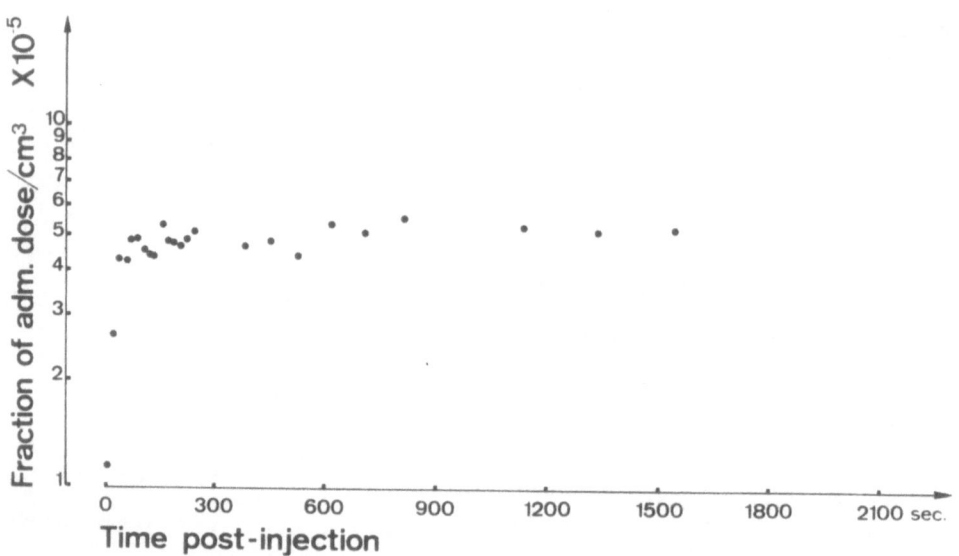

Fig. 1b: 13NH3 time activity curve observed over a retroperitoneal dysgerminoma. After the initial rapid rise no clearance
of the tracer is noted during the time of observation.

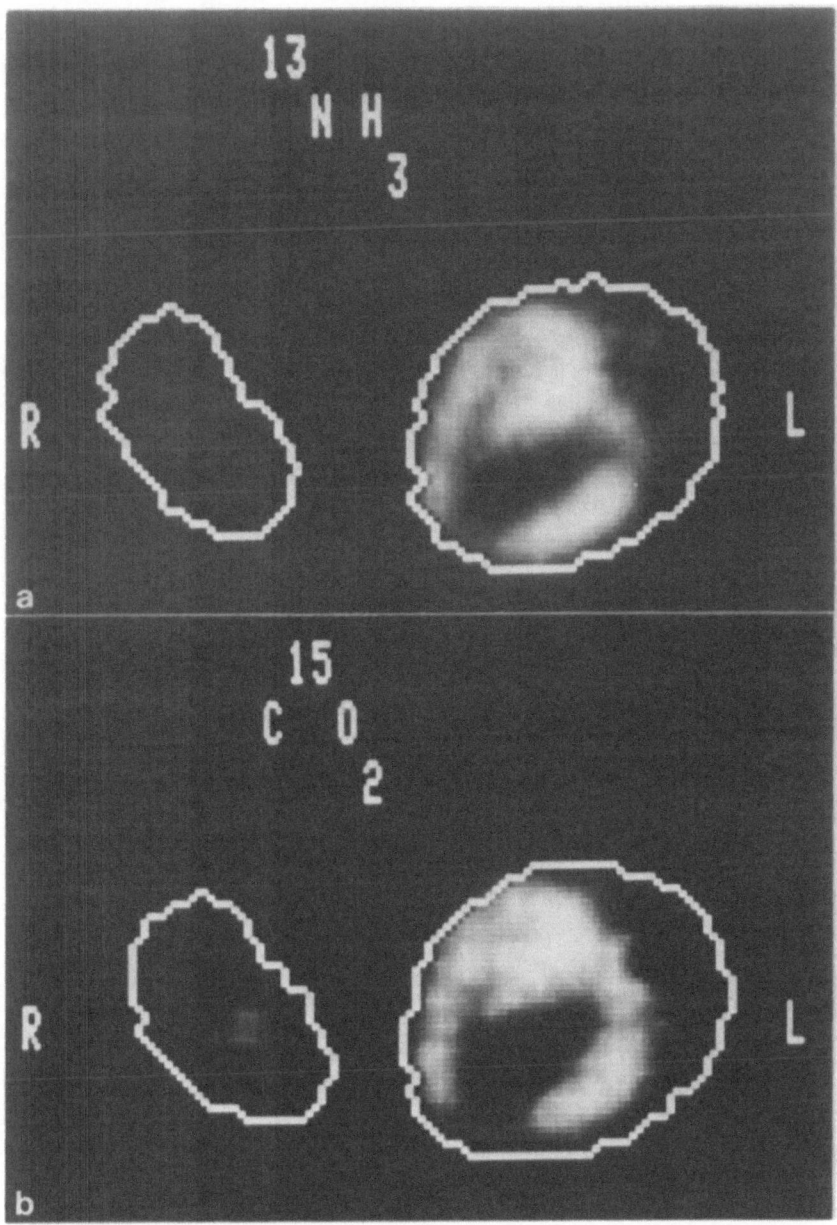

Fig. 2   (first part, continued on next page)

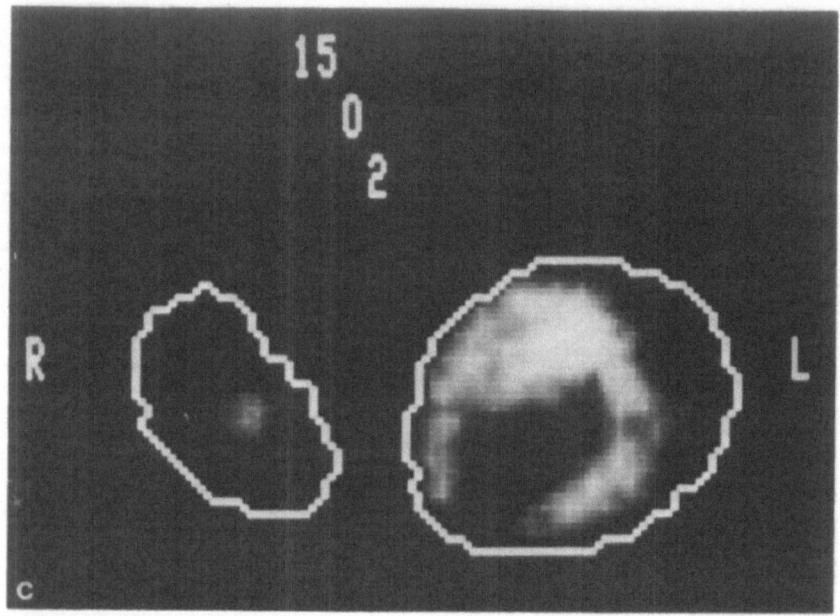

Fig. 2   Comparative PET-picture of a fibrosarcoma of the
inner 2/3 of the left thigh. The images obtained by the C1502 and
1502 steady state inhalation technique correspond very well to the
13N-ammonia scan. A high activity is found mainly at the periphery
of the tumor. A central hypoactive zone is observed.

Our experience with $^{13}NH_3$ in more than 100 cases of various
malignant lesions can be summarized as follows (Schelstraete et al.,
1982):

1. A substantial accumulation of $^{13}NH_3$ - up to 5 times the amount
found in comparable normal tissues - was noted in most tumors, including
breast cancers and their metastases, malignant lymphomas, lung cancers
and their metastases, malignant neck nodes secondary to head and neck
cancers, melanomas, ovarian carcinomas. The highest uptake was noted in
soft tissue sarcomas and osteosarcomas. A remarkable accumulation of
^{13}N-ammonia has also been described in hepatoma (Hayashi et al.,
1985).

2. An inhomogeneous tracer distribution was often observed. Several
lesions denoted a central cold area (probably corresponding to a
vascular or necrotic core).

351

3. After a successful radio- or chemotherapeutic treatment $^{13}NH_3$ uptake could be seen to decrease progressively with tumor regression. However, during a radiotherapeutic course, a transient increase of ammonia uptake per cm³ of tissue might be observed. On the contrary, when the treatment had not been successful, $^{13}NH_3$ uptake was found to persist. This can be illustrated by the following example (Fig. 3):

This woman suffered from a bulky non-Hodgkin lymphoma in the right neck. PET scan using 13NH3 showed a high but inhomogeneous tracer uptake by the tumor. Its more voluminous, anterior, part consisted of an annular zone of actively concentrating tissue surrounding a central area with lower activity, perhaps representing a hypovascular core. The posterior part showed a homogeneous high activity. This patient was reinvestigated after several courses of chemotherapy followed by local irradiation. The posterior part which previously concentrated 13NH3 most actively had virtually disappeared, whereas a substantial tracer uptake persisted in the larger anterior part which previously had a hypoactive core. This example seems to illustrate that well perfused tumors, or parts thereof, tend to respond better to radio- and/or chemotherapy than less well perfused ones.

4. No extra uptake of ^{13}N-ammonia has been observed in the few benign tumors we have studied.

In a patient with a well circumscribed mass on the forearm, a high concentration of 13NH3 was found in the tumor which let us suspect a malignant neoplasm. The resected specimen however was described as a benign myxoma. Four months later the patient developed a local recurrence of the tumor which this time was found to be malignant fibrous histiocytoma. In this particular case, one could at least have suspected the malignant nature of the lesion in spite of the benign histological characteristics.

5. On the other hand, exceptionally a malignant neoplasm was observed which did not accumulate $^{13}NH_3$ in spite of obvious growth and an apparently good vascularization. This observation confirms that $^{13}NH_3$ uptake in tumors must be regarded as being governed by a complex interaction of capillary blood flow and the extraction efficiency of the neoplastic cells. Therefore, using the single tracer $^{13}NH_3$, it is not possible to distinguish between respective roles of either component.

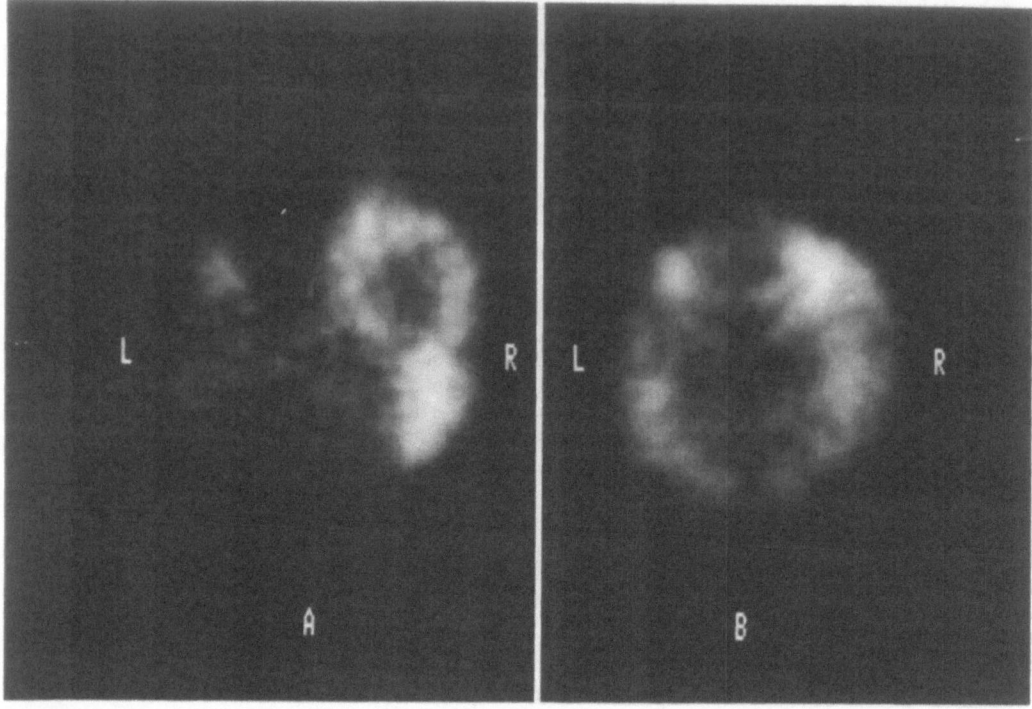

Fig. 3: Cross section through the neck after i.v.injection of
13N-ammonia in a patient with a right-sided non-Hodgkin lymphoma.
A. Before treatment: the bulky anterior part of the tumor consists
   of an annular zone with high tracer uptake, surrounding a
   central "cold" area, probably representing the hypovascular
   core of the tumor. More posterior on the right a less
   voluminous lymph node is seen with a very intense and
   homogeneous 13NH3 uptake.
B. After chemotherapy and local irradiation: the posterior mass
   which concentrated 13NH3 most actively has nearly disappeared,
   whereas a substantial tracer uptake persists in the anterior
   part which previously had a hypoactive core.

II. Studies with ^{11}C-aminocyclopentane carboxylic acid (ACPC)

In an attempt to unravel the complex mechanism of ^{13}NH$_3$
accumulation in malignant tumors, a comparative study was made of the
uptake of ^{13}-ammonia and ^{11}C-ACPC in 28 cases of various neoplasms
(De Vis et al., in press; Schelstraete et al., 1986). ACPC or cycloleucine is a non-natural amino acid which after labeling with ^{11}C has
been introduced as a tumor marker by Hübner et al. (1977, 1981). On
theoretical grounds, the uptake mechanism of ACPC could be expected to
be different from NH$_3$. Although maximum tissue uptake of ACPC is
reached early (by 5 min), its circulating blood level remains quite
stable (at about 20 % of the dose) during the first 20 min after
i.v.injection (Hübner et al., 1977). Therefore, as opposed to NH$_3$,
regional blood flow is not likely to be a decisive factor in tissue
accumulation of this molecule.

Measurements were started 5 min after ^{11}C-ACPC injection. In
general, distribution of ^{13}NH$_3$ and ^{11}C-ACPC in a given tumor was
found to be fairly similar. However, the absolute ACPC concentration in
a given case was often higher as compared to ^{13}NH$_3$ (Table 1).

TABLE 1 Some typical concentrations of ^{11}C-ACPC and ^{13}NH$_3$ in
tumors (expressed in fraction of injected dose/cm^3 x 10^{-5})

	ACPC	NH$_3$	Ratio ACPC/NH$_3$
Osteosarcoma	4.2	2.0	2.1
Synoviosarcoma	3.0	2.0	1.5
Breast cancer	3.5	2.4	1.4
Retrobulb.metast.	4.7	2.9	1.6

Contribution of the intravascular activity has been calculated to be
relatively small (De Vis et al., in press). On the other hand ACPC
uptake was lower in several normal organs, such as the brain, the
moycardium and the liver and kidney (Table 2), whereas the blood

concentration remained much higher. Since ACPC levels in some well perfused organs such as the brain and myocardium did not exceed blood concentration, and since the uptake of ACPC in tumors ranged from levels below up to levels above the blood concentration, tumor cells seemed to be able to selectively control its entrance. As a rule, ^{11}C-ACPC appears superior to [13]NH$_3$ as a tumor tracer because of both its higher accumulation in many neoplastic lesions and its lower uptake in several non neoplastic tissues. Its only disadvantage is its slower blood clearance, which renders it unfit to the exploration of lesions which are adjacent to large blood pools, e.g., the mediastinum. For these sites, [13]NH$_3$ with its rapid blood clearance remains a good alternative.

TABLE 2 Some typical concentrations of ^{11}C-ACPC and [13]NH$_3$ in normal organs (expressed in fraction of injected dose/cm³ x 10^{-5})

	ACPC	NH$_3$	Ratio ACPC/NH$_3$
Cerebral cortex	0.7	2.1	0.3
Myocardium	3.1	5.2	0.6
Liver	4.5	7.0	0.6
Kidney	4.5	11.0	0.4
Muscle	1.1	0.8	1.4
Blood	0.1	3.0	30

In one of our patients ACPC has helped to solve a difficult diagnostic problem.

This patient had been irradiated for a nasopharyngeal carcinoma. Five years later he presented with symptoms which could be due to postradiation necrosis and infection or to tumor recurrence or to a mixture of both possibilities. Several investigations including CT scan had been inconclusive. A 67Gallium-scan was negative, but even if 67Ga-uptake had been present, infection could have been responsible for the positive result. A PET-scan using 11C-ACPC clearly visualized a hot spot at the right side of the nasopharynx (Fig. 4). The definite uptake of ACPC in the suspected area led us to suspect a tumor recurrence, which was confirmed later on.

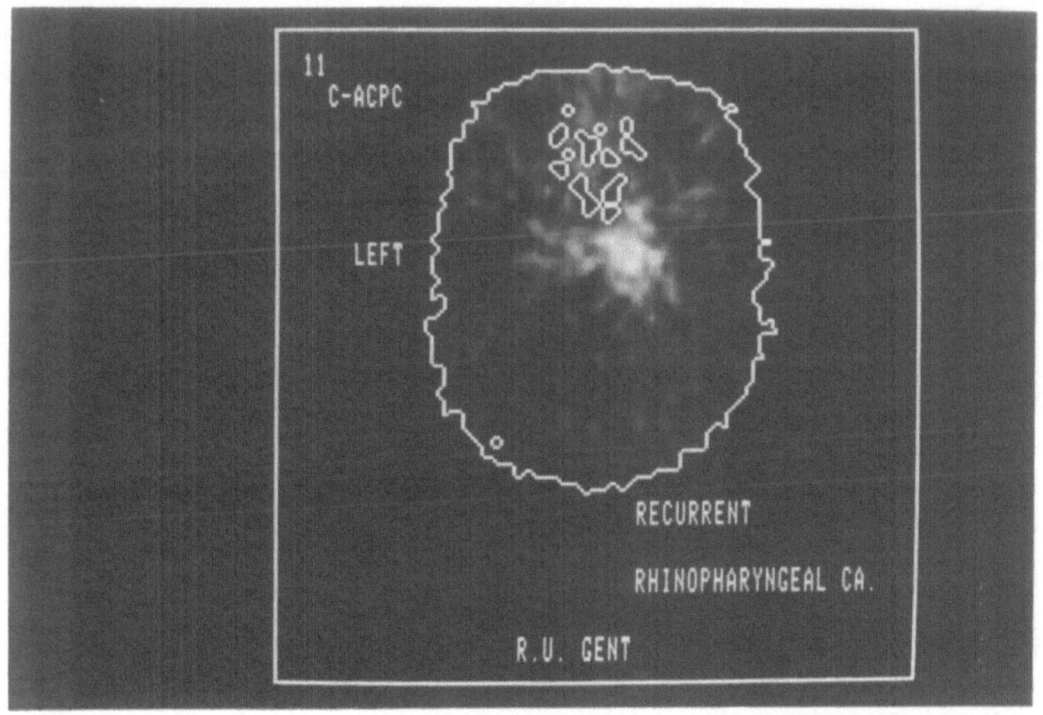

Fig. 4: Recurrence of a nasopharyngeal carcinoma,
demonstrated by PET scan using 11C-ACPC.

In one case of an osteosarcoma of the fibula ^{11}C-ACPC has been
used to follow the responsiveness of the tumor to a preoperative chemo-
therapeutic treatment.

Before treatment, a high ACPC uptake in the tumor was observed (0.000041 of the injected dose per cm³ of tissue). Two and a half months later, after a chemotherapy course, 11C-ACPC uptake in the tumor was found to be even higher than before treatment (0.0000567) (Fig. 5). This was in keeping with the histopathological findings on the resected specimen, which still contained a large number of viable sarcoma cells.

These measurements were performed following the protocol which was elaborated at Memorial Sloan-Kettering Cancer Center to correlate the uptake of an aminoacid (^{13}N-glutamate) with histological changes in tumor tissue in patients undergoing adjuvant preoperative chemotherapy for osteogenic sarcoma (Reiman et al., 1981). To monitor the responsiveness of an osteosarcoma by means of conventional methods is difficult because X-rays and bone scans mainly visualize the calcified part of the tumor. In contrast, uptake of glutamate is assumed to be directly related to the metabolic status of the sarcoma cells. It has been demonstrated by the MSKCC study that regions showing a decrease in ^{13}N uptake of more than 30 % after chemotherapy frequently corresponded with areas of highly necrotic tumor, whereas regions that showed increasing uptake were associated with high residual cell viability at the time of operation. Therefore, the uptake of glutamate appears to be a useful indicator of tumor cell destruction following chemotherapy.

In short term experiments single doses of both radiotherapy and chemotherapy have been shown to reduce the uptake of ^{13}N-glutamate by transplanted tumors, whereas blood flow (as measured by means of ^{11}C-butanol) remained unchanged (Knapp, 1986; Knapp et al., 1986). Thus a decrease in ^{13}N-glutamate uptake appears to be a sensitive indicator of cellular damage, independently of blood flow (Knapp, 1986; Knapp et al., 1986).

In general the primary aim of PET in oncology is not the detection of unknown tumor localizations. Using appropriate tracers PET should be applied to established or suspected cancer sites in order to obtain evidence of the degree of tumor viability, to gather information on the lesion's circulatory and metabolic properties, which might be relevant to an optimal adaptation of treatment modalities, and to monitor the response to various therapeutic interventions by functional criteria.

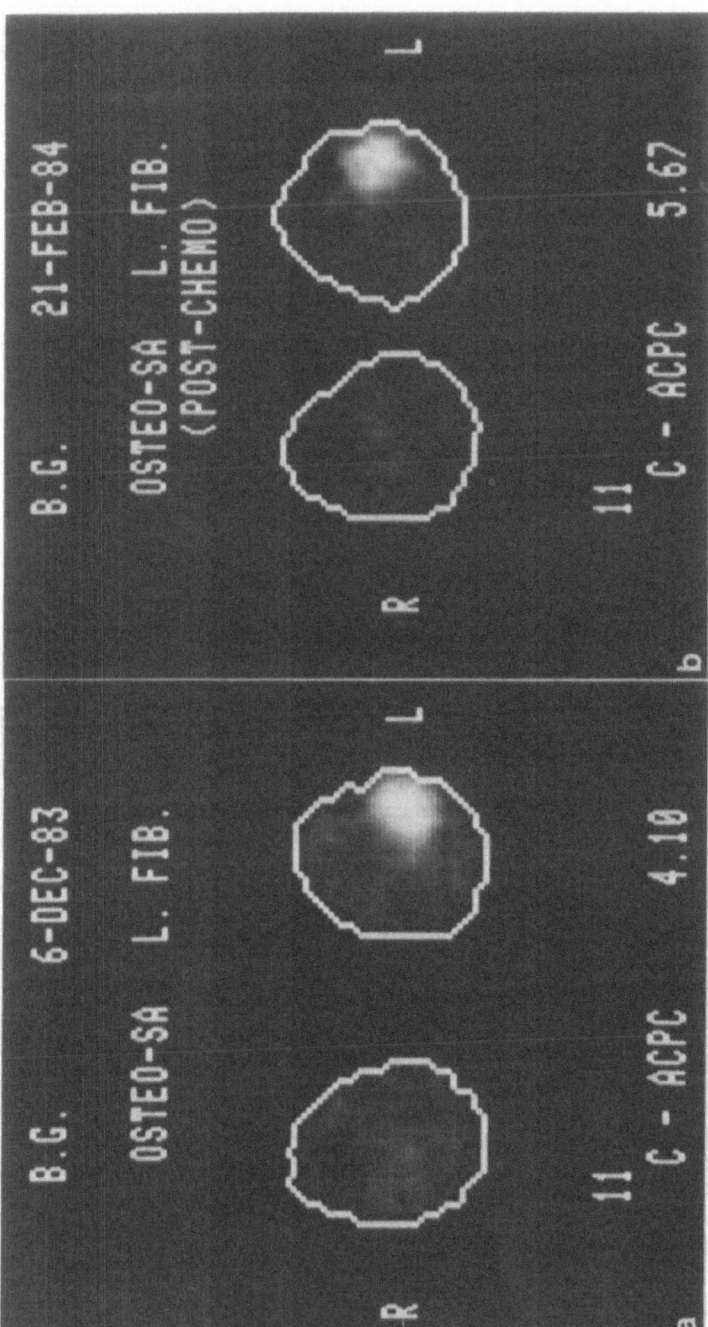

Fig. 5: PET section through the legs in a patient with an osteosarcoma of the left fibula.
a. High uptake of 11C-ACPC in the tumor before treatment (0.000041 fraction of injected dose/cm³).
b. After a 1 1/2 months chemotherapy course tracer uptake had even increased (0.0000567) fraction
of injected dose/cm³). The resected specimen still contained a large number of viable
sarcoma cells.

358

REFERENCES

Ahonen, A., Paul, R., Aho, A. et al. 1985. Differential diagnosis of the bone tumors using fluorodeoxyglucose and three phase 99mTc-DPD scanning. Eur. J. Nucl. Med., 11, A 20.

Beaney, RP 1984. Positron emission tomography in the study of human tumors. Sem. Nucl. Med., 14, 324-341.

Beaney, RP, Lammertsma, A.A., Jones, T. et al. 1984. Positron emission tomography for in vivo measurements of regional blood flow, oxygen utilisation, and blood volume in patients with breast carcinoma. Lancet, I, 131-134.

Brownell, G.L., Kairento, A.L., Swartz, M.R. et al. 1983. Positron emission tomography in study of soft tissue tumors. J. Nucl. Med., 24, P119.

De Vis, K., Schelstraete, K., Deman, J. et al. In press. Clinical comparison of 11C-ACPC (aminocyclopentane carboxylic acid) and 13N-ammonia as tumor tracers. Acta Radiol. Oncol.

Fukuda, H., Matsuzawa, T., Abe, Y. et al. 1982. Experimental study for cancer diagnosis with positron-labeled fluorinated glucose analogs: (18F)-2-fluoro-2-deoxy-D-mannose: a new tracer for cancer detection. Eur. J. Nucl. Med., 7, 294-297.

Fukuda, H., Matsuzawa, T., Ito, M. et al. 1984. Experimental and clinical study of cancer diagnosis with (18F)FDG using positron emission tomography. J. Nucl. Med., 25, P50.

Hayashi, N., Tamaki, N., Yonekura, Y. et al. 1985. Imaging of the hepatocellular carcinoma using dynamic positron emission tomography with nitrogen-13 ammonia. J. Nucl. Med., 26, 254-257.

Hübner, K.F., Andrews, G.A., Washburn, L. et al. 1977. Tumor location with 1-aminocyclopentane (11C) carboxylic acid: preliminary clinical trials with single-photon detection. J. Nucl. Med., 18, 1215-1221.

Hübner, K.F., Krauss, S., Washburn, L.C. et al. 1981. Tumor detection with 1-aminocyclopentane and 1-aminocyclobutane C11-carboxylic acid using positron emission computerized tomography. Clin. Nucl. Med., 6, 249-252.

Kiesewetter, D., Kilbourn, M.R., Landvatter, S.W. et al. 1984. Preparation of four fluorine-18-labeled estrogens and their selective uptakes in target tissues in immature rats. J. Nucl. Med., 25, 1212-1221.

Knapp, W.H. 1986. Production and use of positron-emitting test substances for tumor diagnosis. In "Nuclear Medicine in Clinical Oncology." (Ed. C. Winkler). (Springer, Berlin, Heidelberg, New York, Tokyo). pp. 247-249.

Knapp, W.H., Helus, F., Layer, K. et al. 1986. Nitrogen-13 glutamate uptake and perfusion in Walker 256 carcinosarcoma before and after single-dose irradiation. J. Nucl. Med., 27, 1604-1610.

Kubota, K., Yamada, K., Fukuka, H. et al. 1984. Tumor detection with carbon-11-labeled amino acids. Eur. J. Nucl. Med., 9, 136-140.

Kubota, K., Matsuzawa, T., Ito, M. et al. 1985. Lung tumor imaging by positron emission tomography using C11-L-methionine. J. Nucl. Med., 26, 37-42.

Lieberman, L.M., Wessels, B., Gatley, S.J. et al. 1979. Fluorine-18-5-fluorouracil imaging in humans. J. Nucl. Med., 20, 645.

Lockwood, A.H., McDonald, J.M., Reiman, R.E. et al. 1979. The dynamics of ammonia metabolism in man. J. Clin. Invest., 63, 449-460.

Paul, R., Roeda, R., Johansson, A. et al. 1986. Scintigraphy with (18F)-2-deoxy-D-glucose of cancer patients. Nucl. Med. Biol., 13, 7-12.

Phelps, M.E., Hoffman, E.J., Coleman, R.E. 1976. Tomographic images of blood pool and perfusion in brain and heart. J. Nucl. Med., 17, 603-612.

Reiman, R.E., Huvos, A.G., Benua, R.S. et al. 1981. Quotient imaging with N13-L-glutamate in osteogenic sarcoma. Correlation with tumor viability. Cancer, 48, 1976-1981.

Reiman, R.E., Rosen, G., Gelbard, A.S. et al. 1982. Imaging of primary ewing sarcoma with 13N-L-glutamate. Radiology, 142, 495-500.

Schelbert, H.R., Phelps, M.E., Hoffman, E.J. et al. 1979. Regional myocardial perfusion assessed with N-13 labeled ammonia and positron emission computerized axial tomography. Am. J. Cardiol., 43, 209-218.

Schelstraete, K., Simons, M. Deman, J. et al. 1982. Uptake of 13N-ammonia by human tumors as studied by positron emission tomography. Brit. J. Radiol., 55, 797-804.

Schelstraete, K., Deman, J., Vermeulen, F.L. et al. 1985. Kinetics of 13N-ammonia incorporation in human tumors. Nucl. Med. Comm., 6, 461-470.

Schelstraete, K., De Vis, K., Vermeulen, F.L. et al. 1986. Uptake of 11C-aminocyclopentane carboxylic acid (ACPC) and 13N-ammonia in malignant tumors. A comparative clinical study. In "Nuclear Medicine in Clinical Oncology." (Ed. C. Winkler). (Springer, Berlin, Heidelberg, New York, Tokyo). pp. 250-253.

Shields, A.F., Larson, S.M., Grunbaum, Z. et al. 1984. Short term thymidine uptake in normal and neoplastic tissues: Studies for PET. J. Nucl. Med., 25, 759-764.

Som, P., Atkins, H.L., Bandoypadhyay, D. et al. 1980. A fluorinated glucose analog, 2-fluoro-2-deoxy-D-glucose (F18): nontoxic tracer for rapid tumor detection. J. Nucl. Med., 21, 670-675.

Sordillo, P., Reiman, R.E., Gelbard, A.S. et al. 1982. Scanning with L-(13N)-glutamate. Assessment of the response to chemotherapy of a patient with embryonal rhabdomyosarcoma. Am. J. Clin. Oncol. (CCT), 5, 285-289.

Terpstra, J.W., Vaalburg, A.M.J., Paans, T. et al. 1985. A new production method for Bromine-75 labelled estrogens for positron emission tomography based receptor research. Eur. J. Nucl. Med., 11, A21.

Yonekura, Y., Benua, R.S., Brill, A.B. et al. 1982. Increased accumulation of 2-deoxy-2-(18F) fluoro-D-glucose in liver metastases from colon carcinoma. J. Nucl. Med., 23, 1133-1137.

SOME BIOLOGICAL ASPECTS OF SOFT TISSUE TUMORS
AS STUDIED BY PET

R.P. Beaney

Queen Elizabeth Hospital, Dept. of Radiotherapy,
Birmingham, U.K.

Cancer is one of the major clinical problems we face today; it is the second biggest killer after ischemic heart disease affecting 1 in 5 of us sometime in our life. Anyone working outside the field of positron emission tomography may be forgiven for wondering why more PET work has not been done on cancer. This outsider may be slightly puzzled when he discovers that what little work has been done has dealt with brain tumors. Brain tumors after all account for no more that 9 % of all human tumors. Unfortunately, very little has been done on non-cerebral tumors. The many reasons for this will not be discussed here but include:

a. Many scanners can only accomodate the head.

b. Many scanners are in neurological institutes.

c. The greatest experience has been acquired in brain studies.

d. The tracer kinetic models used are usually derived for brain tissue.

Despite these problems several groups have studied non-cerebral tumors. At the Hammersmith Hospital with its rather limited number of tracers ($^{15}O_2$, $C^{15}O_2$, ^{11}CO and to a lesser extent ^{18}FDG), only basic studies were possible. In some respects this was fortunate because blood flow, the uptake of oxygen and the presence or absence of tumor hypoxia are of immense interest to oncologists.

Other groups have concentrated on metabolic studies using labeled amino acids and hexoses.

It is important to remember that most of the models used are based on normal tissue - usually the brain. One of the major differences between normal and neoplastic tissue is the microvasculature. The microvasculature of tumors in contrast with that of normal tissues demonstrates a wide range of variables that may profoundly affect the manner in which tumor cells respond to insult. Tumor capillaries may be longer, wider, more permeable and have larger intercapillary distances. Blind loops, arteriovenous shunts, and capillary-like vessels lined by tumor cells all contribute to the complex relationship between nutritionally useful blood flow and vascularity.

There is now considerable experimental evidence to support the view that there is intensive glycolysis under both aerobic and anaerobic conditions in tumors. Cancer cells are known to take up sugars and amino acids to a greater extent than normal cells whether this is related to changes in enzyme activity that favor increased metabolism or related to membrane changes that favor increased transport is not fully understood. Indeed there is evidence to suggest that both take place.

With these facts in mind we proceeded to examine several types of tumors which included lymphomas, breast cancer and some rarer cancers and sarcomas.

The blood volume corrected, oxygen-15 steady state inhalation technique was used for the blood flow and oxygen utilization studies. Data was obtained using an ECAT II positron emission tomographic scanner. The spatial resolution of the reconstructed images was 17 mm x 17 mm (FWHM) in the transaxial plane, with a slice thickness of 17 mm.

RESULTS AND DISCUSSION
Blood flow

Of all the tumors studied lymphomas were consistently found to have the highest values for blood flow. Anaplastic tumors appeared to have a slightly higher blood flow than well differentiated ones but the difference was not statistically significant. Fig. 1 compares blood flow in lymphomas with that of carcinomas. Similar findings have been obtained using the xenon washout technique.

It is interesting to postulate a relationship between blood flow and the radio-responsiveness of a tumor. The relationship may be an indirect one with the better perfused tumors having a higher growth fraction.

Blood flow and oxygen consumption

Regional blood flow, oxygen extraction fraction and oxygen utilization were measured in nine patients with carcinoma of the breast. The results are shown in Fig. 2. Regional blood flow was consistently higher in non-necrotic tumor than in normal breast tissue. Oxygen utilization by breast tumors was slightly higher than in normal post-menopausal breast tissue.

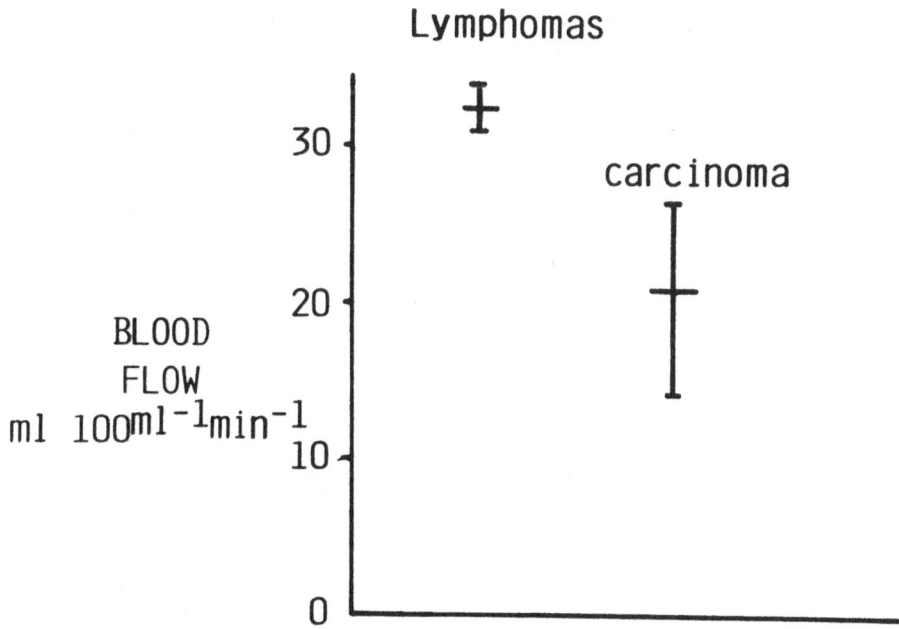

Fig. 1 Comparison of regional blood flow in lymphomas and
   carcinomas.

These findings suggested that there was, at least on a macroscopic
level, no supply-limited impairment of respiration in human breast
cancer (Beaney et al., 1984). Similar findings were obtained for all the
soft tissue tumors found. The main observations were:

1. Blood flow was variable, not only between different tumors but also
   within very large tumors themselves. Values were found ranging from
   virtually zero (in the necrotic center of a large tumor) to values
   greatly in excess of the normal tissue counterpart.

2. The OEF was low, in every tumor studied. This suggested that the
   cells within the tumor capable of influencing the extraction of
   oxygen were overperfused with respect to their oxygen requirements.
   The mean value for all the tumors studied was 0.21 (normal tissue
   0.45).

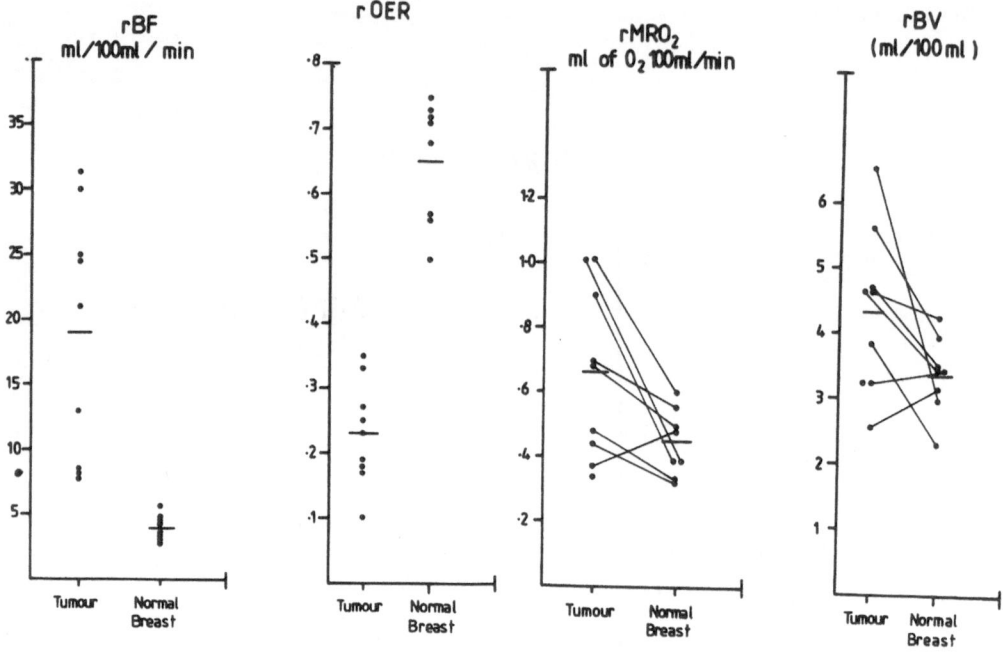

Fig. 2 Regional blood flow, oxygen extraction fraction, oxygen utilization and blood volume in 9 breast tumors and the normal contralateral breast.

3. There was no correlation between rBF and rBV. Tumors are known to contain abnormal blood vessels that may not be nutritionally useful, e.g., arteriovenous shunts. Our PET technique is able to measure blood flow in that part of the microcirculation that is capable of water exchange (and presumably nutrient exchange), and also regional blood volume. It is important to remember that our blood volume measurements cannot differentiate between a few large vessels and many small vessels. Nevertheless, unlike normal tissue, tumors showed no correlation between regional blood flow and regional blood volume.

Of all these findings it was the universally low rOEF in tumors that aroused most interest.

At the outset of this study we hoped a contribution would be made to our understanding of tumor hypoxia. It is commonly accepted that most if not all tumors have appreciable regions that are hypoxic. The reason for this is that the doubling time or growth rate of the tumor cells is much faster than that of the endothelium. This means the tumor cells outgrow their blood supply, the intercapillary distance increases and the tumor tissue develops hypoxic and ultimately anoxic regions.

Now positron emission tomography studies on patients during the early phase after non-hemorrhagic infarction revealed oxygen extraction fractions of around 90 % (Wise et al., 1983). In other words ischemic brain was extracting virtually all the available oxygen from the capillaries. Also in the dog brain reduction of cerebral blood flow was accompanied by a corresponding rise in the fraction of oxygen extracted from the arterial blood in a bid to maintain normal oxidative metabolism.

Returning to tumors; if these tissues had sizable regions of hypoxia due to ischemia, then we would expect to find an elevated rOEF. This has never been found.

The reason for this anomalous finding may lie in the microvasculature. Oxygen is metabolized as it diffuses through tissue. There is a finite distance X_0 at which the partial pressue of O_2 (PO_2) will have fallen to zero. Any cells beyond this region are hypoxic or indeed anoxic. The location of this point, and by that the depth to which O_2 can penetrate into the tissues, depends on the diffusion coefficient K, on the rate of O_2 consumption, $MO_2(C)$, and on the O_2 head of pressure in the capillary, PbO_2, such that

$$X_0 = \sqrt{\frac{2K \cdot PbO_2}{MO_2(C)}}$$

It is evident from this that towards the venous end of the capillary anoxia is reached after a shorter distance. This simple model can be taken further to include radial diffusion into the tissue (Krogh's cylinder), but the principle remains the same and hypoxia is more likely to occur towards the venous end of the capillary.

Normal tissues, e.g., muscle, have remarkable ways of compensating for this; the number of capillaries coursing alongside the muscle fibers increases as we move from the arteriolar to the venular end. Consequently, the capillary density increases as the PO_2 falls, and the distance R into the tissues that must be furnished with O_2 from one capillary decreases (Weibel, 1984).

In tumors, this normal microvasculature is absent, the hypoxic cells lying at the very limit of the diffusion range for oxygen cannot influence the further extraction of oxygen from the capillary. This finding then may account for the OER not being greater than normal. Why then is it usually lower. In brain tumors we think it is because they turn to the anaerobic metabolism of glucose for their energy requirements. In non-necrotic breast tumor they appear to be overperfused for their oxygen requirements despite O_2 consumption being comparable to that of normal breast tissue.

Glucose consumption

Several workers have used glucose or glucose analogues in non-cerebral tumors. Suzuki and Iio (1982) used ^{11}C-glucose for imaging a variety of intrathoracic malignancies. These workers administered orally a photosynthetically produced mixture of ^{11}C-glucose and ^{11}C-fructose, and successfully demonstrated the presence of both lymphomas and bronchogenic cancers. Their qualitative studies were performed with the aid of a modified gamma camera.

Other workers have used (^{18}F)FDG to study tumors of the liver, breast and lung. Nolop et al. (subm.f.publ.) using (^{18}F)FDG studied a group of patients with bronchogenic carcinoma and found that the rate of uptake was significantly higher in tumor tissue compared with normal lung. The results are summarized in Table 1.

TABLE 1 Tumor/normal tissue ratio of 18FDG uptake in a variety of organs.

	Tumor normal tissue ratio of 18FDG
Lung	6.6
Brain	1.04
Colonic metastases in liver	4.0

They also clearly demonstrated hypometabolic regions in the necrotic centers of large tumors, but were unable to demonstrate any correlation between ^{18}FDG uptake and histological type or histological grade of tumor. Increased uptake was noted in involved lymph nodes.

In one breast tumor patient where both $^{15}O_2$ and ^{18}FDG uptake were measured, there was a disproportionate increase in ^{18}FDG uptake in the tumor.

Yonekura et al. (1982) demonstrated increased ^{18}FDG uptake in hepatic metastases from colonic tumors.

Amino acid uptake

Several amino acids, both natural and unnatural, have been labeled with positron emitting radionuclides. These studies remain qualitative or at best semi-quantitative. Animal studies have shown that whereas L-isomers of amino acids have a high affinity for normal pancreas the D-forms localize selectively in tumor tissue. Syrota et al. (1982) using ^{11}C-methionine found decreased pancreatic uptake in chronic pancreatitis and pancreatic carcinoma. Other workers found that pancreatic tumors took up D-L-tryptophan and ^{11}C-ACPC. Kubota et al. (1984) performed a comparative study of 10 ^{11}C-labeled amino acids to find the most useful for cancer detection. They suggested on the basis of their animal studies that ^{11}C-L-methionine and ^{11}C-DL-methyl-ACPC might be the most useful amino acid for the diagnosis of cancer in man. Kubota et al. (1985) used ^{11}C-L-methionine to delineate a bronchogenic carcinoma and found increased uptake in the tumor and involved lymph nodes.

Laughlin et al. (1980) used nitrogen-13 labeled L-glutamate for visualizing a number of human tumors including osteogenic sarcoma, rhabdomyosarcoma, Ewing's sarcoma, malignant fibrous histiocytoma and neuroectodermal tumors. They monitored patients with bone tumors before, during, and after chemotherapy and found a close correlation with other clinical parameters, e.g., serum alkaline phosphatase and ^{99m}Tc-bone scans.

COMMENTS

1. What new information on human disease and its treatment has been provided or is emerging through PET studies?

The importance of the relatively few studies done on soft tissue tumors is to underline or emphasize the fact that the in vitro and animal tumor work relating to glucose metabolism and amino acid metabolism appears to be true. The blood flow studies have emphasized that not all tumors have relatively poor blood supply. The larger ones unquestionably have reduced perfusion in the center.

PET has failed to prove or disprove the presence of hypoxic regions in tumors.

2. What is the role of PET as a clinical diagnostic tool?

It is difficult to place PET in the role of a diagnostic tool. Logistically, so few people will ever have the opportunity to be scanned that it is unlikely (given the present economic climate) that PET will ever seriously challenge the diagnostic role of CT and MRI. A simple chest X-ray and needle biopsy will give more useful information about a lung cancer than a PET scan will. Clinical examination, needle biopsy and routine radiological examination will provide enough information on a breast tumor to satisfy most clinicians.

3. Are the clinical research questions being asked truly relevant?

With respect to the regional blood flow and oxygen uptake studies the answer must be yes. Millions of dollars are spent every year trying to overcome hypoxia in tumors (i.e., high LET radiation, hypoxic cell sensitizers and in the past hyperbaric oxygen). It is just unfortunate that our technique cannot allow us to say there are not hypoxic cells in tumors. All the above maneuvers have been particularly unsuccessful clinically.

When we turn to metabolic studies the answer is not quite so clear. Increased glycolysis in tumors was once a burning issue, today however interest in it clinically can be described as no more than a tiny flicker. If the successful grading of tumors were possible then this might play a role in categorizing tumors. Unfortunately, this avenue of research for most groups has not been particularly successful. At the moment, because of the problems with quantitation, amino acid studies in soft tissue tumors are not clinically relevant.

4. Are there any other clinical research problems that should be tackled?

PET because of its expense and lack of general availability should be used to address major issues. Studies into the basic tumor biology, pathophysiology and radiobiology should continue with a little more emphasis on tumor cell nuclear abnormalities. The technique should also be used to confirm or deny the rationale for any treatment modality. Receptor studies, hormone studies and pharmacokinetic studies should all be tackled.

Combining CT, MR spectroscopy, MR imaing and PET studies, although a rather frightening concept, is likely to reap considerable benefit for all those involved.

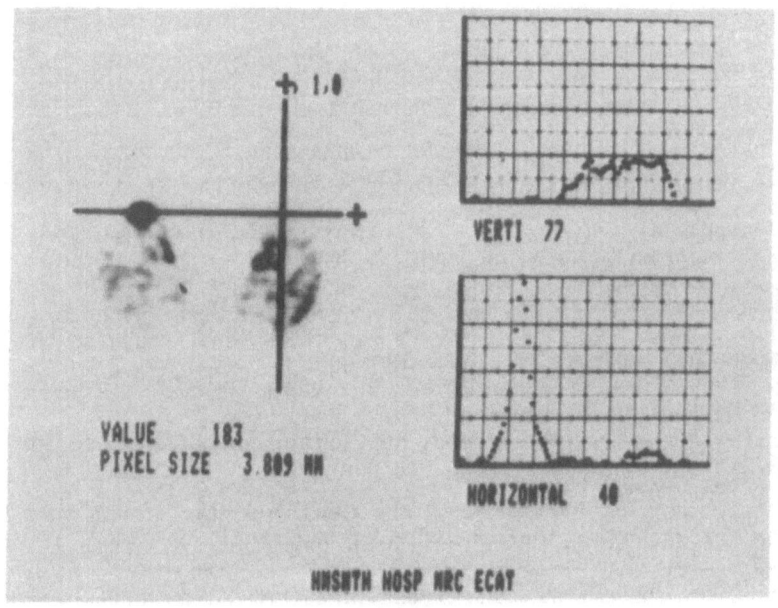

Fig. 3   PET rBF scan image with histogram plot taken through the coordinates marked. The scan was taken through mid-thigh (normal volunteer). The muscle was heated to 40°C and the skin kept at 37°C by a fan. Blood flow through the heated region was approximately 8 times higher than normal resting muscle.

5. What is the role of PET in proving and quantifying the efficacy of therapy?

This question is closely linked with the former. With the multi-modality approach to cancer today employing surgery, radiotherapy, drug

370

therapy, hormone manipulation, hyperthermia and immunotherapy, it is
sometimes easily forgotten that the rationale for some of the combined
modalities have been derived from in vitro work and laboratory animal
studies.

The effects of combining heat (Fig. 3) with radiotherapy on the
micro-vasculature of human tumors and normal tissue has not been
measured correctly. How does hyperthermia or radiotherapy affect tumor
perfusion and hence bioavailability of administered drugs?

REFERENCES

Beaney, R.P., Lammertsma, A.A., Jones, T. et al. 1984. Positron
    emission tomography for in vivo measurement of regional blood
    flow, oxygen utilization and blood volume in patients with breast
    carcinoma. Lancet, I, 131-134.
Kubota, K., Matsuzawa, T., Ido, M. et al. 1985. Lung tumor imaging by
    positron emission tomography using Cll-L-methionine. J. Nucl. Med.,
    26, 37-42.
Kubota, K., Yamada, K., Fudada, H. et al. 1984. Tumor detection with
    carbon-11 labeled amino-acids. Eur. J. Nucl. Med., 9, 136-140.
Laughlin, J.S., Gelbard, A.S., Benva, R.S. et al. 1980. Report on
    compounds labeled with nitrogen-13 or carbon-11 used in cancer
    metabolic studies with quantitative two dimensional scanning and
    PET tomography. IAEA-SM-247, 111, 497-506.
Nolop, K.B., Brudin, L., Rhodes, C.G. et al. (Subm. f. publ.) Glucose
    utilization in vivo by human pulmonary neoplasms.
Suzuki, T., Iio, M. 1982. The clinical application of 11C-glucose for
    diagnosis of lung cancer. Proc. 3rd World Congr. Nucl. Med. Biol.,
    Paris, 2, 2080-2982.
Syrota, A., Duguesnoy, N. Paraf, A. et al. 1982. The role of positron
    emission tomography in the detection of pancreatic disease.
    Radiology, 143, 249-253.
Weibel, E.R. 1984. The pathway for oxygen (chapter 7). Harvard
    University Press, Cambridge. pp. 195-210.
Wise, R.J.S., Bernardi, S., Frackowiak, R.S.J. et al. 1983. Serial
    observations on the pathophysiology of acute stroke. The
    transition from ischemia to infarction as reflected in the
    regional oxygen extraction. Brain, 106, 197-222.
Yonekura, Y., Benva, R.S., Brill, A.B. et al. 1982. Increased
    accumulation of 2-deoxy-2-(18F)-fluoro-D-glucose in liver
    metastases from colon carcinoma. J. Nucl. Med., 23, 1133-1137.

POTENTIAL CLINICAL VALUE OF PET IN ONCOLOGY

J. J. M. van der Hoeven, H. M. Pinedo
Academisch Ziekenhuis, Free University,
Dept. of Oncology, Amsterdam, The Netherlands

The application of positron emission tomography (PET) in oncology is in its infancy. For this reason it is still difficult to evaluate its applicability for the cancer patient.

Although it has been shown that PET is able to detect large breast cancer lesions (Beaney et al., 1984) and primary bronchial carcinomas (Kubota et al., 1985), there are more simple techniques available to detect such tumors. Indeed prior to the introduction of a new diagnostic procedure in clinical medicine its advantages over existing techniques should be proven. Advantages may include a greater resolution, more comfort for the patient, or reduced cost. Research on the effectiveness of PET scanning is useful for the following areas of interest: 1. detection of metastases, 2. differentiation between benign and malignant lesions, 3. evaluation of treatment results, 4. distribution of chemo-therapeutic agents, and 5. prediction of effectiveness of treatment, both chemotherapy and radiotherapy. For most of these areas the value of PET needs to be compared with that of existing diagnostic tools in-cluding CT and MRT. In this paper suggestions will be made how to apply PET as a research tool in each of the areas mentioned above.

Detection of metastases

Clinical staging is critical for decision making in oncology. Patients with local disease will usually receive local treatment, while those with disseminated disease are mostly considered for systemic treatment, mostly chemotherapy. Information considering the extent of disease is particularly of importance in patients with tumors which may be only cured by mutilating surgery such as head and neck cancers, sarcomas and cervical cancer. In the presence of lung metastases amputation of an extremity, laryngectomy or resection of the maxilla will not be considered. A number of relevant clinical situations awaiting more adequate diagnostic techniques than those presently available will be discussed.

At present the most sensitive method for detection of lung metastases is CT scanning, a technique by which lesions with a diameter of only a few millimeters may be detected. Despite preoperative application of a technique with such a low detection limit, a number of patients will develop clinical evidence of metastases following aggressive surgery of the primary tumor. Since the resolution of PET is not as high as that of the CT scan, one may not expect that PET will play a major role in the detection of micrometastases.

In other areas CT scanning still appears to be of limited value for clinical staging. If one considers lung cancer which often involves the mediastinum, CT scan is unable to predict adequately the presence of mediastinal metastases. Brion et al. (1985) conducted a study involving 53 patients in which CT scan findings were compared with those obtained during surgery. While the sensitivity of the CT scan (lesion > 5mm) was 89 %, the specificity was only 47 %. In a study by Libshitz and McKenna (1984) sensitivity was lower (49 %), while specificity was 66 %. A lymph node was considered positive in case of a diameter greater than one centimeter. Also mediastinoscopy, the reliability of which is largely dependent on the skill of the surgeon, failed to detect mediastinal involvement in many cases. Thus, any new technique which proves to be more sensitive and more specific for the detection of mediastinal lymph node metastases would be an important gain.

The clinician is faced with similar diagnostic problems in the design of treatment for patients with urogenital tumors. It is still quite difficult to detect non-invasively metastases in retroperitoneal lymph nodes. Lymphangiography and CT scanning appear to be inadequate in cases with limited lymph node disease, and the final staging is almost always reached after laparotomy.

Breast cancer, a third example in this series, is often treated by surgery. The patient may be considered for radiation of the axillary and parasternal lymph nodes. Although a radioisotope parasternal lymph node scan has been shown to localize the lymph nodes it fails to offer in-formation on the status of the nodes. If PET could distinguish between benign and malign parasternal lymph nodes, many patients would not have to undergo radiation.

One may conclude that clinical staging of tumors is presently often inaccurate. However, because of its relatively low resolution, it is unlikly that any improvement will be offered by PET.

Differentiation between benign and malign tumors

During the follow up of potentially cured cancer patients the clinician may be presented with a mass of unknown origin. Differentiation between cancer, fibrosis and an abscess may be difficult, as the CT scan and gallium scan are not always able to solve this therapeutic dilemma. Testicular cancer and extragonadal germ cell tumors are treated with chemotherapy including cisplatin. The majority of these tumors produce markers including of beta-HCG, alpha-fetoprotein or both. If the markers normalise after chemotherapy with persistence of a residual mass, there may be histological evidence of fibrosis, necrosis, mature teratoma, vital tumor cells or a combination of any of these tissues. For these cases differentiation between malignant and benign lesions by means of PET may prove to be of great value. No investigations have been reported as yet in this area.

Another clinical problem includes the lack of techniques for distinguishing benign naevi from malignant melanoma, lipoma from sarcoma, benign breast lumps and thyroid nodules from breast and thyroid cancer, respectively, and arthrosis from bone metastasis. Sometimes it is possible to establish a diagnosis by fine needle biopsy. Occasionally, however, the clinician may be presented with a true diagnostic and therapeutic dilemma. In such cases of persistent doubt, the lesion will be surgically removed. In patients with a dysplastic naevus syndrome, it is not always possible to remove each suspected mole. It would be less traumatic and most welcome to the patient if the absence of neoplastic disease could be established by a non-invasive technique. The potential role for PET in this area needs to be evaluated.

Distribution of cytostatic agents

Interesting areas of research are studies on distribution of therapeutic agents. It is known that in the case of sarcomas and especially osteosarcomas intraarterial delivery of cisplatin and doxorubicin results in improved tumor response as compared to intravenous administration of the drugs (Jaffe et al., 1984). In addition, there are several case reports showing tumor response after intraarterial 5-fluorouracil in patients with liver metastases of colon cancer failing to respond to intravenous therapy. If one succeeds to synthesize suitable tracers of the drug PET is an effective tool to study its distribution. Some interesting studies have been performed with 11C-BCNU (Tyler et al., 1986). Intraarterial administration of 11C-BCNU achieved concentrations of the drug in the tumor which averaged a 50-fold increase as those obtained after a comparable intravenous doses.

Abe et al. (1983) studied tumor uptake of 18F-5-fluorouracil, 18F-5-fluoridine and 18F-5-fluorodeoxyuridine in animals. It would be of great interest to perform similar studies in man in order to compare tumor uptake of these drugs after intravenous and intraarterial administration. If the tissue concentration of the drug appears to be the same following intraarterial and intravenous administration, one may be able to avoid the invasive technique.

An additional interesting pharmacological problem in oncology is that of multidrug resistance, which has now been studied extensively for doxorubicin and vincristine. A decrease of intracellular drug accumulation has been reported for this phenomenon. However, this can be overcome in vivo by co-administration of calcium channel blockers (Tsuruo et al., 1985). If a suitable tracer of doxorubicin and vincristine can be produced, interesting PET studies could be performed in patients with resistant tumors with and without adding calcium channel blockers.

Prediction of effectiveness of chemotherapy

Unfortunately, chemotherapy is only effective in a limited percentage of patients. Because of its side effects, it would be most helpful to be able to predict which patients will benefit from treatment. It has been established that tumor metabolism changes in case of response to chemotherapy. It seems most timely to perform clinical investigations to delineate whether it is feasible to evaluate tumor response to chemotherapy by performing a PET scan following a test dose of the drug. The relevance of such a study is evident.

Doxorubicin cardiomyopathy

Doxorubicin is a very effective drug in the treatment of several cancers. The dose limiting factor is cardiomyopathy which may develop after a cumulative dose of approximately 500 mg/m². However, in some patients signs of cardiac failure may occur earlier, while others might tolerate a higher dose. At present, the best way to monitor cardiac function is to determine the radioisotope ejection fraction. However, a lack of accuracy has been shown for this method. It is of interest that metabolic changes of the myocardium may be present before the ejection fraction decreases. Since cardiac metabolism can be determined accurately by means of PET, this method should be evaluated for monitoring cardiac function in patients receiving doxorubicin or analogs.

CONCLUSIONS

The role PET might play in oncology is as yet unknown. In the future PET will likely offer more information about tumor metabolism in man. It shows promise for the evaluation of drug biodistribution after different modes of administration. However, before it can be used in the design of cancer treatment, the problems mentioned above need to be solved. It is not very likely that PET will be superior to other diagnostic techniques employed for clinical staging of tumors. Perhaps this would be the case if monoclonal antibodies could be labeled with positron emitting nuclides. For the moment PET is an interesting research tool, but not suitable for clinical practice.

REFERENCES
Abe, Y., Fukuda, H., Ishiwata, K. et al. 1983. Studies on 18F-labeled pyrimidines. Tumor uptakes of 18F-5-fluorouracil, 18F-5-fluorouridine and 18F-5-fluorodeoxyuridine in animals. Eur. J. Nucl. Med., 8, 258-261.
Beaney, R.P., Lammertsma, A.A., Jones, T. et al. 1984. Positron emission tomography for in vivo measurement or regional blood flow, oxygen utilisation and blood pool volume in patients with breast carcinoma. Lancet, 131-134.
Brion, J.P., Depauw, L., Kuhn, G. et al. 1985. Role of computed tomography and mediastinoscopy in preoperative staging of lung carcinoma. J. Comput. Assist. Tomogr., 9, 480-484.
Jaffe, N., Bowman, R., Wang, Y.M. et al. 1984. Chemotherapy for primary osteosarcoma by intraarterial infusion. Cancer Bull., 36, 37-42.
Kubota, K., Matsuzawa, T., Ito, M. et al. 1985. Lung tumor imaging by positron emission tomography using C11 methionine. J. Nucl. Med., 26; 37-42.
Libshitz, H.I., McKenna, R.J. (1984) Mediastinal lymph node size in lung cancer. AJR, 143, 715-718.

Tsuruo, T., Kawabata, H., Naguma, N. et al. 1985. Potentiation of antitumor agents by calcium channel blockers with special referecne to cross resistance patterns. Cancer Chemother. Pharmacol., 15, 16.

Tyler, J.L., Yamamoto, Y.L., Diksic, M. et al. 1986. Pharmacokinetics of superselective intraarterial and intravenous 11C-BCNU evaluated by PET. J. Nucl. Med., 27, 775-780.

BRAIN TUMORS

POSITRON EMISSION TOMOGRAPHY WITH 11-C-METHIONINE IN BRAIN TUMORS: METHIONINE KINETICS, TUMOR DELINEATION, AND FOLLOW-UP STUDIES AFTER THERAPY

K. Ericson*, A. Lilja**, M. Bergström*
*Dept. of Neuroradiology, Karolinska Hospital, Stockholm, Sweden
**Dept. of Diagnostic Radiology, Akademiska Hospital, Uppsala, Sweden

It has become evident that brain tumors cannot always be accurately delineated with computed tomography (CT). This is true for high-grade and in particular for the low-grade tumors - astrocytomas, oligodendrogliomas and oligoastrocytomas classified as Kernohan grade II. These tumors are often seen on CT as more or less ill-defined regions with a reduced attenuation as compared to the surrounding brain tissue. The blood-brain or rather blood-tumor barrier (BTB) is in most cases preserved, and the tumors are therefore not better delineated at contrast-enhanced CT. A more or less well preserved BTB is sometimes also found in anaplastic astrocytomas and glioblastomas. An accurate determination of the extent of the tumor is of value for guiding biopsies, for deciding the type of treatment and for monitoring of the effects of treatment. Furthermore, the degree and character of the contrast enhancement is correlated to some extent to the histologic grading of the tumors since the BTB is more often disrupted in malignant than in benign tumors.

An evident need exists not only for better imaging, but also for methods that reflect the biological behavior of brain tumors. The relative shortcommings of conventional therapy for gliomas, and the development of new treatment, increase further the motives for in vivo studies in patients. Positron emission tomography (PET) with various tracers has been used by several investigators in the evaluation of brain tumors. The results indicate that PET is superior to CT in many respects. The glucose utilization in brain tumors has been studied, and there seems to be a positive correlation between histological degree of malignancy and glycolytic rate (DiChiro et al., 1982, 1984; Patronas et al., 1985). The prediction of degree of malignancy with PET is more accurate than with CT. Furthermore, radionecrosis can be differentiated from tumor recurrence with PET, which is not possible with CT (Patronas et al., 1982). The metabolic demands and supply of brain tumors before and after therapy have been further explored in studies of blood flow, and oxygen and glucose utilization (Rhodes et al., 1983; Beaney, 1984). The low-grade tumors have a glycolytic rate similar to that of normal brain tissue. For delineation of these tumors, therefore, 18-F-fluoro-deoxyglucose and 11-C-glucose are not ideal tracers.

11-C-METHIONINE

11-C-(methyl)-L-methionine (11-C-methionine) has been used for studies of dementia, schizophrenia (Bustany et al., 1985) and brain tumors (Bergström et al., 1983; Ericson et al., 1985; Lilja et al., 1985). To obtain quantitative values of the incorporation of methionine in proteins, a kinetic model has been proposed (Bustany et al., 1985). There has been some discussion on the validity of this model (Phelps et al., 1985). Since methionine is a potent methyl-donor, it has been claimed that the labelled methyl group appears in many metabolic processes other than protein synthesis. On the other hand, there are indications that these other processes do not play a major role during the first hour after administration of the labelled amino acid. Labelling in the carboxyl group, as has been done with leucine and phenylalanine (Phelps et al., 1985), may be a way to avoid these problems. However, the assumptions of the kinetic models designed for normal or near-normal tissue may not necessarily be valid for grossly pathologic tissue as in malignant tumors.

Whatever the fate of the injected tracer, 11-C-methionine has been shown to be of value in the evaluation of intracranial tumors (Lilja et al., 1985). Series of brain tumor patients have been studied in Stockholm and Uppsala in collaboration (Bergström et al., 1983; Ericson et al., 1985; Lilja et al., 1985). In the work to be reviewed below, our aims have been to assess the diagnostic role of PET with 11-C-methionine in studies of brain tumors, in comparison with other radiological and neuropathological data. In order to interpret alterations in amino acid uptake in brain tumor disease, we investigated qualitatively and semi-quantitatively some aspects of 11-C-methionine kinetics in tumor tissue, and made comparisons with normal brain. We have so far mostly used the graphical procedure suggested by Gjedde (1981) and Patlak et al. (1983)

in the analysis of the data. In the clinical use of the PET
examinations, however, the static images have been just as helpful
(Figs. 1 and 2).

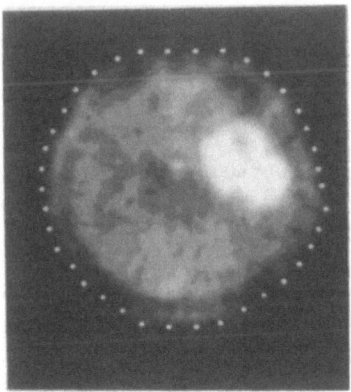

Fig. 1: Anaplastic astrocytoma (grade III) with itense
accumulation of 11-C-methionine.

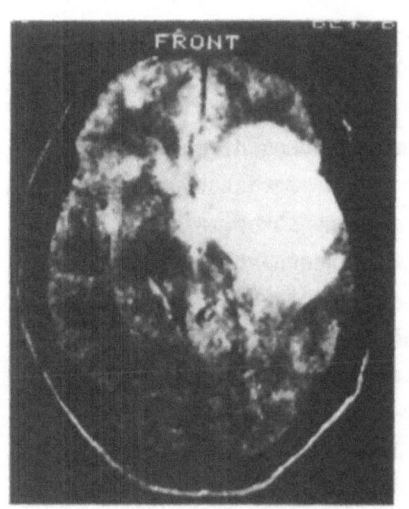 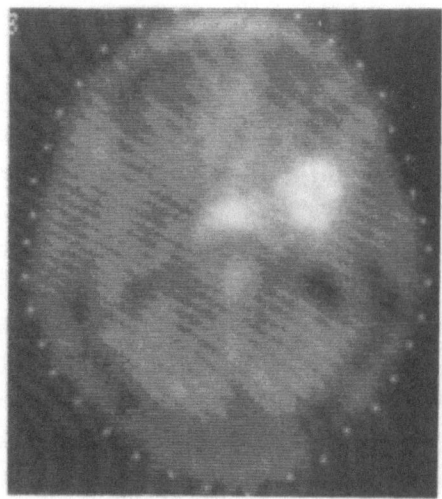

Fig. 2: Astrocytoma (grade II) in the left temporal lobe. a)
T2-weighted MR image shows signal increase in a large area. Tumor
and edema cannot be separated. b) PET with 11-C-methionine
delineates the tumor accurately.

At Karolinska Hospital, about 60 patients with intracranial tumors
have to date been examined with PET using 11-C-methionine. A majority of
the patients (50 %) had low-grade tumors. Twenty-five per cent had anaplastic astrocytomas and only ten per cent had glioblastomas. Less than
15 per cent of the tumors had a methionine accumulation equal to or
lower than that of normal brain tissue. These tumors were all astrocytomas, whereas all oligodendrogliomas and oligo-astrocytomas grade II
had a higher or markedly higher accumulation than the surrounding
tissue. All anaplastic astrocytomas and glioblastomas had considerably
increased methionine accumulation in accordance with previous experience
(Lilja et al., 1985).

The tumor extent as judged by the PET studies correlated very well
with that determined by stereotaxic biopsies in a majority of patients
(Mosskin et al., 1986). There were a few notable exceptions, all in
astrocytomas where the methionine accumulation was concentrated on quite
a small area and the low-attenuating area on CT was large and not quite
corresponding to the PET-findings. In a few such cases we found tumor
cells in regions with normal methionine accumulation. There is no
obvious explanation to this finding. It is probable, though, that these
tumors showed a high accumulation of methionine in an area where the
density of tumor cells was high. These tumors may be supposed to be
growing in an infiltrating manner, and the pathologic metabolism of the
tumor cells may then be masked by the numerous surrounding normal cells
(partial volume effect). Another explanation may be that the degree of
malignancy varies much within the tumor and so does the methionine
accumulation. According to our experience with neuropathological
examinations (Mosskin et al., 1986), the latter hypothesis does not
likely explain the findings. However, these few cases are exceptions. In
the majority of patients, PET with methionine was superior to other
methods used for the delineation even of low-grade tumors.

It should be emphasized that it is usually not possible to base the
tumor grading on PET findings with methionine alone. In most cases, the
combination of findings on CT and PET, however, yielded a correct
diagnosis.

In a group of patients with low-grade gliomas (12 patients), anaplastic astrocytomas (two patients), and meningiomas (two patients), we

followed the radioactivity concentration as a function of time after injection of 11-C-methionine. The evaluation was done regionally in tumor tissue and in anatomically similar regions of non-tumorous brain (Bergström et al., subm. f. publ. A). Plasma radioactivity was sampled at increasing intervals after injection and measured in a well-counter; all values were corrected for labeled plasma proteins (Lundqvist et al., 1985). Using the graphical method of Gjedde (1981) and Patlak et al. (1983), the tissue/plasma radioactivity ratio was plotted versus plasma radioactivity divided by the time integral of plasma radioactivity. In all cases, the graphical analysis was compatible with the assumed model. Rapid equilibration between plasma and tissue took place in a reversible compartment, followed a few minutes later by unidirectional influx of 11-C into an irreversible compartment. Irreversibility was indicated by a linear slope in the plots, occuring from about 5 min after injection to the end of the examination (30-60 min), and was seen both in tumor tissue and in contralateral brain. The magnitude of the slope in the Gjedde/Patlak plots, giving an estimate of the trapping rate of 11-C, was on the average twice as high in tumor tissue as in contralateral brain. The highest rates were seen in an anaplastic astrocytoma and in a meningioma.

In each of five patients with gliomas, PET examinations with 11-C-L-methionine and 11-C-D-methionine were made within a few days (Bergström et al., subm. f. publ. B). Otherwise, the same methodology as above was used. In these five patients, the same relations existed in tumor tissue as in contralateral brain between the estimated accumulation of the L- and D-isomer of 11-C-methionine (on the average, the ratio L-/D- was 2.4).

In another group of five patients with cerebral gliomas, 11-C-methionine was injected on two occasions in each patient. At the first examination, the "cold" plasma amino acid concentrations were not manipulated, while at the subsequent examination an infusion of branched-chain amino acids (BCAA) was given i.v. (Bergström et al., subm. f. publ. C). A total of 10 g of a mixture of amino acids consisting of leucine (70 %), isoleucine (20 %), and valine (10 %) was infused at a constant rate from 45 min before until 50 min after the tracer injection. In four of the patients studied, the accumulation of

11-C-methionine was reduced by about 35 % in tumor tissue as well as in brain when BCAA were infused, as compared with the examinations in the un-altered state. In one patient with a severely disrupted vascular barrier, a reduction of 11-C accumulation was seen only in brain and not in the tumor tissue.

These findings indicate that in brain tumor tissue with an intact vascular barrier, the accumulation of 11-C-methionine is stereo-specific and subject to competitive inhibition. Thus, the uptake of large neutral amino acids across the endothelial "barrier" in glial tumors has similar characteristics, but at a higher level, as that in normal brain, provided the BTB is not grossly disrupted.

GLYCINE

In a few patients, we have utilized another amino acid, 11-C-glycine. The results of this study will be pulished elsewhere, but a few impressions may be given here. Glycine is poorly transported across the normal blood-brain barrier. We were interested to examine whether this also was true for tumors. So far, only a few patients with intracranial tumors have been examined with 11-C-glycine. Some of these patients had anaplastic astrocytomas with an extensive BTB disruption and some had lesions with only a minimal BTB leakage. It appeared that the PET examinations with 11-C-glycine displayed the BTB disrupture much more effectively than did 68-Ga-EDTA. Glycine is a smaller molecule than the EDTA complex. However, the very intense accumulation of glycine may also be explained otherwise. 68-Ga-EDTA diffuses through the leaks in the barrier but is then not utilized. Glycine, however, is leaking through the barrier only to be readily accepted as a substrate. Once across the barrier, the increased demands for glycine of the tumor may be shown. Therefore, glycine also shows the BTB defects much better than EDTA. This explanation is very premature but may serve until some more patients have been examined and a thorough analysis of the kinetics of glycine have been made. In tissue with an intact barrier, glycine was not accumulated, and it therefore seems clear that glycine is of limited value as a tumor tracer.

OTHER TRACERS

Some experiments have shown that a benzodiazepine receptor agonist,

Ro 5-4864, has a tendency to accumulate in experimental lesions known to cause proliferation of glial cells. This stimulated us to use this tracer in the belief that the glial proliferation in astrocytomas then might be shown effectively. The preliminary experience is that not even anaplastic astrocytomas have an increased accumulation of this tracer in comparison with normal brain tissue. On the contrary, although the tracer is an agonist of the peripheral and not the central benzodiazepine receptors, it was accumulating much more in normal tissue than in tumor tissue. However, there seemed to be no specific binding. The results have not yet been fully analyzed, more tumors need to be examined with this tracer in order to fully understand the findings. Suffice it to say that this tracer is not a tumor tracer. In the future other receptors will be studied in the hope that tumors may very well prove to have an abundance of receptors in comparison with normal tissue. This has already been shown to be true with regard to steroid receptors in several types of tumors (Yu et al., 1981).

Recently, 11-C-tyrosine was used in healthy subjects to quantitate the transport across the intact blood-brain barrier. It has not yet been used for tumor studies.

A MODEL FOR METHIONINE UTILIZATION

The kinetic model suggested by Bustany et al. (1985) has been applied with minor modifications to some patients examined at Karolinska Hospital. This study was performed only recently, and the results are therefore preliminary. It was felt, however, that the graphic method of Gjedde and Patlak should be compared with the kinetic model of Bustany. A total of 11 patients have so far been evaluated in this way. We are aware of the fact that processes other than mere protein synthesis may be involved and, therefore, only evaluated the irreversible trapping of the tracer in tissue irrespective of its metabolic fate. In our series, the incorporation rate of methionine was estimated at an average of 0.4 nmol/g/min in normal brain tissue. This value is higher than those obtained by Bustany et al. (1985), who reported values of 0.23 and 0.15 in two series. These discrepancies need further analysis.

Our results are quite similar to those obtained using the graphical method of Gjedde and Patlak (Bergström et al., subm. f. publ. A). This is not surprising since the methods of calculating the net accumulation rate are identical. A larger series of patients is now under study and the reproducibility is also examined. As mentioned above, the static images giving only the relation between uptake in normal and tumorous tissue have been successfully used for the clinical evaluation of PET scans in patients with brain tumors. Some advantages are, however, obtained with the kinetic model. A quantitation of various parameters concerning the methionine distribtuion and trapping enables a more distinct classification of tumor metabolism. Furthermore, the response to treatment may be measured in a more accurate way instead of visual estimates.

STEREOTAXIC DEVICE

In all the patients studied with PET using 11-C-methionine, an individually fabricated plastic helmet was used for the fixation of the patient to the examination table (Bergström et al., 1981). This has enabled reproducibility in the positioning of the patient not only for repeat PET studies, but also in obtaining corresponding slice orientation at CT, angiography, stereotaxic biopsies and radiation treatment. In the majority of tumor patients studied with PET at our hospital, stereotaxic biopsies are guided by the PET findings rather than by CT. However, it is often important to relate the isotope accumulation to the anatomical information obtained with CT. In some instances, a stereotaxic angiography using the same helmet fixation was performed to establish the proximity of the biopsy targets to large intracranial vessels.

FOLLOW-UP EXAMINATIONS

A few patients treated with radiation therapy and surgery underwent repeat PET studies about two years after treatment. The preliminary impression from these patients is that methionine accumulation tends to normalize after irradiation. This is in contrast with the results reported by Lilja et al. (1985). However, the latter series comprised only high-grade tumors examined 1.5-6 months after treatment, and the results may have reflected the low efficacy of radiation therapy in malignant gliomas.

In a further investigation with 11-C-methionine, a patient who developed a glioma recurrence during a time period of 5.5-7.5 years after surgery and irradiation, was studied. Apart from a recurrent tumor part evident already by CT, high tracer uptake in a distand region permitted the delineation of another large, diffusely growing tumor part. The latter tumor component was not possible to diagnose as a tumor by CT alone. A detailed histopathological examination showed exact correspondence with the findings at PET.

A larger series of patients studied early and late after irradiation is now in progress. The results of limited follow-up studies so far indicate that PET with 11-C-labeled amino acids may be valuable in solving some of the great difficulties currently encountered in the CT evaluation of post-therapeutic states.

PET AND MR

Magnetic resonance imaging (MR) appears to be a very sensitive technique for the detection of pathologic changes of brain tissue. However, it is often difficult or impossible to distinguish between tumor and peritumoral edema on MR. Some improvement was achieved by using special pulse sequences, especially in low-grade gliomas (Tovi et al., in press), and in the presence of a blood-brain barrier disruption, intravenously administered contrast media proved useful. Still, many tumors cannot be accurately delineated. Our experience with MR in comparison with PET is very limited, but so far PET has been superior (Figs. 2 and 3). Without doubt, these comparative studies will enable a better understanding of the MR information and optimization of the pulse sequences to be used in the MR examination of intracranial tumors.

The rapid distribution within minutes of 11-C-methionine to brain and tumor tissue, followed by continuous trapping of 11-C-, nearly always without loss of radioactivity, as well as the irradiation effects in low-grade gliomas, favor the view that high tumor uptakes of 11-C-methionine reflect a significant synthesizing or metabolic activity in tumor cells. It therefore seems highly meaningful to further explore amino acid utilization in tumor tissue. Although still used as a research tool, PET has been of obvious practical value in the clinical management of patients with intracranial tumors. In the long run, it is hoped that the PET findings will aid in selecting a treatment adjusted to the biologic character of the individual tumor.

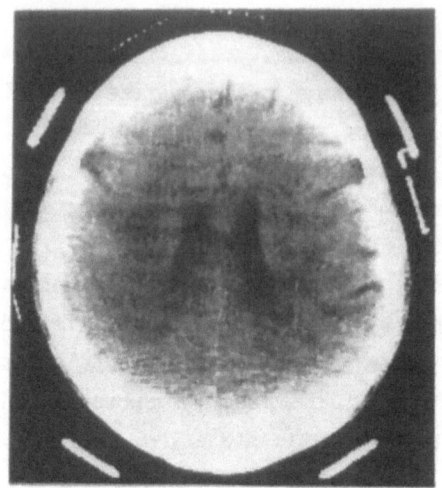

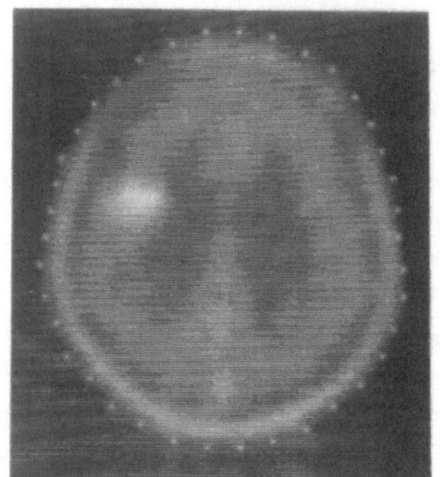
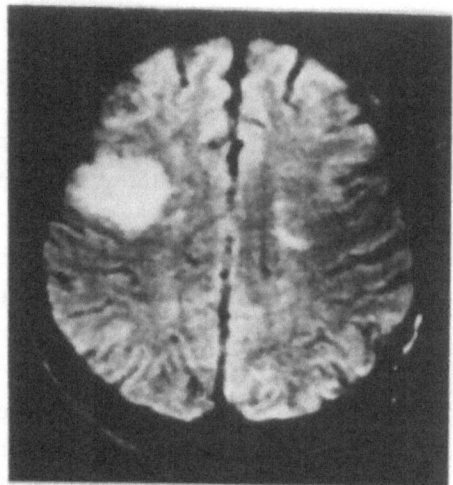

Fig. 3: Astrocytoma (grade II), barely visible as a low-density lesion on contrast-enhanced CT (a). PET with 11-C-methionine (b), the true extent of the tumor is better shown than on T2-weighted MRI (c).

REFERENCES

Beaney, R.P. 1984. Positron emission tomography in the study of human
tumors. Sem. Nucl. Med., 14, 424-441.
Bergström, M., Boethius, J., Eriksson, L. et al. 1981. Head fixation
device for reproducible position alignment in transmission CT and
positron emission tomography. J. Comput. Assist. Tomogr., 5, 136-
141.
Bergström, M., Collins, V.P., Ehring, E. et al. 1983. Discrepancies in
brain tumor extent as shown by computed tomography and positron
emission tomography using 68-Ga-EDTA, 11-C-glucose and 11-C-
methionine. J. Comput. Assist. Tomogr., 7, 1062-1066.
Bergström, M., Ericson, K., Hagenfeldt, L. et al. Subm. f. publ. C.
Methionine accumulation in glioma and normal brain tissue studied
with positron emission tomography - competition with branched
amino acids.
Bergström, M., Lundqvist, H., Ericson, K. et al. Subm. f. publ. B.
Comparison of the accumulation kinetics of L-(methyl-C-11)-
methionine and D-(11-C-methyl)-methionine in brain tumors studied
with positron emission tomography.
Bergström, M. Mosskin, M., Ericson, K. et al. Subm. f. publ. A.
Accumulation kinetics of 11-C-D-glucose, (methyl-11-C)-L-
methionine and 68-Ga-EDTA in brain tumors measured with positron
emission tomography.
Bustany, P., Henry, J.F., Rotrou J. de et al. 1985. Correlations
between clinical state and positron emission tomography
measurement of local protein synthesis in Alzheimer's dementia,
Parkinson's disease, schizophrenia and gliomas. In "The
Metabolism of the Human Brain Studied with Positron Emission
Tomography". (Eds. T. Greitz et al.). (Raven Press, New York). pp.
241-249
DiChiro, G., Brooks, R.A., Patronas, N.J. et al. 1984. Issues in the in
vivo measurement of glucose metabolism of human central nervous
system tumors. Ann. Neurol., 15, 138-146.
DiChiro, G., DeLaPaz, R.L., Brooks, R.A. et al. 1982. Glucose
utilization of cerebral gliomas measured by 18F-fluorodeoxyglucose
and positron emission tomography. Neurology, 32, 1323-1329.
Ericson, K., Lilja, A. Bergström, M. et al. 1985. Positron emission
tomography (PET) using 11-C-methionine, 11-C-glucose and 68-Ga-
EDTA in the examination of supratentorial tumors. J. Comput.
Assist. Tomogr., 9, 683-689.
Gjedde, A. 1981. High- and low-affinity transport of D-glucose from
blood to brain. J. Neurochem., 36, 1463-1471.
Lilja, A., Bergström, K., Hartvig, P. et al. 1985. Dynamic study of
supratentorial gliomas with L-methyl-11-C-methionine and positron
emission tomography. AJNR, 6, 505-514.
Lundqvist, H., Stalnacke, C.G., Langström, B. et al. 1985. Labelled
metabolites in plasma after i.v. administration of 11-C-methyl-L-
methionine. In "The Metabolism of the Human Brain Studied by
Positron Emission Tomography". (Eds. T. Greitz et al.). (Raven
Press, New York). pp. 233-240.
Mosskin, M., Collins, V.P., Bergström, M. et al. 1986. Positron
emission tomography with 11-C-methionine of intracranial tumors
compared with histology of multiple biopsies. (Abstract). XIII
Symp. Neuroradiologicum, Stockholm, Sweden.

Patlak, C.S., Blasberg, R., Fenstermacher, J.D. 1983. Graphical
    evaluation of blood-to-brain transfer constants from multiple-time
    uptake data. J. Cereb. Blood Flow Metabol., 3, 1-7.
Patronas, N.J., DiChiro, G., Brooks, R.A. et al. 1982. Work in
    progress: (18F)-fluorodeoxyglucose and positron emission
    tomography in the evaluation of radiation necrosis of the brain.
    Radiology, 144, 885-889.
Patronas, N.J., DiChiro, G., Kufta, C. et al. 1985. Prediction of
    survival in glioma patients by means of positron emission
    tomography. J. Neurosurg., 62, 816-822.
Phelps, M.E., Barrio, J.R., Huang, S.C. et al. 1985. Measurement of
    cerebral protein synthesis in man with positron computerized
    tomography: Model, assumptions and preliminary results. In "The
    Metabolism of the Human Brain Studied with Positron Emission
    Tomography". (Eds. T. Greitz et al.). (Raven Press, New York). pp.
    215-232.
Rhodes, C.G., Wise, R.J.S., Gibbs, J.M. et al. 1983. In vivo
    disturbance of the oxidative metabolism of glucose in human
    cerebral gliomas. Ann. Neurol., 14, 614-626.
Tovi, M., Thuomas, K.A., Bergström, K. et al. In press. Tumor
    delineation with MRI in gliomas: A comparison with PET and CT.
    Acta Radiol.
Yu, Z.Y. Hatam, A., Bergström, M. et al. 1981. CT findings and gluco-
    corticoid receptors in intracranial lesions with edema. J. Comput.
    Assist. Tomogr., 5, 619-624.

DOPAMINE RECEPTORS IN PITUITARY ADENOMAS AND EFFECT OF BROMOCRIPTINE TREATMENT - EVALUATION WITH PET AND MRI

C. Muhr, M. Bergström, P.O. Lundberg, K. Bergström,
K.A. Thuomas, B. Langström

Dept. of Neurology and Diagnostic Radiology, University Hospital,
and Dept. of Chemistry, Uppsala University,
Uppsala, Sweden

Pituitary adenomas are as a rule benign tumors that can originate from immature pituitary stem cells or from one of the more specialized hormone producing cell types. Accordingly, the classification of pituitary adenomas is dominantly based on the type of hormonal activity or lack of such. Hormone serum/plasma levels will often provide an indication of the probable adenoma type. In some cases, however, this information is not sufficient for differentiation, and only fine needle biopsy with cytological evaluation including immunocytochemistry can adequately diagnose the cell types in the tumor. The importance of a proper classification can be illustrated by the different choices of treatment available for the two most common types of pituitary adenomas - prolactinomas and null cell adenomas (hormonally inactive adenomas) (Kovacs et al., 1984). Most of the prolactinomas will respond well to dopamine agonist treatment whereas the null cell adenomas are rarely affected by such treatment. The positive response to dopamine agonist treatment in prolactinomas, a rapid reduction in serum prolactin and tumor shrinkage, has been shown to be dopamine receptor mediated. In the normal pituitary gland the prolactin secreting cells, the lactotrophs, contain dopamine-D2 receptors through which dopamine from the hypothalamus exerts its regulatory inhibitory effect. The exact mechanism behind the dopamine agonist's effect on prolactinomas is not known.

Positron emission tomography (PET) is a technique for in vivo tracer kinetic studies using compounds labeled with short-lived radionuclides like ^{11}C. PET provides tomographic images demonstrating the regional distribution of the radiotracer. We have previously shown that PET with the administration of ^{11}C-labeled N-methylspiperone can visualize and quantify dopamine-D2 receptor binding in pituitary adenomas (Muhr et al., 1986). Furthermore, we have demonstrated high accumulation of ^{11}C-labeled methionine and bromocriptine in these tumors (Muhr et al., 1984, 1985). It is of great interest to be able to demonstrate and quantify D2-receptors in pituitary adenomas in the characterization of these tumors, and to relate this to the effect of dopamine agonist treatment. We used the potentials of PET to measure in vivo D2-receptor binding and amino acid metabolism in the tumors. Patients were treated with bromocriptine and the effect of this treatment was recorded with PET as well as with MRI (magnetic resonance imaging).

PATIENTS

A total of 26 patients with a pituitary adenoma were included in the studies. There were 10 females and 16 males, age range 27-76 years. All the pituitary adenomas were large; with extrasellar extension. 12 of the patients had a prolactinoma, in 4 of these the serum prolactin levels were 42-151 µg/l and in 8 patients 840-6700 µg/l (normal < 20 µg/l). The remaining 10 patients were classified to have a null cell adenoma without any signs of hormonal hyperproduction. In most of the patients, the diagnoses were verified by fine needle biopsy or by operation with histopathological examination including immunocyto-chemistry. DNA analysis was also performed. In patients with a pituitary insufficiency, substitution was given for adrenal, thyroid, and also in a few patients for gonadal insufficiency.

Four different studies were performed with partially overlapping patient groups.
1) One group consisting of 15 patients was studied with PET using dopamine D2-ligands. All the 8 prolactinomas in this group and some of the null cell adenomas were followed up with PET after bromocriptine treatment.
2) A second group consisting of 5 prolactinomas and 4 hormonally in-active tumors was examined with PET using (^{11}C)-L-methionine before and at follow-up after bromocriptine treatment.
3) A third group was investigated with PET using D- and L-methionine in order to evaluate the amino acid metabolism in the pituitary adenomas.

There were 4 patients with hormonally inactive tumors in this group.
4) A fourth group of 15 patients including 11 prolactinomas were treated
with bromocriptine retard injection (50 mg i.m.) and examined with MRI
before and at regular intervals for follow-up.

METHODS

In the PET studies, a 3-slice positron camera (Scanditronix PC-384
B) with a resolution of 8 mm and a slice thickness of 11 mm was used. The
radiolabeled substance was administered i.v. in a dose of 40-200 MBq. A
dynamic sequence of images was obtained starting at the time of injection and continuing for up to 70 min. During all the PET procedures,
the patient's head was fixated using a special fixation system to enable
exact and reproducible positioning (Bergström et al., 1981). Multiple
blood samples were taken to measure the plasma radioactivity.

PET included studies with ^{11}C-labeled dopamine-D2 ligands, two
dopamine agonists, N-methylspiperone and raclopride (a substituted
benzamide) (Farde et al., 1985), and the dopamine agonist bromocriptine.
In order to separate specific from non-specific binding, a repeated
PET study with protection of the D2-receptors was performed. Haloperidol
was thus given in a dose of up to 3.75 mg i.v. one hour before the administration of the radiolabeled ligand.

Amino acid metabolism was evaluated using ^{11}C-labeled L-methionine, and the free distribution of amino acids was examined with the
metabolically inactive stereoisomer ^{11}C-D-methionine. In the reconstructed images, regions of interest were outlined to represent solid
tumor tissue, cerebellar and normal cortical brain tissue. The radioactivity concentration within these regions of interests was calculated
and the tracer kinetics was analyzed according to a graphical technique of Gjedde (1981) and Patlak et al. (1983). Thus, the radioactivity concentration in the tissue was divided by the radioactivity
concentration in a reference medium, which was plasma in the methionine
studies and cerebellum in the dopamine-D2 ligand studies. This ratio was
plotted against a normalized time simulating constant reference
radioactivity.

MRI studies were performed using a 0.5 Tesla superconductive magnet
(Siemens Magnetom), with coronal, sagittal and axial planes, and with
T1-, T2- and proton density-weighted images (spin echo sequences

TR/TE 500/35 ms, 1500/35 ms and 1500/90 ms). The signal intensity within the tumor was measured as was the tumor size. Areas with different signals suggestive of cyst formation were recorded. Patients were examined with MRI before and at 1 and 6 weeks, and at approximately 3, 6, and 12 months after bromocriptine treatment. The MRI findings were compared with those obtained by CT.

RESULTS

In the dopamine ligand studies, all the prolactinomas with highly elevated serum prolactin showed a very high receptor binding in the tumors (Figs. 1-3). The specific binding obtained by subtraction of the two studies made before and after haloperidol protection was comparable to and in some tumors even higher than that found in striatum. The null cell adenomas showed no or slight D2-receptor binding. In two of the patients, the clinical findings favored a prolactinoma, although the serum prolactin levels were only moderately elevated. In these patients, an intermediate receptor binding was found amounting to 1/3 of that of striatum. There was in all cases a good qualitative correlation between the tumor D2-receptor binding of ^{11}C-N-methylspiperone and ^{11}C-raclopride. The kinetic plot with ^{11}C-N-methylspiperone showed a continous linear increase with time in the prolactinomas, suggesting irreversible trapping of the tracer without signs of dissociation. With ^{11}C-raclopride, the initial increase leveled off and approached a constant value (Fig. 3), which reflects the relatively rapid dissociation known to occur with raclopride. Bromocriptine showed a kinetic pattern similar to that of raclopride, but with a much smaller fraction of specific binding. High accumulation of bromocriptine in the tumor was observed in all cases.

The amino acid metabolism in the tumor, measured by ^{11}C-L-methionine, was higher in the prolactinomas than in the null cell adenomas. In the prolactinomas, the amino acid metabolism was 3.5 times higher than in cerebellum, and in the null cell adenomas 2.8 times higher than in cerebellum. In the follow-up of bromocriptine treatment, using ^{11}C-L-methionine, all the prolactinomas showed a marked decrease in amino acid metabolism (Fig. 4). The amino acid metabolism in these tumors was reduced by 60 % as a result of treatment. The null cell adenomas, however, showed no effect of treatment and the pre- to posttreatment ratios in these tumors ranged from 0.9 to 1.1.

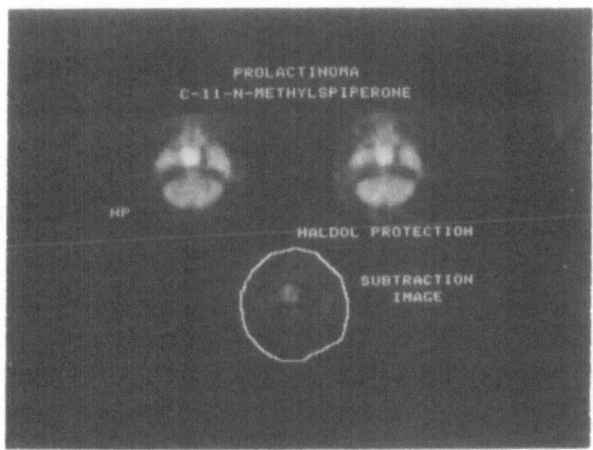

Fig. 1: A patient with a prolactinoma examined with 11C-
N-methylspiperone, showing high D2-receptor binding in the tumor
(upper left). The upper right image was obtained after haloperidol
protection and shows a marked reduction in tumor uptake. The lower
image shows the subtraction of the images obtained without and with
protection.

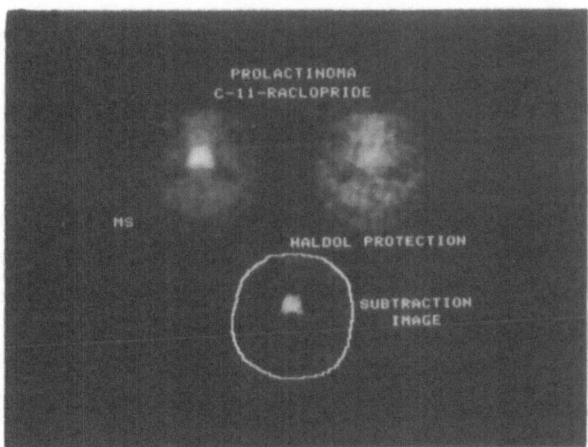

Fig. 2: A patient with a prolactinoma examined with 11C-raclo-
pride. The high uptake in the tumor (upper left) is blocked by
haloperidol (upper right). The lower image shows the subtraction of
the images obtained before and after protection.

PROLACTINOMA RACLOPRIDE

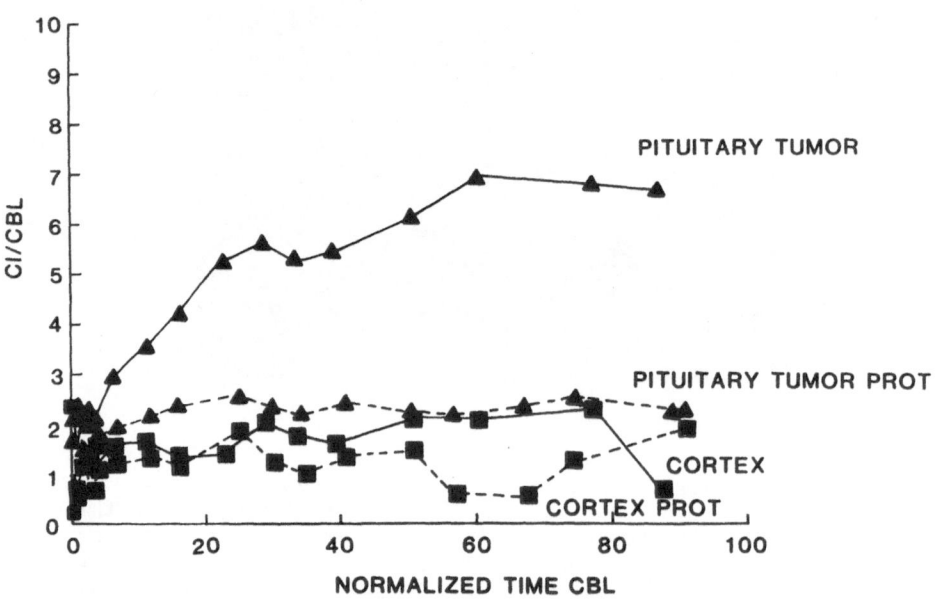

Fig. 3: Accumulation kinetics of 11C-raclopride in a prolactinoma (▲) and cortex (■). Broken lines indicate the result
after protection with haloperidol of the D2-receptors. A large
amount of D2-receptor binding is illustrated by the significant
decrease in the tumor after protection.

The four patients examined with ^{11}C-L- and D-methionine showed a
uniform pattern. With D-methionine, tumor-to-plasma ratio of radioactivity increased rapidly during the first few minutes, whereafter the
ratio assumed a constant level of about 12 with no signs of irreversible
trapping of the tracer. With L-methionine, however, the ratio of tumor
to plasma radioactivity increased linearly with time throughout the
whole experiment. The slope was 2.5 times higher than that of cerebellum,
calculated according to the described graphical procedure. The conclusion
from this study with D- and L-methionine is that D-methionine is rapidly
distributed within the tumor tissue, but it is not incorporated in the
protein synthesis. L-methionine on the other hand is rapidly distributed
in the tumor and also to a large proportion irreversibly trapped in the

metabolic processes. The difference between L- and D-methionine uptake is given by the slope of the L-methionine plot and can be used as a quantitative value of amino acid metabolism.

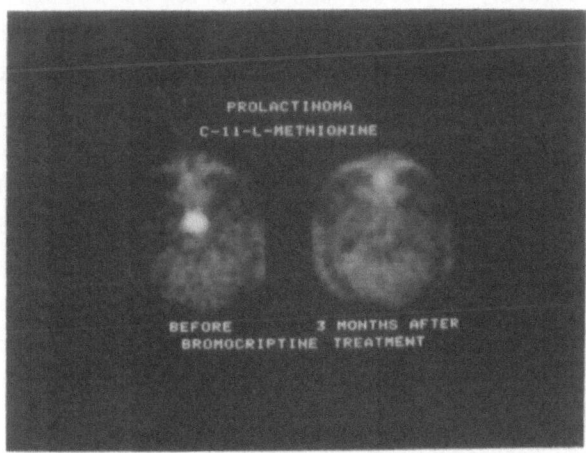

Fig. 4: A patient with a prolactinoma examined with 11C-L-methionine before (left) and 3 months (right) after bromocriptine treatment. A 60 % decrease in the amino acid metabolism is seen after treatment.

Serum prolactin was normalized in 6 of 11 patients with pro-lactinoma already within the first 24 hours after the injection of bromo-criptine retard. In the 5 remaining patients, serum prolactin levels were reduced significantly. After six weeks (in 2 patients with 2 in-jections after 12 weeks), oral bromocriptine treatment was given at a dose of 5-15 mg/day. One patient reacted with a blood pressure fall, otherwise no adverse side effects of bromocriptine retard injections were noticed. In the five patients with visual field defects, a rapid normalization was observed. One patient with a prolactinoma and rapid visual deterioration was subacutely operated on without bromocriptine treatment.

Ten of the 11 prolactinomas treated with bromocriptine retard in-jection showed a decrease in tumor volume as observed at follow-up, 6 weeks to 3 months later. In one patient with a large cystic prolactinoma, the cyst increased in size during the treatment, and visual fields showed increasing defects. In this patient, a fine needle puncture by the trans-sphenoidal route was performed to aspirate the cyst content. The visual fields were immediately restored, and at follow-up 3 months later, no increase in tumor growth was noticed. Three patients had unchanged tumor size - all had a null cell adenoma. In 5 patients with a prolactinoma, a cystic-necrotic area was observed after bromocriptine treatment, and in some patients, the cyst formation was successively enlarging with time, while the overall tumor mass was decreasing. During the follow-up with MRI, consistent changes in relaxation time were observed, with an increase in the T1 and T2-relaxation times of the tumor as compared to white matter during the first month. This tendency was then succeeded by a slight decrease in relaxation times.

DISCUSSION

With the new techniques of PET and MRI it has been possible to evaluate dopamine-D2 receptor properties in vivo in pituitary adenomas, to evaluate amino acid metabolism and to measure tumor size and tissue inhomogeneity within the tumor. The same parameters were also recorded during bromocriptine treatment. This study allows us to correlate the pretreatment status of the tumor with effects of dopamine agonist treatment. In spite of the limited number of patients a few clear tendencies were observed.

Patients with prolactinomas with high serum prolactin levels were characterized at PET by high D2-receptor binding and high amino acid metabolism. These patients responded to bromocriptine treatment with a marked reduction in the amino acid metabolism, and in most of the tumors a considerable tumor shrinkage was noticed. The serum prolactin levels were normalized or significantly decreased in all prolactinomas. The effect on serum prolactin levels of bromocriptine retard lasted for at least 6 weeks.

A group of null cell adenomas was characterized by minimal or lack of D2-receptor binding. The amino acid metabolism was lower than in the prolactinomas. With few exceptions these tumors did not respond to bromocriptine treatment - neither with changes of amino acid metabolism nor with tumor volume.

There also seems to exist an intermediate group with normal or slightly elevated serum prolactin levels, which demonstrate slight to moderate D2-receptor binding at PET. The follow-up time is still too short for any conclusions as to the bromocriptine treatment effect in these tumors.

Some prolactinomas with highly elevated serum prolactin levels do not respond to bromocriptine treatment. It is concievable but not yet demonstrated that some of these may have a high receptor density. Functional alterations of the receptors have been suggested. In these patients, PET may provide valuable information regarding the existence and properties of D2-receptors. With ^{11}C-bromocriptine it was possible to follow the distribution of the drug within the tumors, and thus to validate that the drug had full access to the receptor-containing cells.

The receptor binding studies performed in this study result in a quantitative value of receptor binding capacity, which includes both receptor density and receptor association constant. Separation of these two factors necessitates multiple studies with different specific activities and a ligand that reaches receptor binding equilibrium. Raclopride with relatively rapid dissociation fullfills these criteria, and Scatchard plots in vivo are possible (Farde et al., 1985). It might be of interest to determine the receptor dissociation constant and the correlation with treatment effects, although in vitro studies on samples from human pituitary adenoma tissue have not demonstrated differences in the dissociation constant (Bression et al., 1980).

The delineation of the pituitary adenomas was better with MRI than with CT, and inhomogeneities within the tumor were noticed in several cases by MRI but not with CT. MRI was also superior to CT in revealing changes of size and changes within the tumor as a result of bromocriptine treatment, i.e., the evolution of cystic-necrotic transformations as well as changes in relaxation times.

ACKNOWLEDGEMENTS

This work was supported by grants from the Swedish Medical Research Council (nr B86-39X-07004-02A3), the Swedish Medical Society, and the Swedish Cancer Society.

400

REFERENCES

Bergström, M., Boethius, J., Eriksson, L. et al. 1981. Head fixation
    device for reproducible position alignment in transmission CT and
    positron emission tomography. J. Comput. Assist. Tomogr., 5, 136-
    141.
Bression, D., Brandi, A.M., Martres, M.P. et al. 1980. Dopaminergic
    receptors in human prolactin-secreting adenomas: a quantitative
    study. J. Clin. Endocrinol. Metab., 5, 1037-1043.
Farde, L., Ehrin, E., Eriksson, L. et al. 1985. Substituted benzamides
    as ligands for visualization of dopamine receptor binding in the
    human brain by positron emission tomography. Proc. Natl. Acad.
    Sci., 82, 3863-3867.
Gjedde, A. 1981. High- and low-affinity transport of D-glucose from
    blood to brain. J. Neurochem., 36, 1463-1471.
Kovacs, K., Horvath, E., McComb, D.J. 1984. The fine structure of
    pituitary tumors. In "Ultrastructure of Endocrine Cells and
    Tissues". (Ed. Motta). (M. Nijhoff Publ., Boston, The Hague,
    Dordrecht, Lancaster). pp. 89-113.
Muhr, C., Bergström, M., Lundberg, P.O. et al. 1986. Dopamine receptors
    in pituitary adenomas: PET visualization with 11C-N-methyl-
    spiperone. J. Comput. Assist. Tomogr., 10, 175-180.
Muhr, C., Lundberg, P.O., Antoni, G. et al. 1985. 11C-bromocriptine
    uptake in pituitary adenomas. In "Prolactin. Basic and Clinical
    Correlates". (Eds. McLeod, Thorner, Scapagnini). (Fidia Research
    Series, Vol. 1, Liviana Press, Padova). pp 729-737.
Muhr, C., Lundberg, P.O., Antoni, G. et al. 1984. The uptake of 11C-
    labeled bromocriptine and methionine in pituitary tumors studied
    by positron emission tomography (PET). In "Trends in Diagnosis and
    Treatment of Pituitary Adenomas". (Eds. Lamberts, Tilders, Van der
    Veen, Assies). (Free University Press, Amsterdam). pp. 151-155.
Patlak, C.S., Blasberg, R.G., Fenstermacher, J.D. 1983. Graphical
    evaluation of blood-to-brain transfer constants from multiple-time
    uptake data. J. Cereb. Blood Flow Metabol., 3, 1-7.

Respondent to Brain Tumors:

INTERPRETATION OF TRACER UPTAKE IN BRAIN TUMORS

A. Gjedde

Medical Physiological Dept. A, The Panum Institute,
University of Copenhagen, Copenhagen, Denmark

In conventional kinetic models, the brain consists of a number of compartments corresponding to the different states of the labeled tracer. The compartments reflect the fate of the tracer and represent a specific theory of the biochemistry of the brain. Compartments are volumes in which the concentration of the tracer or its derivatives everywhere is the same, separated by interfaces where concentration gradients are steep.

Normally, the interfaces are cell membranes or chemical reactions involving proteins that function as transport molecules, receptors, or enzymes. The first interface that tracers meet is the endothelium of brain capillaries. For polar tracers, the concentration difference between the two sides of the endothelium is so great that the endothelial barrier frequently is the only significant barrier. To these compounds, the brain is an organ of only two compartments, the vascular compartment and the interstitial space.

The number and definition of compartments relevant to each new tracer must be known before attempts can be made to quantify the rate-limiting steps between them. Only the most insurmountable barriers are "visible" experimentally. Hence, the individual barriers of a series of rate-limiting steps can be distinguished only if their permeabilities are not too different.

By analyzing the brain uptake of inert polar tracers as a function of time, the permeability of the endothelium to the tracers can be determined by autoradiography or positron tomography. The transfer of a tracer, applied at time zero, from one compartment to the next follows a simple expression of preservation of mass which is applicable to most of the problems that arise in autoradiography or positron emission tomography and emcompasses both Fick's law of diffusion and Fick's principle, as well as the kinetic theories of enzyme-substrate and receptor-ligand interactions, the "indicator diffusion" method of Crone (1963), and the blood flow method of Kety and Schmidt (1945),

$$J(t) = \frac{dM2(t)}{dt} = k1 \; V1 \; C1(t) - k2 \; V2 \; C2(t) \qquad (1)$$

where J(t) is the net flux from compartment 1 to compartment 2 and M2(t)
therefore the net gain of tracer in compartment 2 at the time T. V1 and
V2 are the actual volumes of compartments 1 and 2, and k1 and k2
descriptive transfer coefficients. The interpretation of k1 and k2
depends on the process being studied and must be based on the definition
of the compartments analyzed in the study.

C1(t) and C2(t) are the concentrations of the tracer or its
metabolites in the two compartments and need not refer to the same
chemical species. The elements of the product of k, V, and C can be
combined as required for each problem. The product of k1 and V1 defines
a clearance, K1, and the product of V2 and C2(t) defines a mass, M2(t),
as measured in autoradiography or positron tomography.

Equation (1) can be solved for the total amount of tracer in the
two compartments,

$$M(T) = K1 \int_0^T C1(t) \; dt - k2 \int_0^T M2(t) \; dt + V1 \; C1(T) \qquad (2)$$

When solved for K1,

$$K1 = \frac{M(T) + k2 \displaystyle\int_0^T M2(t) \; dt - V1 \; C1(T)}{\displaystyle\int_0^T C1(t) \; dt} \qquad (3)$$

When k2 M2(t) is negligible compared to K1 C1(t) (i.e., very little
backflux), equation (3) is the simplest solution of the "integral"
equation, first introduced as the indicator fractionation or
"microsphere" method in 1956 by Sapirstein who advocated the use of
labeled potassium to measure blood flow, except in brain where K1 is a
measure of the capillary permeability rather than of blood flow.

Schaefer et al. (1976) used labeled butanol to measure blood flow
in the rat brain and advocated using labeled butanol and a labeled test

tracer together to also calculate the fraction of extracted test tracer, as originally reported by Oldendorf (1970). However, unlike Oldendorf (1970), Schaefer et al. (1976) actually determined the integral in equation (3) by continuous, automatic withdrawal of arterial blood. This is a kind of mechanical integration without the blood curve, adopted by Gjedde et al. (1975) from Scheinberg and Stead (1949) for use with the Kety-Schmidt method and also used by Sasaki and Wagner (1971) to determine blood flow in the rat brain with microspheres. The experience with automated integration led directly to the "slope-intercept" or "Patlak" solution of equation (1) discussed below as equation (4) (Gjedde, 1981; Patlak et al., 1983).

The problem was that calculation of K1 according to equation (3) on the basis of a single measurement of M2(t) required both negligible backflux and a known or negligible product of V1 and C1(T). The product of V1 and C1(T) can be measured with a second tracer which remains in plasma but backflux can not easily be ruled out on the basis of a single measurement ("autoradiographic mode").

Alternatively, with the same number of experiments and a single tracer, both K1 and V1 can be estimated by terminating the experiments at different times after administration of the tracer. In positron emission tomography this is made possible by simply following the accumulation, i.e., (M(t), as a function of time. In small animals, however, this can be accomplished only by normalization of individual observations in a large series of experiments.

Normalization is the division of the radioactivity in brain by the plasma concentrations of tracer obtained in individual experiments. The equation for this "dynamic" mode of the integral method is a rearrangement of equation (2) in which the radioactivity in brain is expressed as a distribution volume by dividing the radioactivity in brain by the radioactivity in blood (or plasma) (Gjedde, 1981),

$$\frac{M(T)}{C1(T)} = K1 \left\{ \frac{\int_0^T C1(t)\ dt - \frac{k2}{K1} \int_0^T M2(t)\ dt}{C1(T)} \right\} + V1 \qquad (4)$$

Linearity of a graph of the M(T)/C1(T) ratio ("volume") as a function of the normalized integral ("slope-intercept plot") is proof of absent backflux. The requirement for absent backflux is a very low k2/K1 ratio and/or a negligible integral of M2(t) compared to the integral of C1(t), i.e., low tissue/blood concentration ratios.

The normalized integral has unit of time but the values are not equal to real time. Only when the concentration of the tracer is constant in time is the value of the normalized integral equal to real time. Sarna et al. (1977) measured the brain endothelial permeability to sodium by equation (4) by keeping the concentration of 22-sodium constant in blood. Hence, in that experiment, the values of the normalized integral corresponded to real time.

Fig. 1 illustrates another experiment with this method in which the initial accumulation of 150-labeled oxygen in the human brain was recorded by positron emission tomography of two patients in vivo. The value of K1 is the initial slope of the two curves, corresponding to the time during which backflux was negligible.

Since the initially extracted fraction of labeled oxygen, i.e., the ratio between K1 and the blood flow, is a function of the (infinitely high) endothelial permeability of oxygen, the volume of distribution in blood (made very large by the binding to hemoglobin), and the mean transit time of blood through the tissue (equal to the blood volume divided by the blood flow), the extracted fraction must increase when the transit time falls and decline when the transit time rises.

The rate of initial influx of oxygen has been reported to equal the rate by which oxygen in normal brain tissue is turned into water by electron capture (Mintun et al., 1984). This has the interesting consequence that blood-brain transfer of oxygen in normal tissue must be rate-limiting for oxygen consumption and hence that tissue oxygen levels must be close to zero. However, interpretation of extraction fractions of oxygen are less certain in abnormal tissue in which transit times of blood may change.

Table 1 lists some of the many ions and polar and non-polar non-electrolytes that have been studied with this method, including protein-bound tracers, amino acids, hexoses, blood flow tracers, and receptor ligands such as flunitrazepam, isopropylamphetamine, and the dopamine D2 receptor ligand N-methylspiperone (NMSP).

TABLE 1 Unidirectional blood-brain clearances of common tracers

Tracer	K_1 (ml/100 g/min)		Ref
iodoantipyrine	83.0		a
water	81.0	flow-limited	a
flunitrazepam	67.0	uptake	a
iodoisopropylamphetamine	42.0*		b
fluorodeoxyglucose	30.6		c
deoxyglucose	28.3		c
oxygen	26.5*	high intermediate	d
D-glucose	18.6	uptake	c
N-methylspiperone	17.1*		e
3-O-methylglucose	17.0		c
phenylalanine	15.1		f
tryptophan	10.7		f
leucine	10.0		f
tyrosine	9.7		f
histidine	9.2	low intermediate	f
methionine	8.0	uptake	f
isoleucine	7.7		f
valine	4.4		f
threonine	3.0		f
potassium	0.8		g
mannitol	0.2		h
L-glucose	0.1	diffusion limited	h
sucrose	0.08	uptake	h
sodium	0.08		g
chloride	0.05		g
protein-bound indium	0.01		h

*measured in humans
a) Gjedde et al., 1983
b) Kuhl et al., 1982
c) Fuglsang et al., 1986
d) Gjedde et al., 1987
e) Wong et al., 1986
f) Bodsch and Gjedde, 1987
g) Smith and Rapoport, 1986
h) Gjedde, 1983

Oxygen-15 in Human Cortex

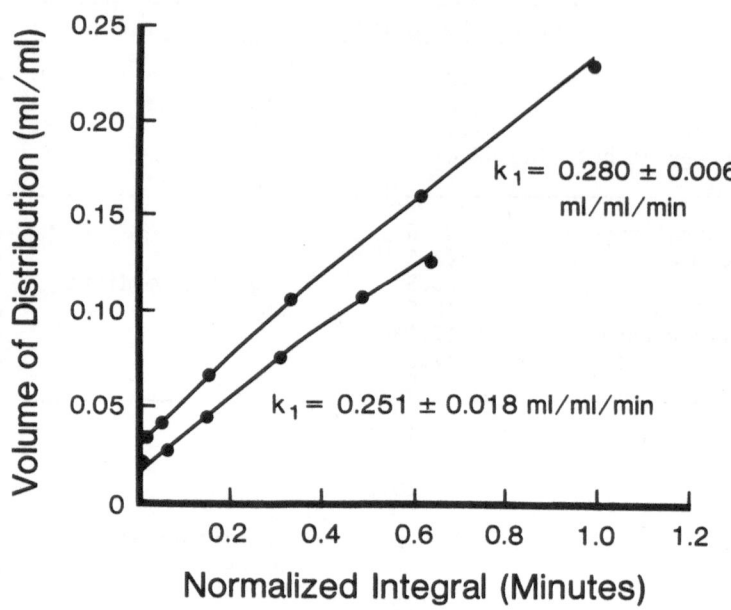

Fig. 1: Brain uptake of 15-0-labeled oxygen during the first minute after single breath inhalation by two patients. The abscissa is the normalized time integral and the ordinate the distribution volume in brain, calculated as the ratio between the radio-activities in brain and blood (after Meyer et al., 1987).

Fig. 2 compares the continued brain uptake of the lipophilic compounds iodoantipyrine, water, and flunitrazepam. Iodoantipyrine and water approach the steady-state between blood and brain dictated by equation (4) in the presence of significant backflux. The uptake of flunitrazepam, on the other hand, continues unabated. We must conclude that labeled flunitrazepam is not inert. It interacts in some manner with the tissue to escape the build-up in the interstitial fluid that leads to the steady-state. This hypothetical interaction is described as "trapping" or "binding".

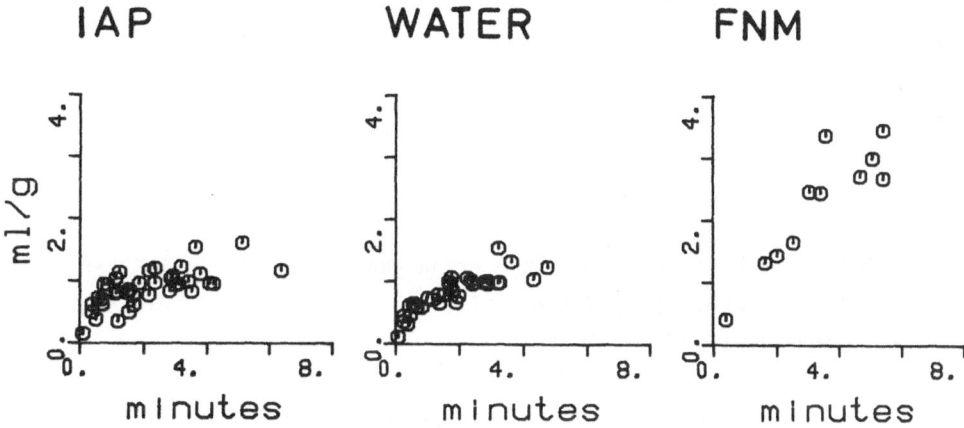

Fig. 2: Brain uptake of 14C-labeled iodoantipyrine, 3H-labeled water, and 3H-labeled flunitrazepam in rats. Abscissae and ordinates as in Fig. 1 (after Gjedde et al., 1983).

The trapping can be described by an additional compartment in brain that reflects transport into the intracellular space, binding to receptors, or conversion by chemical reactions that sequester the label for a shorter or longer time. In the compartmental analysis, this possibility is represented by a transfer coefficient (k3) leading into the additional compartment, and a transfer coefficient (k4) leading out of the compartment.

Entry into the additional compartment competes with the likelihood of transfer back into compartment 1. This competition is described by two differential equations.

$$\frac{dM2(t)}{dt} = K1\ C1(t) - (k2 + k3)\ M2(t) + k4\ M3(t) \qquad (5)$$

$$\frac{dM3(t)}{dt} = k3\ M2(t) - k4\ M3(t) \qquad (6)$$

where M2(t) and M3(t) represent the exchangeable (compart ient 2) and trapped (compartment 3) quantities of tracer. The complete solution to the equations is (Gjedde, 1982),

$$\frac{M(T)}{C1(T)} = K\left\{\frac{\displaystyle\int_0^T C1(t)\ dt - \frac{k2\ k4}{K1\ k3}\int_0^T M3(t)\ dt}{C1(T)}\right\} + re\ \frac{M2(T)}{C1(T)} + V1 \qquad (7)$$

where M(T) is the sum of M1(T), M2(T), and M3(T); K is the uni-directional clearance of the tracer into the third compartment, equal to the product of k3 and Vf where Vf is the distribution volume K1/ (k2+k3); and re is the kinetic "drag" coefficient equal to the ratio k2/(k2+k3).

The fundamental assumption underlying the modified solution by Sokoloff et al. (1977) and its later applications, for example to the analysis of radioligand uptake in brain, is the absence of significant backflux from compartment 3 to compartment 1. This assumption is confirmed when the "slope-intercept plot" of M(T)/C1(T) versus the normalized integral is linear. The requirement for this linearity is that the term k2 k4/K1 k3 and/or the integral of M3(t) are very small compared to the integral of C1(t), and that M2(T)/C1(T) has reached a constant ratio (steady-state). When these requirements are fulfilled, then the following variations of the solution are of special interest:

First, the coefficient k3 may be negligible compared to k2, as discussed above. Second, k3 may be of the same order of magnitude as k2. The propensities for backflux and binding are then equally great. On the average, half of the tracer molecules enter the third compartment and the remaining half return to compartment 1 (e.g., the vascular

compartment). The rate of net transfer to the third compartment is only
50 % of the rate of initial uptake, and the inclination of the line of
net uptake is only 50 % of the slope of the line of initial uptake. The
fraction that net uptake represents of the rate of initial uptake is
1-re where re is the kinetic "drag" coefficient referred to above.

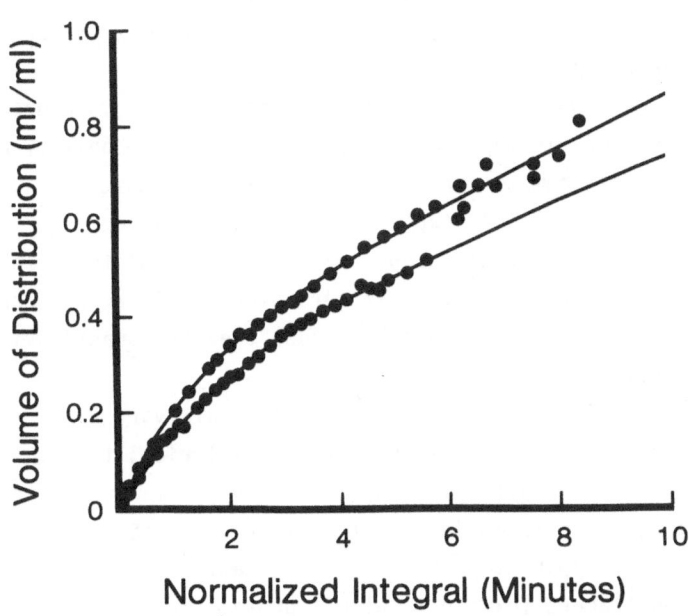

Oxygen-15 in Human Cortex

Fig. 3: Brain uptake of 150-labeled oxygen during the first 4
minutes after single breath inhalation. Note two phases of uptake.
Abscissa and ordinate as in Fig. 1 (after Meyer et al., 1987).

Fig. 3 illustrates the two phases of the brain uptake of 150-
labeled oxygen recorded in human brain in vivo after a single inhalation
of the tracer. Similar dual-phase uptake is characteristic of deoxyglucose, certain amino acids, for example methionine, as well as of
oxygen and radioligands such as NMSP and isopropylamphetamine.

In normal brain tissue, it is generally safe to assume that the initial phase must reflect delivery across the capillary endothelium but it is often impossible to identify the reaction that controls the entry into the third and later compartments. If the endothelium is no barrier, as in heart, muscle, lung, mesentery, and many brain tumors, the rate-limiting steps observed in tracer studies are very much in doubt. Heart and muscle cell membrane transport of hexoses is slow in the absence of insulin stimulation. Since the most impenetrable barriers are the most visible, biochemical reactions inside heart and muscle cells, such as hexokinase activity, are probably not easily distinguished. In these cells, deoxyglucose uptake may reflect cell membrane transport rather than phosphorylation.

Third, it is possible that the coefficient k3 be much greater than the coefficient k2. In this case, the statistical probability of transfer back into compartment 1 is very small and most molecules enter the third compartment. This explains the apparently continued uni-directional uptake of flunitrazepam by the binding to the receptors of the GABA/benzodiazepine complex. Tracers like flunitrazepam behave as "chemical" or "fluid microspheres" because they are quantitatively trapped in brain.

The endothelia of tumor capillaries in brain vary from discontinuous (sinusoids and fenestrated capillaries) through continuous but permeable (like capillaries in muscle and heart) to continuous and impermeable, as also found in normal brain tissue. Since normal brain capillaries have apparent permeabilities to amino acids and the tightly protein-bound tracers (oxygen is also a protein-bound tracer) that differ by three orders of magnitude, changes of the fundamentally different uptake of these compounds must reflect different alterations of the endothelium.

Increases of the uptake of protein-bound tracers probably reflect fenestrations or increased junctional leakiness. Increases of the initial uptake of amino acids probably reflect increases of the endothelial surface area or specific modulations of the transport capacity, while increases of the net uptake of amino acids reflect a metabolic change, often but not always associated with protein synthesis. For these reasons, changes of the uptake of amino acids probably occur earlier in the development of a tumor than changes in the uptake of protein-bound tracers.

REFERENCES

Bodsch, W., Gjedde, A. 1987. Exchange diffusion of large neutral amino acids from blood to brain. XIII Intern. Symp. on Cerebral Blood Flow and Metabol., Montreal, Quebec, June 20-25.

Crone, C. 1963. The permeability of capillaries in various organs as determined by use of the "indicator diffusion" method. Acta Physiol. Scand., 58, 292-305.

Fuglsang, A., Lomholt, M., Gjedde, A. 1986. Blood-brain transfer of glucose and glucose analogs in newborn rats. J. Neurochem., 46, 1417-1428.

Gjedde, A., Caronna, J.J., Hindfeldt, B. et al. 1975. Whole-brain blood flow and oxygen metabolism in the rat during nitrous oxide anesthesia. Am. J. Physiol., 229, 113-118.

Gjedde, A. 1981. High- and low-affinity transport of D-glucose from blood to brain. J. Neurochem., 36, 1463-1471.

Gjedde, A. 1982. Calculation of glucose phosphorylation from brain uptake of glucose analogs in vivo: A re-examination. Brain Res. Rev., 4, 237-274.

Gjedde, A. 1983. Modulation of substrate transport to the brain. Acta Neurol. Scand., 67, 3-25.

Gjedde, A., Drewes, L.R., Christensen, B. 1983. Comparison of flunitrazepam, water and iodoantipyrine transfer across the blood-brain barrier. J. Cereb. Blood Flow Metabol., 3, (Suppl. 1), S73-S74.

Gjedde, A., Meyer, E., Hakim, A.M. 1987. Blood-brain transfer of labeled oxygen. XIII Intern. Symp. on Cerebral Blood Flow and Metabolism, Montreal, Quebec, June 20-25.

Kety, S.S., Schmidt, C.F. 1945. The determination of cerebral blood flow in man by the use of nitrous oxide in low concentrations. Am. J. Physiol., 143, 53-66.

Kuhl, D.E., Barrio, J.R., Huang, S.C. et al. 1982. Quantifying local cerebral blood flow by N-isopropyl-p-(I123)iodoamphetamine (IMP) tomography. J. Nucl. Med., 23, 196-203.

Meyer et al. 1987. Private Communication.

Mintun, M.A., Raichle, M.E., Martin, W.R.W. et al. 1984. Brain oxygen utilization measured with O-15 radiotracers and positron emission tomography. J. Nucl. Med., 25, 177-187.

Oldendorf, W.H. 1970. Measurement of brain uptake of radiolabeled substances using a tritiated water reference. Brain Res., 24, 372-376.

Patlak, C., Blasberg, R.G., Fenstermacher, J.D. 1983. Graphical evaluation of blood-to-brain transfer constants from multiple-time uptake data. J. Cereb. Blood Flow Metabol., 3, 1-7.

Sapirstein, L.A. 1956. Fraction of the cardiac output of rats with isotopic potassium. Circ. Res., 4, 689-692.

Sarna, G.S., Bradbury, M.W.B., Cavanagh, J. 1977. Permeability of the blood-brain barrier after portocaval anastomosis in the rat. Brain Res., 138, 550-554.

Sasaki, Y, Wagner, H.N. Jr. 1971. Measurement of the distribution of cardiac output in unanesthetized rats. J. Appl. Physiol., 30, 879-884.

Schaefer, J.A., Gjedde, A., Plum, F. 1976. Regional cerebral blood flow using n-(14C)butanol. Neurology, 26, 394.

412

Scheinberg, P., Stead, E.A. Jr. 1949. The cerebral blood flow in male
    subjects as measured by the nitrous oxide technique. Normal values
    for blood flow, oxygen utilization, glucose utilization, and
    peripheral resistance, with observations on the effect of tilting
    and anxiety. J. Clin. Invest., 28, 1163-1171.
Smith, Q.R., Rapoport, S.I. 1986. Cerebrovascular permeability
    coefficients to sodium, potassium, chloride. J. Neurochem., 46,
    1732-1742.
Sokoloff, L., Reivich, M., Kennedy, C. et al. 1977. The
    (14C)deoxyglucose method for the measurement of local cerebral
    glucose utilization: Theory, procedure, and normal values in the
    conscious and anesthetized albino rat. J. Neuroch., 28, 897-916.
Wong, D.F., Gjedde, A., Wagner, H.N. Jr. 1986. Quantification of neuro-
    receptors in the living human brain. I. Irreversible binding of
    ligands. J. Cereb. Blood Flow Metabol., 6, 137-146.

SUMMARY of Discussion on Soft Tissue and Brain Tumors

R. Paul, Medical Cyclotron Laboratory, Turku Medical Cyclotron Project, Turku University Central Hospital, Turku, Finland

Although PET has not established itself as a routine imaging technique for oncological clinical purposes, there were several presentations that showed that PET has imminent clinical potential. Thus, it has been found that 11-C-methionine can be used to assess the spread and therapeutic response to treatment of prolactinomas. For this, we do not have to know precisely the fate of the 11-C-label, i.e. we can get clinically valuable data on tumor spread and treatment response by quantifying radioactivity in the tomographic image; exact knowledge of the amino acid metabolism of the tumor is not necessary. Also, 11-C-methionine has been found to be an excellent agent for delineation of tumor extent of astrocytomas. This tumor-localizing capability of 11-C-methionine is used clinically for localizing the exact site of stereotactic biopsies.

Decrements in the uptake of 13-N-NH-3 in treated soft tissue tumors and osteosarcomas indicate a good therapeutic response, whereas unchanged uptake is associated with a poor response. Also, the synthetic amino acid 1-aminocyclopenthane carboxylic acid (cycloleucine) is taken preferentially up by tumors, and this uptake is not related to blood flow, as measured by 13-N-HN-3.

Tumor blood flow, blood volume, oxygen utilization and glucose consumption can be measured with PET. The metabolic rate of glucose in tumors was not specifically addressed at the workshop, but the question of tumor oxygen utilization was extensively discussed. It has been found that the blood flow and blood volume of breast cancer tissue are quite variable from one patient to another, and also within the same tumor of a patient. In contrast to this, a low oxgen extraction fraction has been a common finding to all tumors. This observation generated some discussion related to tumor cell hypoxia. In view of overwhelming clinical evidence speaking in favor of the existence of hypoxic cells in tumors, it was asked whether a low oxygen extraction fraction as measured with PET excludes the possibility that there is true cell hypoxia, maybe on a level below the resolution of the PET device. It was maintained that the absence of vasoregulation may lead to labeled oxygen never reaching the hypoxic tumor cells. Not all participants agreed to this idea, and it was even stated that the hypothesis of hypoxic tumor cells may be a fallacy. PET has not thus far been able to resolve this important question.

Clinically the finding of a high variability in blood flow may be of value in selecting patients with tumors susceptible for treatment by hyperthermia. Tumors with a low blood flow could thus respond better to hyperthermia than tumors with a high flow. Clearly, clinical PET-trials are in order here.

Interesting studies have been carried out with 68-Ga-EDTA in brain tumors. The studies were performed before surgery; specimens of brain tumors were studied histologically in order to investigate vascular pathology and the extent of blood-brain barrier derangement as measured with 68-Ga-EDTA. There was a good correlation between the K-1 and the histologically measured vascular surface. The study shows that modelling can be improved by accessory techniques such as morphometry. Quantification of blood-brain barrier rupture by a generator-produced radiopharmaceutical is, of course, also of importance when discussing clinical applications and clinical accessibility of PET.

There appears to be a pathognomonic finding for cavernous hemangiomas - these tumors, which may be difficult to differentiate from malignant neoplasms by conventional techniques, are characterized by enhanced 68-Ga-EDTA uptake and low 11-C-methionine accumulation. In no malignant cerebral tumor has this pattern been found.

Differentiation between malignant and non-malignant tissue is also crucial when evaluating residual findings after radiotherapy of tumors. Residua may be due to radionecrosis or recurrence. This distinction may be made by 11-C-cycloleucine and 11-C-methionine, as reported at the workshop. There is, however, a notable lack of well-controlled, large series on this issue, as, alas, on several other oncological patient studies with PET. Thus far it appears that only cerebral tumors have been studied sufficiently well for potential clinical applications. I refer to 18-FDG studies and studies on blood flow, oxygen extraction, and blood volume.

A prerequisite for competent use of PET for tumor studies is that we know tumor metabolism. An adequate knowledge of tumor metabolism yields productive models, which, in turn, are necessary when quantitative metabolic data is to be extracted from PET studies. We are only in the process of obtaining such knowledge, and much of the clinical potential of PET will be realized later.

Although PET studies of cerebral tumors have been carried out for as long as other brain studies, the time is still not ripe for attempts at standardizing studies of cerebral tumors - or other tumors, for that matter - by PET. This was evidenced by the decision not to establish a task group for recommendations for standardization of oncological PET studies. The reason for this is also clear: tumors are a heterogenous group of metabolically altered tissues. We still do not know enough about tumor metabolism in general or cerebral tumor in particular to be able to fully utilize the in vivo metabolic data of PET. Still, clinically unique data may be generated by tumor PET studies as shown by the presentations at the workshop.

Discussion of the Summaries of the Respondents

T. Jones, MRC Cyclotron Unit, Hammersmith Hospital, London, United
Kingdom

The respondents were asked to summarise what they saw as the output
of PET studies and the future clinical applications of this investigative speciality. However, before the summaries were delivered, the
opportunity was taken for a frank and open discussion between the
delegates. They were asked to comment on what had been presented and
whether or not the workshop had met its goals. A singular feature of
this discussion by committed exponents of PET was a highlighting of the
problems and short comings of the field:
The speakers had shown difficulty in addressing the questions, as
they had been posed at the beginning of the meeting, of overall clinical
efficacy. They tended to confine themselves to selective items of data
rather than the broader clinical issues. Most had presented as
PETologists rather than clinicians using PET to ask questions in the
broader medical context. Little attention had been paid to the use of
PET for assessing the efficacy and mechanism of therapeutic regimes.
Those clinicians with experience of patho-physiological data produced
with PET still appear restrained in the use of this information to
change therapeutic approaches. Many studies were still no more than
ranging shots and there is a lack of tight protocols. Indeed there seems
to be difficulties in asking appropriate clinical questions and an air
of "potential values". In some instances it is a methodology looking for
application. This picture is compounded by there being still comparatively little quantitative data being produced. In this regard the
groups need to concentrate on collecting more data, standardising
methods of measurement and where possible, co-ordinating intergroup
effort. Some of the non PET experts present had difficulty in
visualising the full scope of PET in the future. In response a
projection was made that PET studies could in future be used for the
registration of new pharmaceuticals.
Concern was shown over the practical aspects of co-ordinating PET
studies with the results of other physiological monitoring. Also there
was a danger that some groups will install a cyclotron and PET scanner
without being aware of the many logistical problems that have to be
overcome in effecting PET studies.
It was emphasised that data of clinical PET studies should not be
presented in isolation but in the context of clinical problems. On the
other hand, meetings where clinical PET data were presented alongside
basic biological studies would be fruitful with both clinical and basic
science respondents present.
Dr. Freund, Düsseldorf, reponded to the presentations on the use of
PET in neurology. He was convinced that PET has already provided new
information in cerebral ischemia and could be used when selecting
patients for specific therapeutic trials. Practical use could rest on
distinguishing regrowth of cerebral tumors within areas of brain with
tissue necrosis. The use of selective ligands to investigate movement
and emotional disorders showed promise but emphasised the need for
highly selective protocols of study. It was stressed that PET offered an
opportunity to answer original elementary neurophysiological questions
on the sequence of connections in the brain that respond to specific
activations. However, to realise this the need was stressed for better
methods for localising data recorded within the brain.

Dr. Farde, Stockholm, discussed the application of PET in psychiatry. There was a danger that since there was a "hunger" for a biological finding in schizophrenia then PET may be misused. He stressed that a change in receptor activity does not give information on disease mechanism. Schizophrenia is a group of diseases and PET may offer a means for subgrouping patients. Correlating the degree of receptor binding to the clinical effects of drugs was proving most interesting. Anti-psychotic effect had been shown to correlate with specific degrees of receptor occupancy. This could lead to the tailoring of pharmaceuticals for clinical management using PET techniques. Here in the future they may help in the management of individual patients.

Dr. Lösse, Düsseldorf, responded to the presentations on the use of PET in cardiology. He commented that most studies had concentrated on angina and myocardial infarctions. It was felt that other diseases, especially cardiomyopathy should be studied as here there were signs of myocardial ischemia in the absence of occluded coronary arteries. He stressed that heterogeneity of such a clinical condition presents a problem for systemic investigations. In heart failure, the opportunity was offered to use PET for research of tissue receptor activity. In more well defined cardiological studies there were indications that PET would be used as a clinical diagnostic tool. However, he emphasised that what was needed was a means of predicting complications that might arise following thrombolysis.

Dr. Huchon, Paris, highlighted some of the new patho-physiology that had been uncovered in pulmonary studies using PET. He emphasised that these were relevant since there were no good animal models of many human respiratory diseases. In the future PET should be used in asthma and interstitial lung disease to study receptor activities and the effect of mediators on these.

Dr. van der Hoeven, Amsterdam, discussed the use of PET in oncology. It was clear that PET would not be used for detecting small metastatic tumors but that it was good for showing the extension of the tumor. It may be possible to differentiate tumors with PET and presentations had shown that it was possible to determine a tumor's response to treatment. PET could be used to delineate the distribution of chemo-therapeutic agents and offers a means for determining the optional route for a drug's administration.

SUMMARY of Discussion on Strategy for the Future

D. Comar, CEA-CEN/Saclay, Département de Biologie, Gif-sur-Yvette, France

As it occurred at the two preceding workshops held at Hammersmith Hospital and Service Hospitalier Frédéric Joliot, Orsay, a general consent appeared on the aim and usefulness of these European meetings. A strong will for having future workshops and task groups on PET was revealed. Thus, the following proposals to the EEC were made:

1. Organisation of two task groups.

    Measurement of regional myocardium perfusion in humans by PET. Validation and standardization of the technique (P. Camici and O. Parodi, Pisa, and A. Syrota, Orsay).

    Guidelines for the implementation and use of PET measurements of cerebral energy metabolism and haemodynamics in cerebrovascular diseases (W.-D. Heiss, Cologne, J.C. Baron, Orsay, and R. Frackowiak, London).

2. Organisation of a fourth workshop in 1987 on ligand-receptor measurement by PET and modelisation.

    This workshop would be held in Louvain and organized by C. Beckers, Brussels.

3. Concerted actions.

    Many proposals were made for concerted actions or exchanges of scientists between European groups. However, it was noted that COMAC-BME has no budget to support research or exchanges. Proposals should be presented to the Stimulation Program Department of the EEC.

PARTICIPANTS

Dr. S.M. AQUILONIUS
University Hospital
Dept. of Neurology
S-750 14 Uppsala 14, Sweden

Dr. J.C. BARON
CEA
Département de Biologie
Service Hospitalier Frédéric Joliot
Hôpital d'Orsay
F-91406 Orsay, France

Dr. R.P. BEANEY
Dept. of Radiotherapy
Queen Elizabeth Hospital
Edgbaston
Birmingham, United Kingdom

Prof. Dr. C. BECKERS
Université Catholique de Louvain
Faculté de Médecine
Centre de Médecine Nucléaire
U.C.L. 54.30
Avenue Hippocrate 54
B-1200 Brussels, Belgium

Prof. Dr. M. BERGER
Zentralinst.f.Seelische Gesundheit
J5
6800 Mannheim 1, FRG

Dr. M. BERGSTRÖM
University Hospital
Dept. of Neurology
S-750 14 Uppsala 14, Sweden

Dr. P. BUSTANY
Centre Hospitalier Regional
et Universitaire de Caen
Lab. de Pharmacologie et
des Explorations Fonctionnelles B
Av. de la Cote de Nacre
F-14033 Caen, France

Dr. P. CAMICI
CNR/Institute of Clinical Physiology
Via P. Savi 8
I-56100 Pisa, Italy

Dr. D. COMAR
CEA-CEN/Saclay
Département de Biologie
F-911 91 Gif-sur-Yvette Cedex, France

Dr. J.C. DEPRESSEUX
Université de Liège
Centre de Recherches du Cyclotron
B 30, Sart Tilman
B-4000 Liège 1, Belgium

Dr. K. Ericson
Karolinska Hospital
Dept. of Neuroradiology
S-104 01 Stockholm, Sweden

Dr. L. FARDE
Karolinska Hospital
Dept. of Psychiatry
S-104 01 Stockholm, Sweden

Prof. Dr. L.E. FEINENDEGEN
Institut für Medizin
der Kernforschungsanlage Jülich GmbH
Postfach 1913
5170 Jülich 1, FRG

Dr. R.S.J. FRACKOWIAK
MRC Cyclotron Unit
Hammersmith Hospital
150 Ducane Road
London W12 OHS, United Kingdom

Prof. Dr. H.J. FREUND
Neurologische Universitätsklinik
Moorenstr. 5
4000 Düsseldorf, FRG

Dr. A. GJEDDE
Medical Physiology Dept. A
The Panum Institute
University of Copenhagen
Blegdamsvej 3C
DK-2200 Copenhagen, Denmark

Dr. A.M. GOFFINET
Université de Louvain
Faculté de Médecine
Lab. de Tomographie par Positrons
Chemin du Cyclotron, 2
B-1348 Louvain-la-Neuve, Belgium

Dr. I. HEBOLD
Max-Planck-Institut für
neurologische Forschung
Ostmerheimer Str. 200
5000 Köln 91, FRG

420

Dr. H.-J. HEINEN
DFVLR-FDG
Projektträgerschaft
Forschung im Dienste der Gesundheit
Südstr. 125
5300 Bonn 2, FRG

Prof.Dr.W.-D. HEISS
Max-Planck-Institut für
neurologische Forschung
Ostmerheimer Str. 200
5000 Köln 91, FRG

Dr. K. HERHOLZ
Max-Planck-Institut für
neurologische Forschung
Ostmerheimer Str. 200
5000 Köln 91, FRG

Dr. HERZOG
Institut für Medizin der
Kernforschungsanlage Jülich GmbH
Postfach 1913
5170 Jülich 1, FRG

Dr.J.J.M. van der HOEVEN
Academisch Ziekenhuis
Free University
Dept. of Oncology
De Boelelaan 1117
1007 MB Amsterdam, The Netherlands

Dr. G. HUCHON
Hopital Laennec
Clinique de Pneumo-
Phtisiologie
42, rue de Sèvres
F-Paris 75007, France

Dr. J.M.B. HUGHES
RPMS Dept. of Medicine
Ducane Road
London W12 OHS, United Kingdom

Dr. F. IANNOTTI
Istituto di Neurochirurgia
la Facoltà di Medicina e Chirurgia
Ospedale C.T.O.
Viale Colli Aminei 21
I-80131 Napoli, Italy

Dr. Terry JONES
MRC Cyclotron Unit
Hammersmith Hospital
Ducane Road
London W12 OHS, United Kingdom

Dr. C. De LANDSHEERE
Université de Liège
Centre de Recherches du Cyclotron
B 30, Sart Tilman
B-4000 Liège 1, Belgium

Dr. K.L. LEENDERS
MRC Cyclotron Unit
Hammersmith Hospital
Ducane Road
London W12 OHS, United Kingdom

Prof. Dr. G.L. LENZI
III Clinica Neurologica
Dept. of Neurological Sciences
Viale Università, 30
I-00185 Rome, Italy

Dr. A. LILJA
Diagnostic Radiology
Section on Neuroradiology
Akademiska Sjukhuset
S-751 85 Uppsala, Sweden

Prof. Dr. B. LÖSSE
Universitätsklinik Düsseldorf
- Kardiologie -
Moorenstr. 5
4000 Düsseldorf, FRG

Prof. Dr. A. MASERI
RPMS Hammersmith Hospital
Ducane Road
London W12 OHS, United Kingdom

Dr. B. MAZIERE
Service Hospitalier Frédéric Joliot
Hopital d'Orsay
F-91406 Orsay, France

Dr. C. MUHR
University Hospital
Dept. of Neurology
S-750 14 Uppsala 14, Sweden

Dr. R.M. MURRAY
University of London
Institute of Psychiatry
De Crespigny Park, Denmark Hill
London, SE5 8AF, United Kingdom

Dr. O. PARODI
Istituto di Fisiologia, Clinica del CNR
c/o Università di Pisa
Via Savi 8
I-56100 Pisa, Italy

Dr. R. PAUL
Medical Cyclotron Laboratory
Turku Medical Cyclotron Project
Turku University Central Hospital
SH Building, Room B 206
SF-20520 Turku, Finland

Dr. G. PAWLIK
Max-Planck-Institut für
neurologische Forschung
Ostmerheimer Str. 200
5000 Köln 91, FRG

Dr. Y. SAMSON
Service Hospitalier Frédéric Joliot
Hopital d'Orsay
F-91406 Orsay, France

Dr. K. SCHELSTRAETE
Dept.of Radiotherapy & Nuclear Medicine
University Hospital
De Pintelaan 185
B-9000 Ghent, Belgium

Prof. Dr. Dr. O. SCHOBER
Med. Hochschule Hannover
Abt. Nuklearmedizin
Konstanty-Gutschow-Str. 8
3000 Hannover 61, FRG

Dr. F. SCHUIER
Neurologische Universitätsklinik
Moorenstr. 5
4000 Düsseldorf, FRG

Dr. Jordi SETOAIN
C E T I R
Londres, 6
08029 Barcelona, Spain

Dr. W. SKUPINSKI
C.E.E.
DG XII/F/2 (SDM 2/47)
200 rue de la Loi
B-1048 Brussels, Belgium

Dr. H. SOCHOR
Kardiolog. Univ.-Klin. Wien
Garnisongasse 13
A-1090 Wien, Austria

Dr. W. STAFFEN
Max-Planck-Institut für
neurologische Forschung
Ostmerheimer Str. 200
5000 Köln 91, FRG

Prof. Dr. G. STÖCKLIN
Institut für Chemie
der Kernforschungsanlage Jülich GmbH
Institut 1 - Nuklearchemie
Postfach 1913
5170 Jülich, FRG

Dr. A. SYROTA
CEA, Département de Biologie
Service Hospitalier Frédéric Joliot
Hopital d'Orsay
F-91406 Orsay, France

Prof. Dr. H. TILLMANNS
Medizinische Universitätsklinik
Innere Medizin III
6900 Heidelberg, FRG

Dr. R. WAGNER
Max-Planck-Institut für
neurologische Forschung
Ostmerheimer Str. 200
5000 Köln 91, FRG

Prof. Dr. L. WIDEN
Karolinska Institute
Dept. of Clin. Neurophysiology
S-104 01 Stockholm, Sweden

Dr. K. WIENHARD
Max-Planck-Institut für
neurologische Forschung
Ostmerheimer Str. 200
5000 Köln 91

Dr. F.A. WIESEL
Karolinska Hospital
Dept. of Psychiatry and Psychology
P.O. Box 60 500
S-104 01 Stockholm, Sweden

Dr. H.G. WIESER
Universitätsspital
Neurologie/EEG
Frauenklinikstr. 26
CH-8091 Zürich, Switzerland

Dr. P. ZIFFLING
Max-Planck-Institut für
neurologische Forschung
Ostmerheimer Str. 200
5000 Köln 91, FRG